TAKING SIDES

Clashing Views on Controversial

Issues in Drugs and Society

SIXTH EDITION

TAKING SIDES

Clashing Views on Controversial

Issues in Drugs and Society

SIXTH EDITION

Selected, Edited, and with Introductions by

Raymond Goldberg
State University of New York College at Cortland

McGraw-Hill/Dushkin
A Division of The McGraw-Hill Companies

To Norma, Tara, and Greta

Cover image: © 2004 by PhotoDisc, Inc.

Cover Art Acknowledgment
Charles Vitelli

Manufactured in the United States of America

Sixth Edition

456789BAHBAH54321

Library of Congress Cataloging-in-Publication Data
Main entry under title:
Taking sides: clashing views on controversial issues in drugs and society/selected, edited, and
with introductions by Raymond Goldberg.—6th ed.
Includes bibliographical references and index.
1. Drug abuse—Social aspects. I. Goldberg, Raymond, *comp.*
362.29
0-07-287304-3
ISSN: 1094-7566

Printed on Recycled Paper

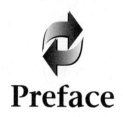

Preface

One of the hallmarks of a democratic society is the freedom of its citizens to disagree. This is no more evident than on the topic of drugs. The purpose of this sixth edition *of Taking Sides: Clashing Views on Controversial Issues in Drugs and Society* is to introduce drug-related issues that (1) are pertinent to the reader and (2) have no clear resolution. In the area of drug abuse, there is much difference of opinion regarding drug prevention, causation, and treatment. For example, should drug abuse be prevented by increasing the enforcement of drug laws or by making young people more aware of the potential dangers of drugs? Is drug abuse caused by heredity, personal characteristics, or environment? Is drug abuse a medical, legal, or social problem? Should events such as rave parties be prohibited because of possible drug use? Are self-help groups the most effective treatment for drug abusers?

There are many implications to how the preceding questions are answered. For example, if addiction to drugs is viewed as hereditary rather than as the result of flaws in one's character or personality, then a biological rather than a psychosocial approach to treatment will be pursued. If the consensus is that the prevention of drug abuse can be achieved by eliminating the availability of drugs, then more money and effort will be allocated for interdiction and law enforcement than for education. If drug abuse is viewed as a legal problem, then prosecution and incarceration will be the goal. If drug abuse is identified as a medical problem, then abusers will be given treatment. However, if drug abuse is deemed a social problem, then energy will be directed at underlying social factors, such as poverty, unemployment, health care, and education. Not all of the issues have clear answers. One may favor increasing penalties for drug violations *and* improving treatment services. And it is possible to view drug abuse as a medical *and* social *and* legal problem.

The issues debated in this volume deal with both legal and illegal drugs. Although society seems more interested in debating issues about illegal drugs, it is quite pertinent to address issues related to legal drugs because they cause more deaths and disabilities. No one is untouched by drugs, and everybody is affected by drug use and abuse. Billions of tax dollars are channeled into the war on drugs. Thousands of people are treated for drug abuse, often at public expense. The drug trade spawns crime and violence. Medical treatment for illnesses and injuries resulting from drug use and abuse creates additional burdens to an already extended health care system. Disabled children whose mothers used drugs while pregnant are entering schools, and teachers are expected to meet the educational needs of these children. Ritalin is prescribed to several million students to deal with their lack of attention in the classroom. Drunk drivers represent a serious threat to public health and safety while raising the cost of everyone's automobile insurance. The issues debated here are not whether drug abuse is a problem but what should be done to rectify this problem.

Many of the issues contained in this volume have an immediate impact on the reader. For example, Issue 3, *Will a Lower Blood Alcohol Level for Drunk Driving Reduce Automobile Accidents?* will likely affect the amount of alcohol that people consume before driving. Issue 14, *Should Nonsmokers Be Concerned About the Effects of Secondhand Smoke?* is relevant to both smokers and nonsmokers because restrictions on smoking are discussed. Issue 10, *Do the Advantages of Psychiatric Medicines Outweigh Their Disadvantages?* is important because millions of people have been diagnosed with depression or some other type of mental illness. And the question *Should Marijuana Be Legal for Medicinal Purposes?* (Issue 9) may become relevant for many readers or their loved ones someday.

Plan of the book In this sixth edition of *Taking Sides: Clashing Views on Controversial Issues in Drugs and Society*, there are 38 selections dealing with 19 issues. Each issue is preceded by an *introduction* and followed by a *postscript*. The purpose of the introduction is to provide some background information and to set the stage for the debate as it is argued in the "yes" and "no" selections. The postscript summarizes the debate and challenges some of the ideas brought out in the two selections, which can enable the reader to see the issue in other ways. Included in the postscripts are additional suggested readings on the issue. The issues, introductions, and postscripts are designed to stimulate readers to think about and achieve an informed view of some of the critical issues facing society today. Internet site addresses (URLs), which should prove useful as starting points for further research, have been provided at the beginning of each part. Also, at the back of the book is a list of all the *contributors to this volume*, which gives information on the physicians, professors, authors, and policymakers whose views are debated here.

Taking Sides: Clashing Views on Controversial Issues in Drugs and Society is a tool to encourage critical thinking. In reading an issue and forming your own opinion, you should not feel confined to adopt one or the other of the positions presented. Some readers may see important points on both sides of an issue and may construct for themselves a new and creative approach. Such an approach might incorporate the best of both sides, or it might provide an entirely new vantage point for understanding.

Changes to this edition This sixth edition represents a significant revision. Five of the 19 issues are completely new: *Should We Be Concerned About "Club Drugs"?* (Issue 4); *Are Athletes Who Use Anabolic Steroids Engaging in High-Risk Behavior?* (Issue 7); *Do the Advantages of Psychiatric Medicines Outweigh Their Disadvantages?* (Issue 10); *Do Consumers Benefit When Prescription Drugs Are Advertised?* (Issue 13); and *Do Alcohol Advertisements Influence Young People to Drink More?* (Issue 19). For 11 of the issues retained from the previous edition, one or both selections were replaced to reflect more current points of view: Issue 1 on drug decriminalization; Issue 2 on whether or not more emphasis should be put on stopping the importation of drugs; Issue 3 on lowering the blood alcohol level for drunk driving; Issue 6 on the basis of drug addiction; Issue 8 on the adverse effects of smoking; Issue 11 on caffeine; Issue 12 on Ritalin; Issue 14 on the effects of secondhand smoke; Issue 15 on total abstinence for alcoholics; Issue 17 on employee drug testing; and Issue 18 on drug abuse treatment. In all, there are 23 new selections.

A word to the instructor   An *Instructor's Manual With Test Questions* (multiple-choice and essay) is available through the publisher for the instructor using *Taking Sides* in the classroom. A general guidebook, *Using Taking Sides in the Classroom*, which discusses methods and techniques for integrating the pro-con approach into any classroom setting, is also available. An online version of *Using Taking Sides in the Classroom* and a correspondence service for Taking Sides adopters can be found at http://www.dushkin.com/usingts/.

   Taking Sides: Clashing Views on Controversial Issues in Drugs and Society is only one title in the Taking Sides series. If you are interested in seeing the table of contents for any of the other titles, please visit the Taking Sides Web site at http://www.dushkin.com/takingsides/.

Acknowledgments   I am grateful to my students and colleagues, who did not hesitate to share their perceptions and to let me know what they liked and disliked about the fifth edition. In addition, without the editorial staff at McGraw-Hill/Dushkin, this book would not exist. The insightful and professional contributions of Ted Knight, managing editor, were most valuable. His thoughtful perceptions and encouragement were most appreciated. In no small way can my family be thanked. I am grateful for their patience and support.

Raymond Goldberg
State University of New York College at Cortland

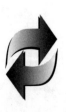

Contents in Brief

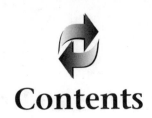

Contents

Ethan A. Nadelmann, director of the Lindesmith Center, maintains that the war on drugs has been futile and counterproductive. Current laws, says Nadelmann, exacerbate problems related to drug use. Eric A. Voth, chairman of the International Drug Strategy Institute, contends that the war on drugs is not a failure and that legalizing drugs would worsen drug-related problems. He maintains that a restrictive yet compassionate approach toward drug use is the best policy to adopt.

Barry R. McCaffrey, former director of the Office of National Drug Control Policy, argues that the importation of drugs into the United States must be stopped to reduce drug use and abuse. He maintains that a coordinated international effort is needed to combat the increased production of heroin, cocaine, and marijuana. Ted Galen Carpenter, vice president of defense and foreign policy studies for the Cato Institute, asserts that the United States has corroborated with foreign governments that have profited from the drug trade. He recommends that the federal government re-examine its role of cooperation with other governments, especially those involved in the drug trade.

Professor of economics Thomas S. Dee supports a .08 blood alcohol concentration (BAC) level for drunk driving. He maintains that alcohol-related fatalities are lower in those states that have adopted a .08 BAC. Dee concludes that an estimated 1,200 fewer deaths would result from the adoption of such a limit. The General Accounting Office (GAO) states that the evidence supporting the beneficial effects of establishing a lower blood alcohol level for drunk driving is inconclusive. The GAO maintains that the government's methods for determining the effectiveness of a lower blood alcohol level are faulty and that rates for drunk driving have declined regardless of changes in BAC legal limits.

Issue 4. Should We Be Concerned About "Club Drugs"? 62

YES: **Eric Sigel,** from "Club Drugs: Nothing to Rave About," *Contemporary Pediatrics* (October 2002) 64

NO: **Jacob Sullum,** from "Sex, Drugs and Techno Music," *Reason* (January 2002) 75

Assistant professor of pediatrics Eric Sigel argues that club drugs such as Ecstasy, GHB, Rohypnol, and Special K are dangerous. Their use, especially at rave parties, allows participants to overlook social barriers and helps individuals to relate better to others. Sigel cautions that some drugs that are taken at rave parties, especially GHB, have led to date rape. Jacob Sullum, a senior editor at *Reason* magazine, contends that the effects of drugs such as Ecstasy, particularly with regard to sexual behavior, are exaggerated. He refers to the history of marijuana and how it too was deemed a drug that would make people engage in behaviors in which they would not typically engage. Sullum maintains that the public's reaction to club drugs is unjustified.

Issue 5. Should Pregnant Drug Users Be Prosecuted? 86

YES: **Paul A. Logli,** from "Drugs in the Womb: The Newest Battlefield in the War on Drugs," *Criminal Justice Ethics* (Winter/Spring 1990) 88

NO: **Drew Humphries,** from *Crack Mothers: Pregnancy, Drugs, and the Media* (Ohio State University Press, 1999) 95

Paul A. Logli, an Illinois prosecuting attorney, argues that it is the government's duty to enforce every child's right to begin life with a healthy, drug-free mind and body. Logli maintains that pregnant women who use drugs should be prosecuted because they may harm the life of their unborn children. Researcher Drew Humphries argues that the prosecution of women who use drugs while pregnant has resulted from overzealous efforts on the part of a handful of state prosecutors. Humphries asserts that the prosecution of pregnant drug users is unfair because poor women are more likely to be the targets of such prosecution and that these cases do not hold up to legal standards.

Issue 6. Is Drug Addiction a Choice? 108

YES: **Jeffrey A. Schaler,** from *Addiction Is a Choice* (Open Court, 2000) 110

NO: **Alan I. Leshner,** from "Addiction Is a Brain Disease," *Issues in Science and Technology* (Spring 2001) 117

Psychotherapist Jeffrey A. Schaler maintains that drug addiction should not be considered a disease, a condition over which one has no control. He states that diseases have distinct characteristics and that drug addiction does not share these characteristics. Classifying behavior as socially unacceptable does not prove that it is a disease, according to Schaler.

Alan I. Leshner, former director of the National Institute on Drug Abuse, contends that drug addiction is not a failure of will nor a sign of weak character. One's initial use of drugs may be voluntary, he says, but over time one cannot stop through force of will alone. Leshner states that biological and chemical changes within the brain are important components in drug addiction.

Physician William N. Taylor opposes athletes using anabolic steroids due to the tremendous risks associated with the drugs. He argues that rather than helping themselves, many athletes are shortening their athletic careers because of the adverse effects of anabolic steroids and that many of the harmful effects of steroids may not be known for years. Charles E. Yesalis, a professor of health policy and administration, exercise, and sport science; acquisitions editor Michael S. Bahrke; and exercise physiologist James E. Wright argue that some of the effects associated with the use of anabolic steroids are not as bad as reported. Yesalis et al. acknowledge that there are problems with the use of steroids, but they assert that those problems are exaggerated. They also maintain that many of the problems related to steroids come from the lack of regulation of these drugs; the quality of illegally purchased anabolic steroids is questionable.

PART 2   DRUGS AND SOCIAL POLICY   149

Robert A. Levy, a senior fellow at the Cato Institute, and Rosalind B. Marimont, a mathematician and scientist, contend that the government distorts and exaggerates the dangers of cigarette smoking. They argue that cigarette smoking is harmful but that the misapplication of statistics about smoking should be regarded as "junk science." Alicia M. Lukachko and Elizabeth M. Whelan, assistant director of public health and president, respectively, of the American Council on Science and Health, contend that cigarette smoking has been the leading cause of disease and death over the last four decades. They argue that Levy and Marimont's methodology is haphazard and unscientific.

Professor of psychiatry Lester Grinspoon contends that, despite the fact that the majority of Americans support marijuana use for medical purposes, the federal government is suppressing its medical use for fear that it may become more acceptable for recreational use. He believes that pharmaceutical companies may develop commercial alternatives but questions the effectiveness of these alternatives. James R. McDonough, director of the Florida Office of Drug Control, agrees that compounds in marijuana, such as THC, may have the potential to be medically valuable. However, smoked marijuana has not been proven to be of medicinal value. In addition, there are existing, approved drugs that are more effective for conditions that may be helped by marijuana use.

Physician Bruce M. Cohen maintains that psychiatric medicines are beneficial in that they enable individuals with a variety of illnesses to return to normal aspects of consciousness. He argues that people with conditions such as anxiety, depression, and psychosis respond very well to medications and that these types of drugs have been utilized successfully for hundreds of years. Physician Ronald W. Dworkin questions whether the increase in the use of psychiatric drugs, especially antidepressant drugs, results from more people needing these drugs or from physicians' becoming more aggressive in diagnosing people as depressed. Dworkin expresses concern that antidepressant drugs are being prescribed for everyday conditions such as unhappiness and boredom.

Writer Nell Boyce states that caffeine is more addictive than most people realize. Boyce maintains that caffeine not only causes dependency but also has a myriad of other effects. Caffeine raises blood pressure, a factor leading to heart disease, and there is also evidence that caffeine consumption during pregnancy involves some risk for the fetus. Registered dietitians Edith Howard Hogan and Betsy A. Hornick and social worker Ann Bouchoux contend that there are numerous misconceptions related to caffeine. They maintain that caffeine has not been proven to cause hyperactivity nor attention deficit disorder (ADD) among children; neither has it been proven that caffeine causes heart disease, fibrocystic breast disease, nor some forms of cancer. They conclude that mental alertness and physical performance may be improved by caffeine use.

Writer Jonathan Leo contends that the tremendous increase in the number of prescriptions written for Ritalin is due to the millions of dollars spent by pharmaceutical companies on promoting the drug. Leo contends that the basis for prescribing Ritalin to children is based on bad science. He argues that the evidence does not support a biological foundation for attention deficit/hyperactivity disorder (ADHD). Writer Michael Fumento disputes the idea that Ritalin is overprescribed and asserts that there are many myths associated with Ritalin. He maintains that Ritalin does not lead to abuse and addiction, and he concludes that Ritalin is an excellent medication for ADHD.

Merrill Matthews, Jr., a health policy adviser with the American Legislative Exchange Council, argues that the advertising of prescription drugs directly to consumers will result in better-informed consumers. Additionally, communication between doctors and patients may improve because advertising increases patients' knowledge about drugs. Writer Anne B. Brown asserts that drug advertising has resulted in an increase in the number of visits by patients to their physicians. She also expresses concern that many consumers may not have the clinical or pharmacological background to adequately comprehend information in drug advertisements.

The U.S. Department of Health and Human Services identifies numerous health consequences associated with secondhand smoke. Secondhand smoke is a human carcinogen, accounting for 3,000 lung cancer deaths annually, and it also causes bronchitis, pneumonia, middle ear diseases, asthma, and heart disease. Statisticians J. B. Copas and J. Q. Shi argue that research demonstrating that secondhand smoke is harmful is biased. They contend that the findings of many studies exaggerate the adverse effects of secondhand smoke.

Professor of health Thomas Byrd maintains that Alcoholics Anonymous (AA) provides more effective treatment for alcoholics than psychiatrists, members of the clergy, or hospital treatment centers. Byrd contends that AA is the most powerful and scientific program, in contrast to all other therapies. Journalist Heather Ogilvie states that a number of studies support the concept that alcoholics can learn to drink moderately. Abstinence is not the only option for alcoholics, she argues, although it is important for alcoholics to identify the treatment that is best for them.

In their review of various studies, David Vlahov, professor of epidemiology and medicine, and Benjamin Junge, evaluation director for the Baltimore Needle Exchange Program, found that needle exchange programs successfully reduced the transmission of the virus that causes acquired immunodeficiency syndrome (AIDS). In addition, many people who participated in needle exchange programs reduced their drug use and sought drug abuse treatment. The Office of National Drug Control Policy, an executive agency that determines policies and objectives for the U.S. drug control program, sees needle exchange programs as an admission of defeat and a retreat from the ongoing battle against drug use, and it argues that compassion and treatment are needed, not needles.

Writer Todd Nighswonger supports workplace drug testing because most people between ages 18 and 49 who use illicit drugs work full time. Also, drug-using employees are more than three times more likely to be involved in a workplace accident and five times more likely to submit a claim for worker's compensation. Authors Leslie Kean and Dennis Bernstein oppose drug testing because many employees, especially African Americans, falsely test positive for drugs. As a result, too many employees with false positive findings are unfairly discharged.

Social science research analyst Bernadette Pelissier and her colleagues found that males and females in federal prisons who were provided with drug treatment, as well as some type of follow-up treatment, were less likely to be rearrested or to test positive for drugs than others who were not provided with drug treatment. Psychology professor Robert Apsler questions the effectiveness of drug abuse treatment. He also questions whether or not drug addicts would go for treatment if services were expanded.

Professors of communication Sandi W. Smith and Charles K. Atkin and Ph.D. candidate Thomas Fediuk assert that advertisements for alcoholic beverages are perceived as appealing and influential by young people. The ads consistently portray alcohol use as humorous and fun, and actors in the advertisements are perceived as sociable, romantic, adventurous, and relaxed. The secretary of health and human services contends that the research demonstrating a link between alcohol advertisements and actual drinking behavior among young people is inconsistent. Young people whose alcohol use is affected by alcohol advertisements may be predisposed to alcohol use in the first place, says the secretary, concluding that alcohol advertisements essentially reinforce behavior.

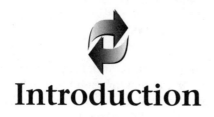

Introduction

Drugs: Divergent Views

Raymond Goldberg

An Overview of the Problem

Very few topics generate as much debate and concern as drugs. Drug use, either directly or indirectly, affects everyone. Drugs and issues related to drugs are evident in every aspect of life. There is much dismay that drug use and abuse cause many of the problems that plague society. Individuals, families, and communities are adversely affected by drug abuse, and many people wonder if the very fabric of society will continue to experience decay because of drugs. The news media are replete with horrific stories about people under the influence of drugs committing crimes or perpetrating violence against others, of people who die senselessly, of men and women who compromise themselves for drugs, and of women who deliver babies that are addicted to or impaired by drugs. In some countries drug cartels have a major impact on government. Clearly, one does not need to be a drug user to experience its effects.

From conception until death, almost everyone is touched by drug use. For example, stimulants such as Ritalin are prescribed for children so that they can learn or behave better in school. Some college students take stimulants so that they can stay up late to write a term paper or lose a few pounds. Many teenagers take drugs to cope with daily stresses and increasing responsibilities or because they want to be accepted by their friends. For many people, young and old, the elixir for relaxation may be sipped, swallowed, smoked, or sniffed. Some people who live under poverty-stricken conditions anesthetize themselves with drugs as a way to escape from their unpleasant environment. On the other hand, some individuals who seem to have everything immerse themselves in drugs, possibly out of boredom. To contend with the ailments that accompany getting older, the elderly often rely on drugs. Many people use drugs to confront their pains, problems, frustrations, and disappointments. Others take drugs simply because they like their effects or out of curiosity. And some people just want to experience more happiness in their lives. This last concern is debated in Issue 10, which examines whether or not medicinal drugs should be prescribed to alter people's consciousness and to make them happy.

Background on Drugs

Despite one's feelings about drug use, drugs are an integral part of society. The popularity of various drugs rises and falls with the times. For example, according to annual surveys of 8th-, 10th-, and 12th-grade students in the United States, the use of LSD and marijuana increased throughout the 1990s despite a decline in use throughout the 1980s (Johnston, O'Malley, and Bachman, 2002). Especially alarming is the fact that the largest increase in drug use in the 1990s occurred among 8th-grade students. One particular drug whose popularity increased significantly in the late 1990s is Ecstasy. And although many types of drugs declined in use in 2002, Ecstasy and other "club drugs" remain popular with many young people. Issue 4 looks at whether or not we should be concerned about club drugs.

Understanding the history and the role of drugs in society is critical for addressing drug-related problems. Drugs have been used throughout human history. Alcohol played a significant role in the early history of the United States. According to Lee (1963), for example, the Pilgrims landed at Plymouth Rock because they ran out of beer. Marijuana use dates back nearly 5,000 years, when the Chinese Emperor Shen Nung prescribed it for medical ailments like malaria, gout, rheumatism, and gas pains. Ironically, 5,000 years after marijuana was first used medicinally, its medical value remains a matter of contention. Some issues simply refuse to go away. Hallucinogens have existed since the beginning of humankind and have been used for a variety of reasons, including to enhance beauty or to cast spells on enemies. Furthermore, about 150 of the estimated 500,000 different plant species have been used for hallucinogenic purposes (Schultes and Hofmann, 1979).

Opium, from which narcotics are derived, was written about extensively by the ancient Greeks and Romans; opium is even referred to in Homer's *Odyssey* (circa 1000 B.C.). In the Arab world opium and hashish were widely used (primarily because alcohol was forbidden). The Arabs were introduced to opium through their trading in India and China. Arab physician Avicenna (A.D. 1000) wrote an extremely complete medical textbook in which he describes the benefits of opium. Ironically, Avicenna died from an overdose of opium and wine. Eventually, opium played a central role in a war between China and the British government.

The most commonly consumed drug throughout the world is caffeine. More than 9 out of every 10 Americans drink beverages that include caffeine. Coffee dates back to A.D. 900, when, to stay awake during lengthy religious vigils, Muslims in Arabia consumed coffee. However, coffee was later condemned because the Koran, the holy book of Islam, described coffee as an intoxicant (Brecher, 1972). Drinking coffee became a popular activity in Europe, although it was banned for a short time. In the mid-1600s, coffeehouses were prime locations for men to converse, relax, and do business. Medical benefits were associated with coffee, although England's King Charles II and English physicians tried to prohibit its use. Many claims have been made regarding the safety of caffeine. Issue 11 discusses whether or not the consequences of caffeine outweigh its benefits.

Coffeehouses served as places of learning. For a one-cent cup of coffee, one could listen to well-known literary and political leaders (Meyer, 1954). Lloyd's of London, the famous insurance company, started around 1700 from Edward Lloyd's coffeehouse. However, not everyone was pleased with these "penny universities," as they were called. In 1674, in response to the countless hours men spent at the coffeehouses, a group of women published a pamphlet titled *The Women's Petition Against Coffee,* which criticized coffee use. Despite the protestations against coffee, its use proliferated. Today, more than 325 years later, coffeehouses are still flourishing as centers for relaxation and conversation.

Coca leaves, from which cocaine is derived, have been chewed since before recorded history. Drawings found on South American pottery indicate that coca chewing was practiced before the rise of the Incan Empire. The coca plant was held in high regard: considered a present from the gods, it was used in religious rituals and burial ceremonies. When the Spaniards arrived in South America, they tried to regulate coca chewing by the natives but were unsuccessful. Cocaine was later included in the popular soft drink Coca-Cola. Another stimulant, amphetamine, was developed in the 1920s and was originally used to treat narcolepsy. It was later prescribed for treating asthma and for weight loss. Today the stimulant Ritalin is given to approximately 6 million school-age children annually to address attention deficit disorders. Some people contend that too many children are given Ritalin, while others assert that not enough students are receiving the drug. The question of whether or not Ritalin is being overprescribed is debated in Issue 12.

Minor tranquilizers, also called "antianxiety drugs," were first marketed in the early 1950s. The sales of these drugs were astronomical. Drugs to reduce anxiety were in high demand. Another group of antianxiety drugs are benzodiazepines. Two well-known benzodiazepines are Librium and Valium; the latter ranks as the most widely prescribed drug in the history of American medicine. Xanax, which has replaced Valium as the minor tranquilizer of choice, is one of the five most prescribed drugs in the United States today. Minor tranquilizers are noteworthy because they are legally prescribed to alter one's consciousness. Mind-altering drugs existed prior to minor tranquilizers, but they were not prescribed for that purpose. In many instances consumers request prescription drugs from their physicians after seeing them advertised in the media. Is it a good practice for people to encourage their physicians to prescribe drugs that they saw advertised? This is the focus of Issue 13.

Combating Drug Problems

The debates in *Taking Sides: Clashing Views on Controversial Issues in Drugs and Society* confront many important drug-related issues. For example, what is the most effective way to reduce drug abuse? Should laws preventing drug use and abuse be more strongly enforced, or should drug laws be less punitive? How can the needs of individuals be met while ensuring that the greater good of society is served? Should drug abuse be seen as a public health problem or a legal problem? Are drugs an American problem or an international problem? The debate over whether the drug problem should be fought nationally or internationally is addressed in Issue 2. Many people argue that America would benefit most by focusing its attention on stopping the proliferation of drugs in other countries.

Others feel that reducing the demand for drugs should be the primary focus. If federal funding is limited, should those funds go to reducing the demand for drugs or stopping their importation?

One of the oldest debates concerns whether or not drug use should be decriminalized. In recent years this debate has become more intense because well-known individuals such as political analyst William F. Buckley, Jr., and economist Milton Friedman have come out in support of changing the drug laws. For many people the issue is not whether drug use is good or bad but whether or not people should be punished for taking drugs. Is it worth the time and expense for law enforcement officials to arrest nonviolent drug offenders? One question that is basic to this debate is whether drug decriminalization would cause more or less damage than keeping drugs illegal. Issue 1 addresses this question.

In a related matter, should potentially harmful drugs be restricted even if they may be of medical benefit? Some people are concerned that currently illegal drugs that are used for medical reasons may be illegally diverted. Yet most people agree that patients should have access to the best medicine available. In referenda in numerous U.S. states, voters have approved the medical use of marijuana. Is the federal government consistent in allowing potentially harmful drugs to be used for medical purposes? For example, narcotics are often prescribed for pain relief. Is there a chance that patients who are given narcotics will become addicted? Issue 9 debates whether or not marijuana has a legitimate medical use. Issue 6 looks at whether drug addiction is based on heredity or whether it is a choice that people make.

A major emphasis in society today is on competition, especially athletic competition. With a win-at-all-cost mentality, many athletes try to gain an edge by taking performance-enhancing drugs. The issue of whether or not athletes who use anabolic steroids are engaging in high-risk behavior is discussed in Issue 7.

Many of the issues debated in this book deal with drug prevention. As with most controversial issues, there is a lack of consensus on how to prevent drug-related problems. For example, Issue 5 debates whether or not prosecuting women who use drugs during pregnancy will affect drug use by other women who become pregnant. On the other hand, will pregnant women who use drugs avoid prenatal care because they fear prosecution? Will newborns be better served if pregnant women who use drugs are charged with child abuse? Are such laws discriminatory, since most of the cases that are prosecuted involve poor women?

Some people contend that drug laws discriminate not only according to social class but also according to age and ethnicity. Many drug laws in the United States were initiated because of their association with different ethnic groups. Opium smoking, for example, was made illegal after it was associated with Chinese immigrants (Musto, 1991). Cocaine became illegal after it was linked with blacks. And marijuana was outlawed after it was linked with Hispanics.

Drug-related issues are not limited to illegal drugs. Tobacco and alcohol are two pervasive legal drugs that generate much debate. For example, are the adverse effects of smoking exaggerated (Issue 8)? Should nonsmokers be concerned about the effects of secondhand smoke (Issue 14)? Should alcoholics totally abstain from alcohol, or can they learn to drink moderately (Issue 15)? A fourth issue relating to legal drugs deals with whether or not the legal blood alcohol concentration limit for driving while intoxicated should be lowered (Issue 3).

Gateway Drugs

Drugs like inhalants, tobacco, and alcohol are considered "gateway" drugs. These are drugs that are often used as a prelude to other, usually illegal, drugs. Inhalants are composed of numerous products, from paints and solvents to glues, aerosol sprays, petroleum products, cleaning supplies, and nitrous oxide (laughing gas). Inhalant abuse in the United States is a relatively new phenomenon. It seems that until the media starting reporting on the dangers of inhalant abuse, its use was not particularly common (Brecher, 1972). This raises questions regarding the impact of the media on drug use. Issue 19 explores the related question of how alcohol advertisements affect alcohol use by young people.

Advertisements are an integral part of the media, and their influence can be seen in the growing popularity of cigarette smoking among adolescents. In the 1880s cigarette smoking escalated in the United States. One of the most important factors contributing to cigarettes' popularity at that time was the development of the cigarette-rolling machine (previously, cigarettes could be rolled at a rate of only four per minute). Also, cigarette smoking, which was considered an activity reserved for men, began to be seen as an option for women. As cigarettes began to be marketed toward women, cigarette smoking became more widespread. As is evident from this introduction, numerous factors affect drug use. One argument is that if young people were better educated about the hazards of drugs and were taught how to understand the role of the media, then limits on advertising would not be necessary.

Drug Prevention and Treatment

Some people maintain that educating young people about drugs is one way to prevent drug use and abuse. Studies show that by delaying the onset of drug use, the likelihood of drug abuse is reduced. In the past, however, drug education had little impact on drug-taking behavior (Goldberg, 2002).

Another way to reduce drug abuse that has been heavily promoted is drug abuse treatment. However, is drug abuse treatment effective? Does it prevent recurring drug abuse, reduce criminal activity and violence, and halt the spread of drug-related disease? Issue 18 examines whether or not drug abuse treatment affects these outcomes. A study by Glass (1995) indicated that methadone maintenance, a treatment for heroin addiction, may have some benefits. But do those benefits outweigh the costs of the treatment? If society feels that treatment is a better alternative to other solutions, such as incarceration, it is imperative to know if treatment works.

Distinguishing Between Drug Use, Misuse, and Abuse

Although the terms *drug, drug misuse,* and *drug abuse* are commonly used, they have different meanings to different people. Defining these terms may seem simple at first, but many factors affect how they are defined. Should a definition for a drug be based on its behavioral effects, its effects on society, its pharmacological properties, or its chemical composition? One simple, concise definition of a drug is "any substance that produces an effect on the mind, body, or both." One could also define a drug by how it is used. For example, if watching television and listening to music are forms of escape from daily problems, then they may be considered drugs.

Legal drugs cause far more death and disability than illegal drugs, but society appears to be most concerned with the use of illegal drugs. The potential harms of legal drugs tend to be minimized. By viewing drugs as illicit substances only, people can fail to recognize that commonly used substances such as caffeine, tobacco, alcohol, and over-the-counter preparations are drugs. If these substances are not perceived as drugs, then people might not acknowledge that they can be misused or abused.

Definitions of misuse and abuse are not affected by a drug's legal status. Drug misuse refers to the inappropriate or unintentional use of drugs. Someone who smokes marijuana to improve his or her study skills is misusing marijuana because the drug impairs short-term memory. Drug abuse alludes to physical, emotional, financial, intellectual, or social consequences arising from chronic drug use. Under this definition, can a person abuse food, aspirin, soft drinks, or chocolate? Also, should people be free to make potentially unhealthy choices?

The Cost of the War on Drugs

The U.S. government spends billions of dollars each year trying to curb the rise in drug use. A major portion of that money goes toward law enforcement. Vast sums of money are used by the military to intercept drug shipments, while foreign governments are given money to help them with their own wars on drugs. A smaller portion of the funds is used for treating and preventing drug abuse. One strategy to eliminate drug use is drug testing. Currently, men and women in the military, athletes, industry employees, and others are subject to random drug testing.

The expense of drug abuse to industries is staggering: Experts estimate that about 14 percent of full-time construction workers in the United States between the ages of 18 and 49 use illicit drugs while at work (Gerber and Yacoubian, 2002). The cost of drug abuse to employers is approximately $171 billion each year (Kesselring and Pittman, 2002). Compared to nonaddicted employees, drug-dependent employees are absent from their jobs more often, and drug users are less likely to maintain stable job histories than nonusers. In its report *America's Habit: Drug Abuse, Drug Trafficking and Organized Crime,* the President's Commission on Organized Crime supported testing all federal workers for drugs. It further recommended that federal contracts be withheld from private employers who do not implement drug-testing procedures (Brinkley, 1986).

A prerequisite to being hired by many companies is passing a drug test. Drug testing may be having a positive effect. From 1987 to 1994 the number of workers testing positive declined 57 percent (Center for Substance Abuse Prevention, 1995). Many companies have reported a decrease in accidents and injuries after the initiation of drug testing (Angarola, 1991). However, most Americans consider drug testing degrading and dehumanizing (Walsh and Trumble, 1991). An important question is, What is the purpose of drug testing? Drug testing raises three other important questions: (1) Does drug testing prevent drug use? (2) Is the point of drug testing to help employees with drug problems or to get rid of employees who use drugs? and (3) How can the civil rights of employees be balanced against the rights of companies? Issue 17 examines whether or not employees should be required to participate in drug testing.

How serious is the drug problem? Is it real, or is there simply an unreasonable hysteria regarding drugs? In the United States there has been a growing intolerance toward drug use during the last 20 years (Musto, 1991). Drugs are a problem for many people. Drugs can affect one's physical, social, intellectual, and emotional health. Ironically, some people take drugs because they produce these effects. Individuals who take drugs receive some kind of reward from the drug; the reward may come from being associated with others who use drugs or from the feelings derived from the drug. If these rewards were not present, people would likely cease using drugs.

The disadvantages of drugs are numerous: they interfere with career aspirations and individual maturation. They have also been associated with violent behavior; addiction; discord among siblings, children, parents, spouses, and friends; work-related problems; financial troubles; problems in school; legal predicaments; accidents; injuries; and death. Yet are drugs the cause or the symptom of the problems that people have? Perhaps drugs are one aspect of a larger scenario in which society is experiencing much change and in which drug use is merely another thread in the social fabric.

References

R. T. Angarola, "Substance-Abuse Testing in the Workplace: Legal Issues and Corporate Responses," in R. H. Coombs and L. J. West, eds., *Drug Testing: Issues and Options* (Oxford University Press, 1991).

E. M. Brecher, *Licit and Illicit Drugs* (Little, Brown, 1972).

J. Brinkley, "Drug Use Held Mostly Stable or Better," *The New York Times* (October 10, 1986).

Drug-Free for a New Century, Center for Substance Abuse Prevention, Substance Abuse and Mental Health Services Administration (1995).

J. K. Gerber and G. S. Yacoubian, "An Assessment of Drug Testing Within the Construction Industry," *Journal of Drug Education* (vol. 32, no. 1, 2002), pp. 53–68.

R. M. Glass, "Methadone Maintenance: New Research on a Controversial Treatment," *Journal of the American Medical Association* (vol. 269, no. 15, 1995), pp. 1995–1996.

R. Goldberg, *Drugs Across the Spectrum* (Wadsworth, 2002).

L. D. Johnston, P. O. O'Malley, and J. G. Bachman, *Monitoring the Future* (National Institute on Drug Abuse, 2002).

R. G. Kesselring and J. P. Pittman, "Drug Testing Laws and Employment Injuries," *Journal of Labor Research* (vol. 32, no. 2, 2002), pp. 293–302.

H. Lee, *How Dry We Were: Prohibition Revisited* (Prentice Hall, 1963).

H. Meyer, *Old English Coffee Houses* (Rodale Press, 1954).

D. F. Musto, "Opium, Cocaine and Marijuana in American History," *Scientific American* (July 1991), pp. 40–47.

R. E. Schultes and A. Hofmann, *Plants of the Gods: Origins of Hallucinogenic Use* (McGraw-Hill, 1979).

J. M. Walsh and J. G. Trumble, "The Politics of Drug Testing," in R. H. Coombs and L. J. West, eds., *Drug Testing: Issues and Options* (Oxford University Press, 1991).

On the Internet . . .

Drug Policy Alliance

Formerly the Drug Policy Foundation, this site is an excellent source of information on drug-related legal issues.

http://www.drugpolicy.org

Office of National Drug Control Policy (ONDCP)

This site provides information regarding the U.S. government's position on many drug-related topics. Funding allocations by the federal government to deal with drug problems are also included.

http://www.whitehousedrugpolicy.gov

Club Drugs.org

Current information about club drugs such as Ecstasy, Rohypnol, ketamine, methamphetamines, and LSD can be accessed through this National Institute on Drug Abuse site.

http://www.clubdrugs.org

DanceSafe

This organization attempts to reduce the harm of the drug Ecstasy by testing pills to determine whether the contents are Ecstasy or some type of adulterant.

http://www.dancesafe.org

National Institute on Drug Abuse (NIDA)

Health risks associated with anabolic steroids and strategies for preventing steroid abuse can be obtained at this location.

http://www.steroidabuse.org

PART 1

Drugs and Public Policy

*D*rug abuse causes a myriad of problems for society: The psychological and physical effects of drug abuse can be devastating; many drugs are addictive; drugs wreak havoc on families; disability and death result from drug overdoses; and drugs are frequently implicated in crimes, especially violent crimes. Identifying drug-related problems is not difficult. What is unclear is the best course of action to take when dealing with these problems.

Three scenarios exist for dealing with drugs: policies can be made more restrictive, they can be made less restrictive, or they can remain the same. The position one takes depends on whether drug use and abuse are seen as legal, social, or medical problems. Perhaps the issue is not whether drugs are good or bad but how to minimize the harm of drugs. The debates in this section explore these issues.

- Should Drugs Be Decriminalized?

- Should the United States Put More Emphasis on Stopping the Importation of Drugs?

- Will a Lower Blood Alcohol Level for Drunk Driving Reduce Automobile Accidents?

- Should We Be Concerned About "Club Drugs"?

- Should Pregnant Drug Users Be Prosecuted?

- Is Drug Addiction a Choice?

- Are Athletes Who Use Anabolic Steroids Engaging in High-Risk Behavior?

ISSUE 1

Should Drugs Be Decriminalized?

YES: Ethan A. Nadelmann, from "Ending the War on Drugs," *Lapis Magazine* (Spring 2001)

NO: Eric A. Voth, from "America's Longest 'War,'" *The World & I* (February 2000)

ISSUE SUMMARY

YES: Ethan A. Nadelmann, director of the Lindesmith Center, maintains that the war on drugs has been futile and conterproductive. He feels that a pragmatic approach is necessary. Current laws, says Nadelmann, exacerbate problems related to drug use.

NO: Eric A. Voth, chairman of the International Drug Strategy Institute, contends that the war on drugs is not a failure and that legalizing drugs would worsen drug-related problems. He maintains that a restrictive yet compassionate approach toward drug use is the best policy to adopt.

In 2002 the federal government allocated nearly \$19 billion to control drug use and to enforce laws that are designed to protect society from the perils created by drug use. Some people believe that the government's war on drugs could be more effective but that governmental agencies and communities are not fighting hard enough to stop drug use. They also hold that laws to halt drug use are too few and too lenient. Others contend that the war against drugs is unnecessary; that, in fact, society has already lost the war on drugs. These individuals feel that the best way to remedy drug problems is to end the fight altogether by ending the criminalization of drug use.

There are conflicting views among both liberals and conservatives on whether or not legislation has had the intended result of curtailing the problems of drug use. Many argue that legislation and the criminalization of drugs have been counterproductive in controlling drug problems. Some suggest that the criminalization of drugs has actually contributed to and worsened the social ills associated with drugs. Proponents of drug legalization maintain that the war on drugs, not drugs themselves, is damaging to American society. They do not advocate drug use; they argue only that laws against drugs exacerbate problems related to drugs.

Proponents of drug decriminalization argue that the strict enforcement of drug laws damages American society because it drives people to violence and crime. These people overburden the court system, thus rendering it ineffective. Moreover, proponents contend that the criminalization of drugs fuels organized crime, allows children to be pulled into the drug business, and makes illegal drugs themselves more dangerous because they are manufactured without government standards or regulations. Hence, drugs may be adulterated or of unidentified potency. Decriminalization advocates also argue that decriminalization would take the profits out of drug sales, thereby decreasing the value of and demand for drugs.

Some decriminalization advocates argue that the federal government's prohibition stance on drugs is an immoral and impossible objective. To achieve a "drug-free society" is self-defeating and a misnomer because drugs have always been a part of human culture. Furthermore, prohibition efforts indicate a disregard for the private freedom of individuals because they assume that individuals are incapable of making their own choices.

People who favor decriminalizing drugs feel that decriminalization would give the government more control over the purity and potency of drugs and that the international drug trade would be regulated more effectively. Decriminalization, they argue, would take the emphasis off of law enforcement policies and allow more effort to be put toward education, prevention, and treatment. Decriminalization advocates assert that most of the negative implications of drug prohibition would disappear.

Opponents of this view maintain that decriminalization is not the solution to drug problems and that it is a very dangerous idea. Decriminalization, they assert, will drastically increase drug use because if drugs are more accessible, more people will turn to drugs. This upsurge in drug use will come at an incredibly high price: American society will be overrun with drug-related accidents, loss in worker productivity, and hospital emergency rooms filled with drug-related emergencies. Drug treatment efforts would be futile because users would have no legal incentive to stop taking drugs. Also, users may prefer drugs rather than rehabilitation, and education programs may be ineffective in dissuading children from using drugs. Advocates of drug decriminalization maintain that drug abuse is a "victimless crime" in which the only person being hurt is the drug user. Decriminalization opponents argue that this notion is ludicrous and dangerous because drug use has dire repercussions for all of society. Drugs can destroy the minds and bodies of many people. Also, regulations to control drug use have a legitimate social aim to protect society and its citizens from the harm of drugs. Decriminalization opponents maintain that criminalization is not immoral nor a violation of personal freedom; rather, criminalizing drugs allows a standard of control to be established in order to preserve human character and society as a whole.

In the following selections, Ethan A. Nadelmann explains why he feels drugs should be decriminalized, while Eric A. Voth describes the detrimental effects that he believes would result from drug decriminalization.

Ethan A. Nadelmann 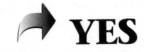 **YES**

Ending the War on Drugs

The failed drug war in this country is an international disgrace. Our overflowing prisons and the easy availability of cheap, hard drugs are sufficient evidence that fresher, saner solutions to the question of drugs in America are available and must be tried. Thankfully, encouraging developments are beginning to appear.

"So what you're saying is, you want to legalize drugs, right?"

That's the first question I'm typically asked when I start talking about drug policy reform. My short answer is, "No, that's not what I'm saying. Legalize marijuana? Yes, I think we need to head in that direction. But no, I'm not suggesting we make heroin and cocaine available the way we do alcohol and cigarettes."

"So what are you recommending?" is the second question. "And what do you mean by drug policy reform?"

Here's the longer answer.

Most drug "legalizers" aren't really drug legalizers. That's the conclusion I've come to after more than a decade of writing about legalization, associating with "legalizers," and being called one myself.

A legalizer, as most Americans apparently understand the term, is someone who believes that heroin, cocaine, and most or all other drugs should be available over the counter—like alcohol or cigarettes. The state might impose heavy taxes as well as strict limits on advertising and places of sale and consumption, and even prohibit sales to minors—but so long as it's available to adults without a prescription, that's legalization.

The truth is, that's not what I'm fighting for. Nor is it the ultimate aim of the philanthropist and financier George Soros, who has played a leading role in funding drug policy reform efforts, nor is it the aim of the great majority of people who devote their time, money, and energies to ending the drug war.

This is not to say there is no such thing as a "legalizer." Milton Friedman, the Nobel Prize–winning economist, and Thomas Szasz, the provocative professor of psychiatry, have argued that total drug legalization is the only rational and ethical way to deal with drugs in our society. Most libertarians and many others agree with them. Szasz and others have even opposed the medical marijuana ballot initiatives and other modest reform efforts as steps backward in the struggle for more sensible drug policies.

Friedman, Szasz, and I agree on many points—that US drug prohibition, like alcohol prohibition decades ago, generates extraordinary harms. It, not drugs per se, is responsible for creating vast black markets, criminalizing millions of otherwise law-abiding citizens, corrupting both governments and societies at large, empowering organized criminals, increasing predatory crime, spreading disease, curtailing personal freedom, disparaging science and honest inquiry, and legitimizing public policies that are both extraordinary and insidious in their racially disproportionate consequences. But by Friedman and Szasz's criteria, and presumably the drug warriors' as well, I'm not a legalizer. I'm not ready to advocate for over-the-counter sale of heroin and cocaine, and not just because that's not a politically palatable argument right now. I'm simply not convinced that outright legalization is the optimal alternative.

There is no drug legalization movement in America. What there is, is a nascent political and social movement for drug policy reform. It consists of the growing number of citizens who have been victimized, in one way or another, by the drug war, and who now believe that our current drug policies are doing more harm than good. Most members of this "movement" barely perceive themselves as such, in part because their horizons only extend to one or two domains in which the harms of the drug war are readily apparent to them.

It might be the judge required by inflexible, mandatory minimum sentencing laws to send a drug addict, or petty dealer, or dealer's girlfriend, or Third World drug courier to prison for a longer time than many rapists and murderers serve.

Or the corrections officer who recalls the days when prisons housed "real" criminals, not the petty, nonviolent offenders who fill jails and prisons these days.

Or the addict in recovery—employed, law abiding, a worthy citizen in every respect—who must travel fifty or a hundred miles each day to pick up her methadone, i.e., her medicine, because current laws do not allow methadone prescriptions to be filled at a local pharmacy.

Or the nurse in the oncology or AIDS unit obliged to look the other way while a patient wracked with pain or nausea smokes her forbidden medicine. Both know, from their own experience, that smoked marijuana works, and that for many people it works better than anything else.

Or the teacher or counselor warned by school authorities not to speak so frankly about drug use with his students lest he violate federal regulations prohibiting anything other than "just say no" bromides.

Or the doctor who fears to prescribe medically appropriate doses of opioid analgesics to a patient in pain because any variations from the norm bring unfriendly scrutiny from government agents and state medical boards.

Or the employee with an outstanding record who fails a drug test on Monday morning because she shared a joint with her husband over the weekend, and is fired.

Or the struggling farmer in North Dakota who wonders why farmers in Canada and dozens of other countries can plant hemp, but he cannot.

Or the conservative Republican who abhors the extraordinary powers of police and prosecutors to seize private property from citizens who have not been convicted of violating any laws, and who worries about the corruption inherent in sending forfeited proceeds directly to law enforcement agencies.

Or the upstanding African American citizen repeatedly stopped by police for "driving while black," or even "walking while black," never mind "running while black."

Some are victims of the drug war, and some are drug policy reformers, but most of them don't know it yet.

The ones who know they're drug policy reformers are the ones who connect the dots—the ones who see and understand the panoply of ways in which our prohibitionist policies are doing more harm than good. We may not agree on what aspect of prohibition is most pernicious—the generation of crime, the corruption, the black market, the spread of disease, the loss of freedom, the burgeoning of prisons, or simply the lies and hypocrisies—and we certainly don't agree on the optimal solutions, but we all regard our current policy of punitive drug prohibition as a fundamental evil in our society.

Most drug policy reformers I know believe that marijuana should be decriminalized, and taxed and regulated, even as we step up our efforts to provide honest and effective drug education rather than ineffective, feel-good programs like DARE.

Most drug policy reformers I know don't want crack or methamphetamine sold in 7-Elevens (to quote one of the more pernicious accusations hurled by former drug czar Barry McCaffrey), but we do favor public health policies proven to reduce the death, disease, crime, and suffering associated with injection drug use and heroin addiction: expanded methadone maintenance treatment; heroin maintenance trials, ready access to sterile syringes, and other harm reduction policies that have proven effective abroad and that should work just as well here.

We believe that responsible doctors should be allowed, and encouraged, to prescribe whatever drugs work best, notwithstanding their feared and demonized status in the eyes of the ignorant and the law.

We believe that people should not be incarcerated for possessing small amounts of any drug for personal use. But we also believe that people who put their fellow citizens at risk by driving while impaired should be treated strictly, and punished accordingly.

We reject drug testing programs that reveal little about whether or not people are impaired in the workplace, but much about what they may have consumed over the weekend.

We believe that those who sell drugs to other adults are not the moral equivalents of violent and other predatory criminals, and should not be treated so by our criminal laws.

These beliefs, these statements of principles and objectives, represent a call for a fundamentally different drug policy. It's not legalization, but it's also not simply a matter of spending more on treatment and prevention and less on interdiction and enforcement. We call it "harm reduction"—a new approach grounded not in the fear, ignorance, prejudice, and vested pecuniary and institutional interests that drive current policies, but rather in common sense, science, public health, and human rights.

Efforts to reform US drug policy obviously confront powerful obstacles. Punitive drug prohibition and a temperance ideology almost as old as the nation itself are deeply embedded in American laws, institutions, and culture. It's our chronic national hysteria, rejuvenated each time a "new" drug emerges, ripe for political posturing and media mania. But America's war on drugs is neither monolithic nor irreversible. Cracks in its façade are increasingly visible, and dissent is popping out all over, even within the headquarters of the war itself.

The former drug czar, retired General Barry McCaffrey, is a case in point. He was almost certainly the best drug czar to date, even if that's not saying much given his competition. Unlike the first drug czar, William Bennett, Mc-Caffrey preferred to leave the rhetoric of war and zero tolerance behind, speaking instead of the drug problem as a cancer in need of treatment. He attacked the relentless incarceration of petty drug offenders, spoke out against New York's draconian Rockefeller drug laws, and even called our prison system "America's internal gulag." McCaffrey defended methadone maintenance treatment, and he at least tried to reduce the billions of dollars wasted on futile air and sea interdiction efforts.

Of course, this is the same drug czar who mangled and mocked the truth on issues like needle exchange, marijuana, and harm reduction policies inside and outside the United States. McCaffrey played a pivotal role in ensuring that the US government remains alone among advanced, industrialized nations in the West in providing not a penny for needle exchange programs to reduce the spread of HIV/AIDS. His efforts to challenge the scientific consensus brought to mind the cigarette companies' last, desperate claims to have found a new study demonstrating that smoking does not cause cancer.

His position on medical marijuana was shameful—mocking patients and doctors, threatening them with prosecution and loss of license, and steadfastly blocking the efforts of state and local authorities to establish responsible, regulated systems of distribution. The murder rate in the Netherlands, he claimed, was twice that of the United States—no apology necessary when told that in 1995 Americans were actually murdered at four times the rate of the Dutch.

McCaffrey was also notorious for his thin skin, which may explain why he studiously avoided any public debate with reformers. His insults and claims were always lobbed from a distance. He was careful to withdraw from televised and other public fora when he learned that patients, doctors, scientists, and others with a critical view had been invited to participate.

As a reformer, I found McCaffrey's dissembling indefensible. But as a political analyst, I could not help but be aware of the political forces that weighed upon him and his office. Political power in the United States increasingly lies in the hands of those who smoked marijuana when they were younger, but that generational shift has yet to influence policy. Far more important, and perhaps distinctly American, is the lingering influence of our rigid anti-drug ideology.

Most Americans have strong doubts about the drug war. They support treatment instead of incarceration for drug addicts. They think marijuana should be legally available for medical purposes. They don't want the government seizing money and property from people who have never been convicted of a crime. They're beginning to have doubts about the cost and meaning of incarcerating almost half a million of their fellow citizens for drug law violations.

So why does the drug war not just persist but keep growing?

Part of the answer lies in what might best be described as a "drug prohibition complex"—to take off on President Eisenhower's farewell warning of the military-industrial complex—composed of the hundreds of thousands of law enforcement officials, private prison corporations, anti-drug organizations, drug testing companies, and many others who benefit economically, politically, emotionally, and otherwise from this evergrowing edifice. Drug prohibition is now big business in the United States.

Equally important is the powerful influence of what might be called the "John Birchers of the drug war." In the 1960's, when anti-communism still represented the American national ideology, the John Birch Society was the most anti-communist of all, ever vigilant for any sign of moderation or detente. The John Birchers of the drug war represent no more than twenty percent of public opinion today, but their political influence far exceeds that of the nation's leading scientists, scholars, and other drug policy experts. Powerful senators and congressmen take their calls, invite them to testify before official hearings, ensure that their organizations are well funded, and act on their advice. Directors of drug treatment and research agencies, fearful of the zealots' wrath, are quick to compromise their own scientific and intellectual integrity. So too was drug czar Barry McCaffrey.

Nonetheless, signs of reform abound. The John Birchers may still be powerful, but they're gradually losing credibility. Marijuana is to them what alcohol was to the temperance warriors of old. And just as the temperance advocates became increasingly shrill and silly as Prohibition stumbled along, so today's anti-drug extremists sound increasingly foolish to the American parent who knows something about marijuana.

The most powerful evidence of reform occurred on Election Day 2000, when voters in five states approved drug policy reform ballot initiatives.

In California, voters overwhelmingly endorsed Proposition 36, the "treatment instead of incarceration" ballot initiative that should result in tens of thousands of non-violent drug possession offenders being diverted from jail and prison into programs that may help them get their lives together. The new law—which received more votes than Al Gore and Ralph Nader combined—may do more to reverse the unnecessary incarceration of non-violent citizens than any other law enacted anywhere in the country in decades.

But it wasn't just California that opted for drug reform. Voters in Nevada and Colorado both approved medical marijuana ballot initiatives, following in the footsteps of California, Oregon, Alaska, Washington state, Maine, and

Washington, DC. In Oregon and Utah, voters overwhelmingly approved (by margins of 2:1) ballot initiatives requiring police and prosecutors to meet a reasonable burden of proof before seizing money and other property from people they suspect of criminal activity—and also mandating that the proceeds of legal forfeitures be handed over not to the police and prosecuting agencies that had seized the property but rather to funds for public education or drug treatment. (The only defeats were in Massachusetts, where voters narrowly defeated a combined forfeiture reform/diversion into treatment initiative, and in Alaska, where voters rejected a far-reaching marijuana legalization initiative.)

These were not the only victories for drug policy reform at the ballot in recent years. California's Proposition 36 was modeled in part on Arizona's Proposition 200, the treatment instead of incarceration initiative that won overwhelmingly in 1996, was gutted by the state legislature in 1997, and reinstituted in 1998 with two voter referenda. In 1998 in Oregon, the first of eleven states to decriminalize marijuana during the 1970s, voters rejected an effort by the state legislature to recriminalize marijuana. Their vote, by a margin of 2:1, could readily be construed as a conservative endorsement of the status quo policy of decriminalization. And in California's Mendocino County, voters [recently] approved a local initiative to decriminalize personal cultivation of modest amounts of marijuana.

What do all these victories for drug policy reform mean? Clearly, more and more citizens realize that the drug war has failed and are looking for new approaches. The votes also suggest that there are limits to what people will accept in the name of the war on drugs. Parents don't want their teenagers to use marijuana, but they also don't want sick people who could benefit from marijuana held hostage to the war on drugs. People don't want drug dealers profiting from their illicit activities, but neither do they want police empowered to take what they want from anyone they merely suspect of criminal activity. Americans don't approve of people using heroin or cocaine, but neither do they think it makes either economic or human sense to lock up drug addicts without first offering them a few opportunities to get their lives together outside prison walls.

So what do we (drug policy reformers) do next? In the case of medical marijuana, three things: enact medical marijuana laws in other states through the legislative process—as Hawaii did . . . with the support of Governor Cayetano; work to ensure that medical marijuana laws are effectively implemented; and try to induce the federal government to stop undermining good faith efforts by state officials to establish regulated distribution systems.

The strategy post-Proposition 36 is somewhat similar. The struggle over implementation of the initiative in California has already begun, with many of its opponents trying either to grab their share of the pie or to tie the process up in knots and thereby undermine support for the new law. Powerful vested interests in the criminal justice business, accustomed to getting their way, did not look kindly on the challenges which Proposition 36 posed to the status quo. If California's new law is implemented in good faith—with minimal corruption of its intentions by those who opposed it—the benefits could be extraordinary, saving taxpayers up to $1.5 billion over the next five years while simultaneously making good drug treatment available to hundreds of thousands of citizens who struggle with drug problems.

Proposition 36 also provides a model—both for initiatives in other states where public opinion favors reform but the legislature and/or the governor are unable or unwilling to comply, and in states like New York, where no ballot initiative process exists to repeal draconian and archaic laws like the infamous Rockefeller drug laws. Our hope is that legislators will derive both inspiration and example from California's initiative.

The initiative victories demonstrated once again that the public is ahead of the politicians when it comes to embracing pragmatic drug policy reforms. But there was also growing evidence . . . that even some politicians are beginning to get it. Hawaii's medical marijuana law was not the only reform bill passed [in 2000]. Three states—North Dakota, Minnesota, and Hawaii—all enacted laws legalizing the cultivation of hemp (to the extent permitted by federal law), and hemp legalization bills are beginning to advance through other state legislatures as well. Vermont was one of eight states that prohibited methadone maintenance treatment, until . . . a law was enacted that may ultimately lead to this treatment being made available not just in specialized clinics but also through public health clinics and private physicians. And, most significantly in terms of potential lives saved, three states—New York, New Hampshire, and Rhode Island—each enacted laws making it easier to purchase sterile syringes in pharmacies. Governors and legislators, including Republican Governor George Pataki, thereby acknowledged the evidence that such laws can help reduce the spread of HIV/AIDS—at no cost to taxpayers.

New Mexico doesn't have the initiative process, but it does have a Republican governor, Gary Johnson, committed to far-reaching drug policy reform. Even before the governor stepped out on this issue, New Mexico was the first state to pass a "Harm Reduction Act" authorizing needle exchange programs throughout the state. Many state Democratic leaders are critical of the war on drugs but wary of the governor. The question is whether bipartisan support for sensible drug reforms can transcend generic partisan hostilities. Our (drug policy reformers') job is to help make that happen.

In Salt Lake City, the new mayor elected [in 2000], Rocky Anderson, gave the boot to the popular but demonstrably ineffective DARE program. He is now following in the footsteps of Baltimore's former three-term mayor, Kurt Schmoke, by making clear that he too supports sensible reforms to reduce the harms of the drug war in his city.

Perhaps it's too early to claim that all this adds up to a national vote of no confidence in the war on drugs. After all, drug war rhetoric still goes down easy in many parts of the country, and Congress has yet to demonstrate any reluctance to enact ever harsher and more far-reaching drug war legislation.

But the pendulum does seem to be reversing direction. The initiatives and recent state legislative victories, the pending reform bills making their way through legislative committees, the governors and mayors beginning to speak out, the rapidly rising anti-war sentiment among African American leaders—are beginning to add up to something new in American politics. Call it a new anti-war movement. Call it a nascent movement for political and social justice. Or simply call it a rising chorus of dissent from the war on drugs. Drug policy reform is clearly gaining around the country.

Let me conclude on a personal note. I have been deeply involved in drug policy reform efforts in the United States and abroad since 1987, first as a professor at Princeton University, then as founder and director of the Lindesmith Center and coordinator of most of the initiatives of George Soros in this area. With the mid-2000 merger of the Lindesmith Center and the Drug Policy Foundation, my colleagues and I are now trying to create the Sierra Club or NAACP or Human Rights Campaign of drug policy reform—a powerful national organization capable of effectively attaining our objectives.

Please support our efforts. America's war on drugs can be brought to an end, but only if millions of Americans give their support and make their voices heard.

Eric A. Voth

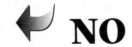 **NO**

America's Longest "War"

Bashing our drug policy is a popular activity. The advocates of legalization and decriminalization repeatedly contend that restrictive drug policy is failing, in the hope that this becomes a self-fulfilling prophecy. An objective look at the history of drug policy in the United States, especially in comparison to other countries, demonstrates that, indeed, our policies are working. What we also see is the clear presence of a well-organized and well-financed drug culture lobby that seeks to tear down restrictive drug policy and replace it with permissive policies that could seriously jeopardize our country's viability.

To understand our current situation, we must examine the last 25 years. The 1970s were a time of great social turmoil for the United States, and drug use was finding its way into the fabric of society. Policymakers were uncertain how to deal with drugs. As permissive advisers dominated the discussion, drug use climbed. The National Household Survey and the Monitoring the Future Survey both confirm that drug use peaked in the late 1970s. Twenty-five million Americans were current users of drugs in 1979, 37 percent of high school seniors had used marijuana in the prior 30 days, and 10. 7 percent of them used marijuana daily. During the same time frame, 13 states embraced the permissive social attitude and legalized or decriminalized marijuana.

In the late 1970s, policymakers, parents, and law enforcement began to realize that our drug situation was leading to Armageddon. As never before, a coordinated war on drugs was set in motion that demanded a no-use message. This was largely driven by parents who were sick of their children falling prey to drugs. The "Just Say No" movement was the centerpiece of antidrug activities during the subsequent years. A solid national antidrug message was coupled with rigorous law enforcement. The results were striking. As perception of the harmfulness of drugs increased, their use dropped drastically. By 1992, marijuana use by high school students in the prior 30 days had dropped to 11.9 percent and daily use to 1.9 percent.

Breakdown in the 1990s

Unfortunately, several major events derailed our policy successes in the early 1990s, resulting in an approximate doubling of drug use since that time. From a national vantage point, a sense of complacency set in. Satisfied that the drug war was won, we lost national leadership. Federal funding for antidrug programs became mired in bureaucracy and difficult for small prevention organizations to obtain. A new generation of drug specialists entered the scene. Lacking experience of the ravages of the 1970s, they were willing to accept softening of policy. The Internet exploded as an open forum for the dissemination of inaccurate, deceptive, and manipulative information supporting permissive policy, even discussions of how to obtain and use drugs. The greatest audience has been young people, who are exposed to a plethora of drug-permissive information without filter or validation.

The entertainment media have provided a steady diet of alcohol and drug use for young people to witness. A recent study commissioned by the White House Office of National Drug Control Policy found that alcohol appeared in more than 93 percent of movies and illicit drugs in 22 percent, of which 51 percent depicted marijuana use. Concurrently, the news media have begun to demonstrate bias toward softening of drug policy, having the net effect of changing public opinion.

The single most dramatic influence, however, came in the transformation of the drug culture from a disorganized group of legalization advocates to a well-funded and well-organized machine. With funding from several large donors, drug-culture advocates were able to initiate large-scale attacks on the media and policymakers. The most prominent funder is the billionaire George Soros, who has spent millions toward the initiation of organizations such as the Drug Policy Foundation, Lindesmith Center, medical-marijuana-advocacy and needle-handout groups, to name a few projects.

A slick strategic shift toward compartmentalizing and dissecting restrictive drug policy has resulted in what is termed the "harm reduction" movement. After all, who would oppose the idea of reducing the harm to society caused by drug use? The philosophy of the harm reduction movement is well summarized by Ethan Nadelmann of the Lindesmith Center (also funded by Soros), who is considered the godfather of the legalization movement:

> Let's start by dropping the "zero tolerance" rhetoric and policies and the illusory goal of drug-free societies. Accept that drug use is here to stay and that we have no choice but to learn to live with drugs so that they cause the least possible harm. Recognize that many, perhaps most, "drug problems" in the Americas are the results not of drug use per se but of our prohibitionist policies. . . .

The harm reduction movement has attacked the individual components of restrictive drug policy and created strategies to weaken it. Some of these strategies include giving heroin to addicts; handing out needles to addicts; encouraging use of crack cocaine instead of intravenous drugs; reducing drug-related criminal penalties; teaching "responsible" drug use to adolescents instead of working toward prevention of use; the medical marijuana movement; and the expansion of the industrial hemp movement.

Softening Drug Policies

The move toward soft drug policy has created some strange bedfellows. On one hand, supporters of liberal policy such as Gov. Gary Johnson of New Mexico have always taken the misguided view that individuals should have a right to use whatever they want in order to feel good. They often point to their own "survival" of drug use as justification for loosening laws and letting others experiment. Interestingly, the governor's public safety secretary quit as a result of being undermined by Johnson's destructive stand on legalization. Libertarian conservatives such as Milton Friedman and William Buckley have attacked drug policy as an infringement of civil liberties and have incorrectly considered drug use to be a victimless event. Societal problems such as homelessness, domestic abuse, numerous health problems, crimes under the influence, poor job performance, decreased productivity, and declining educational levels have strong connections to drug use and cost our society financially and spiritually.

The notion that decriminalizing or legalizing drugs will drive the criminal element out of the market is flawed and reflects a total lack of understanding of drug use and addiction. Drug use creates its own market, and often the only thing limiting the amount of drugs that an addict uses is the amount of money available. Further, if drugs were legalized, what would the legal scenario be? Would anyone be allowed to sell drugs? Would they be sold by the government? If so, what strengths would be available? If there were any limitations on strength or availability, a black market would immediately develop. Most rational people can easily recognize this slippery slope.

Consistently, drug-culture advocates assert that policy has failed and is extremely costly. This is a calculated strategy to demoralize the population and turn public sentiment against restrictive policy. The real question is, has restrictive policy failed? First we should consider the issues of cost. An effective way to determine cost-effectiveness is to compare the costs to society of legal versus illegal drugs. Estimates from 1990 suggest that the costs of illegal drugs were $70 billion, as compared to that of alcohol alone at $99 billion and tobacco at $72 billion. Estimates from 1992 put the costs of alcohol dependence at $148 billion and all illegal drugs (including the criminal justice system costs) at $98 billion.

Referring to the National Household Survey data from 1998, there were 13.6 million current users of illicit drugs compared to 113 million users of alcohol and 60 million tobacco smokers. There is one difference: legal status of the drugs. The Monitoring the Future Survey of high school seniors suggests that in 1995, some 52.5 percent of seniors had been drunk within the previous year as compared to 34.7 percent who had used marijuana. Yet, alcohol is illegal for teenagers. The only difference is, again, the legal status of the two substances.

Results of Legalization

Permissive drug policy has been tried both in the United States and abroad. In 1985, during the period in which Alaska legalized marijuana, the use of marijuana and cocaine among adolescents was more than twice as high as in other parts of the country. Baltimore has long been heralded as a centerpiece for harm reduction drug policy. Interestingly, the rate of heroin use found among arrestees in Baltimore was higher than in any other city in the United States. Thirty-seven percent of male and 48 percent of female arrestees were positive, compared with 6–23 percent for Washington, D.C., Philadelphia, and Manhattan.

Since liberalizing its marijuana-enforcement policies, the Netherlands has found that marijuana use among 11- to 18-year-olds has increased 142 percent from 1990 to 1995. Crime has risen steadily to the point that aggravated theft and breaking and entering occur three to four times more than in the United States. Along with the staggering increases in marijuana use, the Netherlands has become one of the major suppliers of the drug Ecstacy. Australia is flirting with substantial softening of drug policy. That is already taking a toll. Drug use there among 16- to 29-year-olds is 52 percent as compared with 9 percent in Sweden, a country with a restrictive drug policy. In Vancouver in 1988, HIV prevalence among IV drug addicts was only 1–2 percent. In 1997 it was 23 percent, after wide adoption of harm reduction policies. Vancouver has the largest needle exchange in North America.

Clearly, the last few years have witnessed some very positive changes in policy and our antidrug efforts. A steady national voice opposing drug use is again being heard. Efforts are being made to increase cooperation between the treatment and law enforcement communities to allow greater access to treatment. The primary prevention movement is strong and gaining greater footholds. The increases in drug use witnessed in the early 1990s have slowed.

On the other hand, the drug culture has been successful at some efforts to soften drug policy. Medical marijuana initiatives have successfully passed in several states. These were gross examples of abuse of the ballot initiative process. Large amounts of money purchased slick media campaigns and seduced the public into supporting medical marijuana under the guise of compassion. Industrial hemp initiatives are popping up all over the country in an attempt to hurt anti-marijuana law enforcement and soften public opinion. Needle handouts are being touted as successes, while the evidence is clearly demonstrating failures and increases in HIV, hepatitis B, and hepatitis C. Internationally, our Canadian neighbors are moving down a very destructive road toward drug legalization and harm reduction. The Swiss are experimenting with the lives of addicts by implementing heroin handouts and selective drug legalization. In this international atmosphere, children's attitudes about the harmfulness of drugs teeter in the balance.

Future drug policy must continue to emphasize and fund primary prevention, with the goal of no use of illegal drugs and no illegal use of legal drugs. Treatment availability must be seriously enhanced, but treatment must not be a revolving door. It must be carefully designed and outcomes based. The Rand Drug Policy Research Center concluded that the costs of cocaine use could be reduced by $33.9 billion through the layering of treatment for heavy users on top of our current enforcement efforts.

Drug screening is an extremely effective means for identifying drug use. It should be widely extended into business and industry, other social arenas, and schools. Screening must be coupled with a rehabilitative approach, however, and not simply punishment. The self-serving strategies of the drug culture must be exposed. The public needs to become aware of how drug-culture advocates are manipulating public opinion in the same fashion that the tobacco industry has for so many years.

A compassionate but restrictive drug policy that partners prevention, rehabilitation, and law enforcement will continue to show the greatest chance for success. Drug policy must focus on harm prevention through clear primary prevention messages, and it must focus upon harm elimination through treatment availability and rigorous law enforcement.

POSTSCRIPT

Should Drugs Be Decriminalized?

Nadelmann asserts that utilizing the criminal justice system to eradicate drug problems simply does not work. He argues that international control efforts, interdiction, and domestic law enforcement are ineffective and that many problems associated with drug use are the consequences of drug regulation policies. Nadelmann maintains that decriminalization is a feasible and desirable means of dealing with the drug crisis. He adds that there is no mechanism for regulating the use of illegal drugs.

Voth charges that the advantages of maintaining illegality far outweigh any conceivable benefits of decriminalization. He professes that if drug laws were relaxed, the result would be more drug users and, thus, more drug addicts and more criminal activity. Also, there is the possibility that more drug-related social problems would occur. Voth concludes that society cannot afford to soften its position on the criminality of drugs.

Decriminalization proponents argue that drug laws have not worked and that the drug battle has been lost. They believe that drug-related problems would disappear if drugs were decriminalized. Citing the legal drugs alcohol and tobacco as examples, decriminalization opponents argue that decriminalizing drugs would not decrease profits from the sale of drugs (the profits from cigarettes and alcohol are incredibly high). Moreover, opponents argue, decriminalizing a drug does not make its problems disappear (alcohol and tobacco have extremely high addiction rates as well as a myriad of other problems associated with their use).

Many European countries, such as the Netherlands and Switzerland, have a system of legalized drugs, and most have far fewer addiction rates and lower incidences of drug-related violence and crime than the United States. These countries make a distinction between soft drugs (those identified as less harmful) and hard drugs (those with serious consequences). However, would the outcomes of decriminalization in the United States be the same as in Europe? Decriminalization in the United States could still be a tremendous risk because its drug problems could escalate and recriminalizing drugs would be difficult. This was the case with Prohibition in the 1920s, which, in changing the status of alcohol from legal to illegal, produced numerous crime- and alcohol-related problems.

Many good articles debate the pros and cons of decriminalization, including "The Economics of Drug Prohibition and Drug Legalization," by Jeffrey A. Miron, *Social Research* (Fall 2001); "Marijuana, Heroin, and Cocaine: The War on Drugs May Be a Disaster, but Do We Really Want a Legalized Peace?" by Robert Maccoun and Peter Reuter, *The American Prospect* (June 3, 2002); "A Quagmire for Our Time: The War on Drugs," by Peter Schag, *The American Prospect* (August 13, 2001); and "Fighting the Real War on Drugs," by Bill Ritter, *The World & I* (February 2000).

ISSUE 2

Should the United States Put More Emphasis on Stopping the Importation of Drugs?

YES: Barry R. McCaffrey, from *The National Drug Control Strategy: 2001 Annual Report* (January 2001)

NO: Ted Galen Carpenter, from "Washington's Unsavory Anti-drug Partners," *USA Today* (November 2002)

ISSUE SUMMARY

YES: Barry R. McCaffrey, former director of the Office of National Drug Control Policy, argues that the importation of drugs into the United States must be stopped to reduce drug use and abuse. If the supply of drugs being trafficked across American borders is reduced, then there will be fewer drug-related problems. He maintains that a coordinated international effort is needed to combat the increased production of heroin, cocaine, and marijuana.

NO: Ted Galen Carpenter, vice president of defense and foreign policy studies for the Cato Institute, asserts that the United States has corroborated with foreign governments that have profited from the drug trade. He recommends that the federal government reexamine its role of cooperation with other governments, especially those involved in the drug trade.

Since the beginning of the 1990s, overall drug use in the United States has increased. Up to now, interdiction has not slowed the flow of drugs into the United States. Drugs continue to cross U.S. borders at record levels. This point may signal a need for stepped-up international efforts to stop the production and trafficking of drugs. Conversely, it may illustrate the inadequacy of the current strategy. Should the position of the U.S. government be to improve and strengthen current measures or to try an entirely new approach?

Some people contend that rather than attempting to limit illegal drugs from coming into the United States, more effort should be directed at reducing the demand for drugs and improving treatment for drug abusers. Foreign countries would not produce and transport drugs like heroin and cocaine into the United States if there were no market for them. Drug policies, some people maintain, should be aimed at the social and economic conditions underlying domestic drug problems, not at the practices of foreign governments.

Many U.S. government officials believe that other countries should assist in stopping the flow of drugs across their borders. Diminishing the supply of drugs by intercepting them before they reach the user is another way to eliminate or curtail drug use. Critical elements in the lucrative drug trade are multinational crime syndicates. One premise is that if the drug production, transportation, distribution, and processing functions as well as the money-laundering operations of these criminal organizations can be interrupted and eventually crippled, then the drug problem will abate.

In South American countries such as Peru, Colombia, and Bolivia, where coca—from which cocaine is processed—is cultivated, economic aid has been made available to help the governments of these countries fight the cocaine kingpins. An alleged problem is that a number of government officials in these countries are corrupt or fearful of the cocaine cartel leaders. One proposed solution is to go directly to the farmers and offer them money to plant crops other than coca. This tactic, however, failed in the mid-1970s, when the U.S. government gave money to farmers in Turkey to stop growing opium poppy crops. After one year the program was discontinued due to the enormous expense, and opium poppy crops were once again planted.

Drug problems are not limited to the Americas. Since the breakup of the Soviet Union, for example, there has been a tremendous increase in opium production in many of the former republics. These republics are in dire need of money, and one source of income is opium production. Moreover, there is lax enforcement by police officials in these republics.

There are many reasons why people are dissatisfied with the current state of the war on drugs. For example, in the war on drugs, the *casual* user is generally the primary focus of drug use deterrence. This is viewed by many people as a form of discrimination because the vast majority of drug users and sellers who are arrested and prosecuted are poor, members of minorities, homeless, unemployed, and/or disenfranchised. Also, international drug dealers who are arrested are usually not the drug bosses but lower-level people working for them. Finally, some argue that the war on drugs should be redirected away from interdiction and enforcement because they feel that the worst drug problems in society today are caused by legal drugs, primarily alcohol and tobacco.

The following selections address the issue of whether or not the war on drugs should be fought on an international level. Barry R. McCaffrey takes the view that international cooperation is absolutely necessary if we are to stem the flow of drugs and maintain world order. Ted Galen Carpenter argues that an international approach to dealing with drugs has been ineffective because many of the foreign countries receiving U.S. financial aid profit from the drug trade.

Barry R. McCaffrey

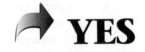 **YES**

The National Drug Control Strategy, 2001

Shielding U.S. Borders From the Drug Threat

Borders delineate the sovereign territories of nation-states. Guarding our country's 9,600 miles of land and sea borders is one of the federal government's most fundamental responsibilities—especially in light of the historically open, lengthy borders with our northern and southern neighbors. The American government maintains three hundred ports-of-entry, including airports where officials inspect inbound and outbound individuals, cargo, and conveyances. All are vulnerable to the drug threat. By curtailing the flow of drugs across our borders, we reduce drug availability throughout the United States and decrease the negative consequences of drug abuse and trafficking in our communities.

In FY 2000, more than eighty million passengers and crew members arrived in the United States aboard commercial and private aircraft. Some eleven million came by marine vessels and 397 million through land border crossings. People entered America on 211,000 ships; 971,000 aircraft; and 139 million trucks, trains, buses, and automobiles. Cargo arrived in fifty-two million containers. This enormous volume of movement makes interdiction of illegal drugs difficult.

Even harder is the task of intercepting illegal drugs in cargo shipments because of the ease with which traffickers can switch modes and routes. Containerized cargo has revolutionized routes, cargo tracking, port development, and shipping companies. As the lead federal agency for detection and monitoring, the Department of Defense [DoD] provides support to law enforcement agencies involved in counter-drug operations. A recent study by the Office of Naval Intelligence indicated that over 60 percent of the world's cargo travels by container. Moreover, vessels carrying as many as six thousand containers—which have the ability to offload cargo onto rail or trucks at various ports-of-entry and then transport it into the heart of the United States—further complicate the interdiction challenge. Drug-trafficking organizations take advantage of these dynamics by hiding illegal substances in cargo or secret compartments. False seals have been used on containers so shipments can move unimpeded through initial ports-of-entry. The United States Customs Service seized more than 1.5 million pounds of illicit drugs in FY 2000—an 11 percent increase over the previous

From Barry R. McCaffrey, Office of National Drug Control Policy, *The National Drug Control Strategy: 2001 Annual Report* (January 2001). Washington, D.C.: U.S. Government Printing Office, 2001. Notes omitted.

year. To counteract this threat, the federal government is constantly seeking new technologies which, together with capable personnel and timely intelligence, facilitate a well-coordinated interdiction plan responsive to changing drug-trafficking trends.

Organizing Against the Drug Threat

The U.S. Customs Service has primary responsibility for ensuring that all cargo and goods moving through ports-of-entry comply with federal law. Customs is the lead agency for preventing drug trafficking through airports, seaports, and land ports-of-entry. Customs shares responsibility for stemming the flow of illegal drugs into the United States via the air and sea. It accomplishes this mission by detecting and apprehending drug-smuggling aircraft and vessels trying to enter the country. The Customs' Air and Marine Interdiction Division provides seamless twenty-four-hour radar surveillance along the entire southern tier of the United States, Puerto Rico, and the Caribbean using a wide variety of civilian and military ground-based radar, tethered aerostats, reconnaissance aircraft, and other detection sensors. In fiscal year 2000, Customs seized 1,442,778 pounds of marijuana, cocaine, and heroin—a 10.1 percent increase over seizures in FY 1999. In addition, Customs has deployed over forty non-intrusive inspection systems as part of its Five-Year Technology Plan. These systems allow for the advanced detection of narcotics and other contraband in various cargo containers, trucks, automobiles, and rail cars. Such technology has been deployed to ports of entry along the southern tier of the U.S. where it assisted in the seizure of over 180,000 pounds of drugs in the past 3 years.

The U.S. Border Patrol [USBP] specifically focuses on drug smuggling between land ports of entry. In FY 1998, the USBP seized 395,316 kilograms of marijuana, 10,285 kilograms of cocaine, and fourteen kilograms of heroin. In addition, this agency made 6,402 arrests of suspected traffickers.

The Coast Guard [USCG] as the lead federal agency for maritime drug interdiction shares responsibility for air interdiction with the U.S. Customs Service. As such, the Coast Guard plays a key role in protecting our borders. Coast Guard air and surface assets patrol over six million square miles of transit zone that stretches from the Caribbean Basin to the eastern Pacific Ocean. In FY 2000, the Coast Guard set a record for the second consecutive year by seizing 132,920 pounds of cocaine—a 19 percent increase over FY 1999. This success has been a result of the service's Campaign Steel Web counterdrug strategy, intelligence, and deployment of non-lethal technologies to counter go-fast smuggling boats. All the armed forces provide support to law-enforcement agencies involved in drug-control operations, particularly in the Southwest border region.

Drug Trafficking Across the Southwest Border

In FY 2000, 293 million people, eighty-nine million cars, four-and-a-half million trucks, and 572,000 rail cars entered the United States from Mexico. More than half of the cocaine on our streets and large quantities of heroin, marijuana, and methamphetamine come across the Southwest border. Illegal drugs are hidden in all modes of conveyance—car, truck, train, and pedestrian. The success that the Border Patrol and Customs have had at and around ports of entry (through innovative enforcement strategies and physical security improvements) have forced smugglers to move through the vast open spaces between official border crossing points. Approximately, fifty percent of the border with Mexico is under the jurisdiction of the federal land management agencies, almost all of that in rugged, remote areas with limited law enforcement presence. Drugs cross the desert in armed pack trains as well as on the backs of human "mules." They are tossed over border fences and then whisked away on foot or by vehicle. Operators of ships find gaps in U.S./Mexican interdiction coverage and position drugs close to the border for eventual transfer to the United States. Small boats in the Gulf of Mexico and eastern Pacific seek to deliver drugs directly to the United States. Whenever possible, traffickers try to exploit incidences of corruption in U.S. border agencies. It is a tribute to the vast majority of dedicated American officials that integrity, courage, and respect for human rights overwhelmingly characterize their service. Rapidly growing commerce between the United States and Mexico complicates the attempt to keep drugs out of cross-border traffic. Since the Southwest border is currently the most porous part of the nation's periphery, we must mount a determined effort to stop the flow of drugs there. At the same time, we cannot concentrate resources along the Southwest border at the expense of other vulnerable regions because traffickers follow the path of least resistance and funnel drugs to less defended areas.

Five principal departments—Treasury, Justice [DOJ], Transportation, State, and Defense—are concerned with drug-control issues along the Southwest border. These agencies have collaborated in six drug-control areas: drug interdiction, anti-money laundering, drug and immigration enforcement, prosecutions, counter-drug support, and counter-drug cooperation with Mexico. During the past decade, the federal presence along the Southwest border expanded. Customs' budget for Southwest border programs increased 72 percent since FY 1993. The number of assigned DEA [Drug Enforcement Agency] special agents increased 37 percent since FY 1990. DoD's drug-control budget for the Southwest border increased 53 percent since FY 1990. The number of U.S. attorneys handling cases there went up by 80 percent since FY 1990. The Southwest Border Initiative enabled federal agencies to coordinate intelligence and operational assignments at Customs, DOJ's Special Operations Division, HIDTA [High Intensity Drug Trafficking Areas], and state and local law-enforcement agencies.

The United States Coast Guard plays a critical role in protecting the maritime flanks of the Southwest Border. Operations *Border Shield* and *Gulf Shield* protect the coastal borders of Southern California and along the Gulf of Mexico from maritime drug smuggling with USCG air and surface interdiction assets. The Coast Guard operations are coordinated, multi-agency efforts that focus on interdiction to disrupt drug trafficking.

All Borders

We must stop drugs everywhere they enter our country—through the Gulf Coast, Puerto Rico, the U.S. Virgin Islands, Florida, the northeastern and northwestern United States, and the Great Lakes. The vulnerability of Alaska, Hawaii, and the U.S. territories must also be recognized. Florida's location, geography, and dynamic growth will continue to make that state particularly attractive to traffickers for the foreseeable future. Florida's six hundred miles of coastline render[ed] it a major target for shore and airdrop deliveries in the 1980s. The state is located astride the drug-trafficking routes of the Caribbean and Gulf of Mexico. The busy Miami and Orlando airports and Florida's seaports—gateways to drug-source countries in South America—are used as distribution hubs by international drug rings. To varying degrees, Florida's predicament is shared by other border areas and entry points.

The Department of Justice's Southern Frontier Initiative focuses law enforcement on drug-trafficking organizations operating along the Southwest border and the Caribbean. *Operation Trinity* resulted in 1,260 arrests, including eight hundred members of the five largest drug syndicates in Mexico and Colombia. DOJ's Caribbean Initiative substantially enhanced its counterdrug capabilities in this region, with more law-enforcement agents, greater communications, and improved interception. A major element of the Coast Guard's comprehensive multi-year strategy (Campaign Steel Web) is "Operation Frontier Shield," which focuses on disrupting maritime smuggling routes into and around Puerto Rico and the U.S. Virgin Islands.

U.S. Seaports

Criminal activity, including the illegal importation of illicit drugs and the export of controlled commodities and drug proceeds, with a nexus to U.S. seaports is a serious problem. In response to the threat that such activities pose to the people and critical infrastructures of the United States and its seaport cities, the Interagency Commission on Crime and Security in U.S. Seaports was created by Executive Memorandum in April 1999. The Commission's report, released in August 2000, provides an overview of criminal activity and security measures at the seaports; an assessment of the nature and effectiveness of ongoing coordination among federal, state, and local governmental agencies; and gives recommendations for improvement. . . .

Reducing the Supply of Illegal Drugs

Since 1993, the United States has emphasized that supply reduction is an essential component of a well-balanced strategic approach to drug control. When illegal drugs are readily available, the likelihood increases that they will be abused. Supply reduction has both international and domestic components. The vast majority of illicit drugs used in the United States are produced outside of our borders. Internationally, supply reduction includes working with partner nations within the source zones to reduce the cultivation and production of illicit drugs through drug-crop substitution and eradication; alternative development and strengthening public institutions; coordinated investigations; interdiction; control of precursors; anti-money laundering initiatives; and building consensus thorough bilateral, regional and global accords. Within the

United States, supply reduction entails regulation (through the Controlled Substances Act), enforcement of anti-drug laws, eradication of marijuana cultivation, control of precursor chemicals, and destruction of illegal synthetic drug laboratories within our borders.

Breaking Cocaine Sources of Supply

Coca, the raw material for cocaine, is grown primarily in the Andean region of South America. Dramatic successes in Bolivia and Peru have been tempered by the continued expansion of coca cultivation in southern Colombia. Despite more than doubling of the coca crop in Colombia between 1995–1999, successes in the rest of the Andes have helped reduce global cultivation by 15 percent. Although crop estimates for 2000 have yet to be finalized, preliminary indications suggest increases in crop production in southern Colombia that may offset eradication efforts and reduced cultivation in Bolivia and Peru.

Bolivia   This South American country has achieved remarkable counternarcotics successes over the past half decade. The current Banzer administration achieved a 55 percent reduction in cultivation between 1995 and 1999. This achievement, which is the result of sustained eradication and law-enforcement efforts combined with extensive alternative crop development, reduced cocaine production in Bolivia from 255 metric tons in 1994 to seventy mts in 1999. Bolivia continues to make rapid progress towards its goal of complete elimination of all illicit coca production by the end of 2002. By the end of 2000, the Chapare region—once one of the world's major suppliers of this illegal drug—will probably cease to produce any commercial level of coca. From a high of 33,900 hectares of coca fields in the Chapare in 1994, the government eliminated all but a thousand hectares by November 2000. Bolivia plans to launch an eradication campaign, preceded by alternative-development programs, in the Yungas within calendar year 2001. As eradication efforts move from the Chapare to the Yungas, the government will leave sufficient forces to monitor the region and destroy any replanted fields. More importantly, USAID [United States Agency for International Development] Bolivia is contributing to alternative-development programs, using both regular and supplemental budgets to turn farmers away from illegal coca in favor of other crops.

In addition to eradication and alternative development, the United States is helping Bolivia pursue an aggressive drug and chemical precursor-interdiction campaign. Increased success in the interdiction of smuggled substances, particularly in the Chapare region, has raised the price of many essential chemicals, forcing Bolivian lab operators to use inferior substitutes, recycled solvents, and a streamlined production process that virtually eliminates the oxidation stage. The result has been radically diminished drug purity to a record low of 47 percent. This development dramatically affected the marketability of Bolivian cocaine in Brazil and elsewhere.

A limiting factor in Bolivia's continued success against illegal coca cultivation will be the government's ability to work with the cocalerias. In Fall 2000, government eradication efforts were beset by civil strife resulting in ten deaths and approximately a hundred injuries. Funnelling alternative-development aid to the Chapare and Yungas will likely determine whether the Banzer government is able to meet its eradication goals.

Peru Like Bolivia, the government of Peru made enormous strides toward eliminating illegal coca cultivation in the past five years. Despite the rehabilitation of some previously abandoned coca fields, 24 percent of Peruvian coca was eliminated in 1999 with an overall reduction of 66 percent over the last four years. Contributing to this figure was a 1999 total of fifteen thousand fewer hectares under manual coca cultivation. Peru's counternarcotics alternative-development program, working through a hundred local governments, seven hundred communities, and fifteen thousand farmers significantly strengthened the social and economic infrastructure in these areas and helped shift the economic balance in favor of licit activities.

In 2000, the government of Peru continued its eradication campaign for coca. The country hoped to eliminate some twenty-two thousand acres (nine thousand hectares) of coca. However, a deteriorating political situation increased discontent among coca growers in the Huallaga valley, and potential spillover from southern Colombia could affect the positive direction in Peru. In November 2000, growers in the central upper Huallaga valley conducted the biggest protests in a decade, slowed eradication efforts, and endangered Peru's ability to meet its eradication objectives. However, with sustained U.S. law enforcement, alternative development, interdiction assistance, and support for eradication, Peru will continue to reduce coca cultivation.

Colombia President [Andres] Pastrana and his reform-minded government took office in August of 1998. Pastrana faced multiple challenges from the outset of his administration. Ongoing, inter-related crises in Colombia threaten U.S. national interests, including: stemming the flow of cocaine and heroin into the United States, support for democratic government and the rule of law, respect for human rights, promoting efforts to reach a negotiated settlement in Colombia's long-running internal conflict, maintaining regional stability, and promoting legitimate trade and investment.

Rapidly growing cocaine production in Colombia constitutes a threat to U.S. security and the well-being of our citizens. Ninety percent of the cocaine entering the United States originates in or passes through Colombia. Over the last decade, drug production in Colombia has increased dramatically. In spite of an aggressive aerial eradication campaign, Colombian cultivation of coca, the raw material for cocaine, has more than tripled since 1992. New information about the potency of Colombian coca, the time required for crops to reach maturity, and efficiency in the cocaine conversion process has led to a revision in estimates of Colombia's 1998 potential cocaine production from 165 metric tons to 435 metric tons. The 1999 figures indicate that both the number of hectares of coca under cultivation and the amount of cocaine produced from those crops continue to skyrocket. Colombian coca cultivation rose 20 percent to 122,500 hectares in 1999; there was a corresponding 20 percent increase in potential cocaine production to 520 metric tons. Left unchecked, these massive increases in drug production and trafficking could reverse gains achieved over the last four years in Peru and Bolivia. Continued expansion of drug production in Colombia is likely to result in more drugs being shipped to the United States. . . .

Breaking Heroin Sources of Supply

The U.S. heroin problem is supplied entirely by foreign sources of opium. Efforts to reduce domestic heroin availability face significant problems. Unlike cocaine, where the supply is concentrated in the Andean region of South America, heroin available in the United States is produced in four distinct parts of the world: South America, Mexico, Southeast Asia, and Southwest Asia. Worldwide potential heroin production was estimated at 287 metric tons in 1999.

Latin America has emerged in recent years as the primary supplier of heroin to the United States. Colombian and Mexican heroin comprises 65 and 17 percent respectively of the heroin seized today in the United States. The heroin industry in Colombia is still young and growing. Reports of some opium poppy fields surfaced in the mid-1980s, but not until the early 1990s was any significant cultivation confirmed. By the mid-1990s, the Colombian heroin industry was producing enough high-purity white heroin to capture the U.S. East Coast market. Between 1995 and 1998, opium production in Colombia was sufficient to support more than six metric tons of heroin annually. In 1999, however, increased cultivation resulted in a larger crop, increasing potential heroin production to nearly eight metric tons.

Today, the Colombian heroin trade closely mirrors the heroin industry in Mexico rather than operations in Southeast or Southwest Asia. Heroin processing labs in Colombia operate on a small scale; heroin production is not dominated by large, well-armed trafficking organizations; there are no multi-hundred-kilogram internal movements of opiate products; and Colombian traffickers rarely attempt to smuggle large shipments of heroin into other countries. Like the Mexican industry , the heroin trade in Colombia services the U.S. market almost exclusively. Production of heroin is more fragmented, with smaller trafficking groups playing a major role. Individual couriers smuggle heroin into the United States daily in small, single-kilogram amounts. In addition, Colombia's heroin industry—like Mexico's—must cope with significant government opium-poppy eradication.

Significant diversion of the essential precursor acetic anhydride suggests that Colombian traffickers are prepared to increase heroin production. In 1999, about ninety-six metric tons of acetic anhydride—six percent of Colombia's legal imports of this chemical for pharmaceutical use—were hijacked or stolen after arriving in Colombia. The illegal diversion of acetic anhydride in 1999 alone would be enough to meet heroin production requirements for the next three to five years.

Low-level opium-poppy cultivation in Venezuela and even more limited growing in Peru currently serve only marginal heroin production but could become the foundation for an expanding opium and heroin industry beyond Colombia. Opium-poppy cultivation in Venezuela is limited to the mountains opposite Colombia's growing area and appears to be a spillover from cultivation on the Colombian side of the border. Since 1994, when a thousand hectares of opium poppy were discovered during a joint U.S.-Venezuelan aerial reconnaissance mission, Caracas has conducted periodic eradication operations that reduced the size of the annual crop to fewer than fifty hectares. The cultivation, harvesting, and processing of Venezuela's poppy crop is done primarily by Colombians who access the growing area from Colombia. Many of the farmers arrested by Venezuelan authorities for growing opium are Colombian nationals. The Venezuelan side of the border is readily accessible from trails and unimproved roads originating in Colombia.

Reports indicate that opium poppy cultivation in Peru over the last several years is nearly negligible. However, the seizure of more than fifty kilograms of opium by police in 1999 suggests that opium production in Peru may be heading for commercial levels. In Peru, Colombian backers provide farmers with poppy seed, teach processing methods, and buy Peruvian opium; most of the opium produced in Peru is reportedly shipped to Colombia. While the cultivation pattern in Peru is similar to that in Colombia, so far there has been no widespread deforestation as there was in Colombia when opium-poppy cultivation virtually exploded.

An intensification of eradication efforts in Colombia significant enough to reduce opium production might spur increased cultivation in Peru and Venezuela. Both governments, however, appear committed to preventing opium cultivation from becoming a significant problem. Successful elimination of opium-poppy cultivation in Venezuela will depend, to a large extent, on Colombia's ability to suppress cultivation on its side of the border and for both Bogota and Caracas to control the mountainous region where Colombian guerrillas operate on both sides of the border. The prospects for significant increases in opium production would be greater in Peru if cultivation were firmly established there because the growing areas are isolated and nearly inaccessible to authorities, making large-scale eradication more difficult.

With long-established trafficking and distribution networks and exclusive markets for black tar and brown powder heroin, Mexico's hold on the U.S. heroin market in the West seems secure. Mexico grows only about two percent of the world's illicit opium, but virtually the entire crop is converted into heroin for the U.S. market. Despite significant historical production in Mexico, local consumption of opium and heroin has never been more than marginal. Unlike in the far larger source countries of Southeast and Southwest Asia, opium-poppy cultivation in Mexico—as in Colombia—occurs year-round because of the favorable climate. With a hundred-day growing cycle, single opium fields in Mexico can yield up to three crops per year although the size and quality of the plants typically depends on seasonal variations. The largest crop is generally achieved in the relatively mild and wet months of December through April. Mexican officials report that many growers are planting new varieties of opium poppy in an effort to increase opium yields.

Opium cultivation and production in Mexico have been relatively stable through most of the 1990s. Between 1993 and 1998, according to the U.S. government's annual imagery-based crop survey, Mexico's opium harvest averaged fifty-four metric tons, allowing Mexican traffickers to produce five to six metric tons of heroin annually. In 1999, a drought in the best growing season reduced opium cultivation and stunted opium-poppy growth in many of the fields where plants reached maturity.

Poppy-crop eradication is the primary constraint against increased opium production. The Mexican Army's manual eradication effort, using more than twenty-thousand soldiers on any given day, is responsible for roughly 75 percent of the eradicated crop each year. The Attorney General's Office (PGR) destroys about one-quarter of the eradicated crop through helicopter aerial fumigation. However, a lack of roads and infrastructure in the remote growing areas makes manual and spray operations difficult and dangerous. Moreover, counterinsurgency operations and disaster-relief missions in recent years overburdened military personnel and may have caused the transfer of some personnel away from eradication efforts. However, this change does not seem to have had an appreciable impact on overall eradication effort. The combination of drought and eradication decreased Mexico's heroin production to slightly more than four metric tons in 1999.

Historically, most of the world's illicit opium for heroin has been grown in the Golden Triangle of Southeast Asia. Burma alone has accounted for more than half of all global production of opium and heroin for most of the last decade. In the absence of sustained alternative crop-substitution programs and consistent narcotics crop-eradication efforts (except in Thailand), only weather fluctuations have had a significant impact on opium-poppy cultivation and production. Major droughts in 1994, 1998, and 1999 caused the region's opium production to plummet.

No other country surpasses Burma in terms of hectares of opium cultivation. However, crop yields are much lower than those in Southwest Asia are. Consequently, even if normal weather conditions were to again prevail in Southeast Asia, Burma would not challenge Afghanistan as the world's leading source of heroin. Although the Burmese government showed both a willingness and capability to ban poppy cultivation in areas under its control the last two years, authorities refrain from entering prime opium-growing areas controlled by ethnic Wa insurgents.

In Thailand, aggressive eradication and crop-substitution programs have reduced opium production to less than one percent of the region's total. Thailand is now a net importer of opium to meet its addicts' demands. Without a meaningful eradication effort of its own and with little change in the status of UN-supported crop-substitution projects, Laos remains the world's third-largest producer of illicit opium. Opium production in that country was less affected by drought than was Burma. Laos accounted for about 12 percent of Southeast Asia's opium production in 1999, as compared to less than 10 percent through most of the 1990s.

The profitability of growing opium poppy as a cash crop and the lack of resources or commitment by regional governments to implement crop substitution, alternative development, or eradication are key factors that predict a significant rebound in opium production within Southeast Asia. The remote location and rugged terrain of poppy-growing areas in Burma and Laos are major obstacles to establishing crop-substitution programs. The lack of transportation infrastructure in most opium-producing regions further complicates crop substitution because farmers have difficulty moving alternative crops to distant markets. Opium buyers, by contrast, typically come to the farmer, saving him a long trek to the nearest village or city. Although significant efforts by transit countries over the past led to the seizure of large amounts of heroin, the key to curbing heroin production and trafficking in Southeast Asia lies with the source countries—particularly Burma.

The explosive growth of opium production and development of an imposing opiate-processing infrastructure in Afghanistan during the 1990s made Southwest Asia the world's leading source of heroin. While Southwest Asian heroin is unlikely to penetrate much of the American market share anytime soon, the region's drug trade significantly affects U.S. strategic interests—including political stability and counterterrorism—in that volatile region. In 1999, Southwest Asia produced an estimated 2,898 metric tons of opium, compared to 1,236 metric tons in drought-stricken Southeast Asia. Afghanistan, whose estimated opium production increased 22 percent from 2,390 metric tons in 1998 to 2,861 metric tons, was solely responsible for Southwest Asia becoming the world's leading source of heroin. By comparison, opium production in Pakistan—the region's other source country—declined by half for the second consecutive year to thirty-seven metric tons.

In the coming decade, additional progress is achievable if governments can cordon off growing areas, increase their commitment, and implement counternarcotics programs. U.S.-backed crop-control programs reduced illicit opium cultivation in Guatemala, Mexico, Pakistan, Thailand, and Turkey. Both Colombia and Mexico have aggressive heroin-control programs. Mexico has destroyed between 60 and 70 percent of the crop each year for the past several years. In Colombia, some eight thousand hectares of poppies were fumigated from the air in 1999. However, little progress is likely if the ruling Taliban in Afghanistan doesn't commit to narcotics control. In Burma, the future is also uncertain as long as the country fails to muster the political will to make inroads against the opium cultivation in areas ruled by the Wa Army.

The United States continues to help strengthen law-enforcement in heroin source countries by supporting training programs, information sharing, extradition of fugitives, and anti-money laundering measures. In addition, America will work through diplomatic and public channels to increase the level of international cooperation and support the ambitious UNDCP [UN International Drug Control Program] initiative to eradicate illicit opium-poppy cultivation in ten years.

Ted Galen Carpenter

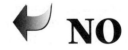 **NO**

Washington's Unsavory Antidrug Partners

American officials have frequently cooperated with unsavory regimes in an attempt to stem drug trafficking, even when Washington has treated those regimes as pariahs on all other issues. A graphic example of that dual approach occurred in May, 2002, when a senior member of the military junta ruling Burma, Col. Kyaw Thein, came to Washington for discussions with Bush Administration officials on ways to improve his government's efforts to eradicate illicit opium production. Kyaw met with Assistant Secretary of State Rand Beers, as well as officials of the Drug Enforcement Administration (DEA), the Justice and Treasury departments, and the White House Office of National Drug Control Policy.

Kyaw's visit was curious on multiple levels. He was a prominent figure in the junta that had strangled Burma's aspirations for democracy and harassed the leader of the democratic forces, Nobel laureate Aung San Suu Kyi, for years. That mistreatment has included placing her under house arrest for nine months—an episode that had just ended in early May. Kyaw's trip was a departure from the ban imposed in 1996 on visits to the U.S. by high-ranking members of the junta. Indeed, Kyaw had been specifically named as being ineligible to receive a visa. Yet, to discuss drug policy, he was now welcome in Washington. His visit could not even be interpreted as a reward to Burma's military leaders for freeing Suu Kyi. Administration officials conceded that the visit had been planned for weeks—long before her release. Yet, the Administration emphasized that the extensive talks with Kyaw did not herald a loosening of the economic sanctions that had been imposed on Burma. Cooperation was to take place on the drug issue alone.

That was not the first time U.S. officials had sought to make an exception to general policy toward Burma in the name of waging the war on drugs. In 1995, Lee P. Brown, director of the White House Office of National Drug Control Policy under Pres. Bill Clinton, led a push for expanded cooperation with the Burmese military to eradicate poppy fields and arrest traffickers. Thomas A. Constantine, director of the DEA; Assistant Secretary of State Robert Gelbard; and Under Secretary of State for Global Affairs Timothy E. Wirth supported Brown's effort. They waged their campaign even though the State Department's most-recent human rights report had concluded that Burma had a highly authoritarian regime that had killed or jailed its political opponents, squelched free speech and demonstrations, and impressed thousands of people into forced labor to assist the military.

Brown summarized his attitude and that of his colleagues on that uncomfortable issue: "I'm very concerned about human rights violations in Burma. But I'm equally concerned about human rights in America and the poison being exported from Burma that ends up on the streets of our cities." In other words, fighting drug trafficking took precedence over any qualms Americans might have about the brutally repressive nature of the Burmese junta. Although Brown did not get his wish entirely, some American cooperation with Burma continued throughout the remainder of the 1990s, despite Washington's overall policy of trying to isolate the military regime.

Throughout the decades since Pres. Richard Nixon first proclaimed a war on drugs in 1971, the U.S. has repeatedly made a "drug war exception" in its foreign policy toward repugnant and repressive regimes. Policy toward Burma has been by no means an aberration. The U.S. adopted a similar approach to Panama's dictator, Manuel Noriega; Peru's authoritarian president, Alberto Fujimori; and even Cuban dictator Fidel Castro. Incredibly, Washington even sought to cooperate with the infamous Taliban regime in Afghanistan and praised its effort to eradicate the cultivation of opium poppies.

When the Taliban announced a ban on opium cultivation in early 2001, U.S. officials were most complimentary. James P. Callahan, director of Asian affairs for the State Department's Bureau of International Narcotics and Law Enforcement Affairs, uncritically relayed the alleged accounts of Afghan farmers that "the Taliban used a system of consensus-building" to develop and implement the edict. That characterization was more than a little dubious, since the Taliban was not known for pursuing consensus in other aspects of its rule. *Los Angeles Times* columnist Robert Scheer was scathing in his criticism of the U.S. response. "That a totalitarian country can effectively crack down on farmers is not surprising," he noted, but Sheer contended that "it is grotesque" for a U.S. official to describe the drug-crop crackdown in such benign terms.

The Bush Administration did more than praise the Taliban's announced ban on opium cultivation. In mid May, 2001, Secretary of State Colin Powell announced a $43,000,000 grant to Afghanistan in addition to the humanitarian aid the U.S. had long been providing to agencies assisting Afghan refugees. Given Callahan's comment, there was little doubt that the new stipend was a reward for Kabul's anti-drug efforts. That $43,000,000 grant needs to be placed in context. Afghanistan's estimated gross domestic product at the time was a mere $2,000,000,000. The equivalent financial impact on the U.S. economy would have required an infusion of $215,000,000,000. In other words, the $43,000,000 was very serious money to Afghanistan's theocratic masters.

To make matters worse, U.S. officials were naïve to take the Taliban edict at face value. The much-touted crackdown on opium poppy cultivation appears to have been little more than an illusion. Despite U.S. and United Nations reports that the Taliban had virtually wiped out the poppy crop in 2000–01, authorities in neighboring Tajikistan reported that the amounts coming across the border were actually increasing. In reality, the Taliban gave its order to halt cultivation to drive up the price of the opium the regime had already stockpiled.

Even if the Taliban had tried to stem cultivation for honest reasons, U.S. cooperation with that regime should have been morally repugnant. Among other outrages, the Taliban government prohibited the education of girls, tortured and executed political critics, and required non-Muslims to wear distinctive clothing—a practice reminiscent of Nazi Germany's edict that Jews must display the Star of David on their clothes. Yet, U.S. officials deemed none of that to be a bar to cooperation with the Taliban on drug policy.

Even if the Bush Administration had not been dissuaded by moral considerations, it should have been by purely pragmatic concerns. In an eerily prescient passage, Sheer noted in May, 2001, "Never mind that Osama bin Laden still operates the leading anti-American terror operation from his base in Afghanistan, from which, among other crimes, he launched two bloody attacks on American embassies in Africa in 1998." Sheer was on the mark when he concluded, "The war on drugs has become our own fanatics' obsession and easily trumps all other concerns."

Washington's approach came to an especially calamitous end in September, 2001, when the Taliban regime was linked to bin Laden's terrorist attacks on the World Trade Center and the Pentagon that killed more than 3,000 people. Moreover, evidence quickly emerged that the Taliban all along had been collecting millions of dollars in profits from the illicit drug trade, with much of that money going into the coffers of the terrorists. Rarely is there such graphic evidence of the bankruptcy of American drug policy.

When it comes to waging the war on drugs, no moral or ideological impediment has seemed sufficient to keep the U.S. government from cooperating with any regime. In recent years, the U.S. has even worked with Fidel Castro on drug matters. As early as 1996, Cuban and U.S. authorities collaborated in the interception and search of a Colombian freighter carrying six tons of cocaine. Cuban officials acted as prosecution witnesses in the trial of the crew in a U.S. court.

In May, 1999, Barry McCaffrey, director of the White House Office of National Drug Control Policy, praised the Cuban government for its cooperation on the drug issue and urged a broader dialogue. He rejected allegations that the Cuban government itself was involved in drug trafficking, even though previous U.S. administrations had cited evidence of such activity. (McCaffrey's exoneration of the Castro regime drew a stinging rebuke from Alberto Hernandez, chairman of the Cuban American National Foundation. "Cooperating with Castro on drugs is like asking Don Corleone to help you fight organized crime in New York," he stated.)

What was striking about Washington's willingness to collaborate with Castro's regime on antidrug activities was that it stood in such sharp contrast to overall American policy toward Cuba. The U.S. had severed diplomatic relations with Castro's communist regime at the beginning of the 1960s and had maintained a far-reaching economic embargo against the island since that time. Indeed, sanctions had actually been tightened during the Clinton years. Although there were scattered voices of dissent, leaders of both the Republican and

Democratic parties strongly endorsed the hard-line policy. Yet, on one issue—drugs—U.S. officials were willing to deviate from the strategy of making the communist autocrat a pariah. Castro's American critics routinely excoriated him for jailing political opponents, suppressing a wide range of freedoms, and turning his country into an economic disaster. His record, in their view, precluded U.S. trade with Cuba and even made it necessary to prevent American tourists from visiting the island. However, none of that apparently was an impediment to collaborating with his security forces in the war on drugs.

The policy of cooperating with the Castro regime on the drug war has drawn praise in two Council on Foreign Relations Task Force reports on policy toward Cuba. In the second, issued in 2001, the Task Force recommended that the U.S. develop "an active program of counternarcotics contacts with Cuban counterparts," and stated that such cooperation should involve "limited exchanges of personnel" with Cuba's security agencies.

On another occasion, McCaffrey reiterated that he thought cooperation with the Castro regime was a splendid idea and urged the Bush Administration to intensify mutual counterdrug activities. Although there is no evidence of an intensification of cooperation under Bush, there is likewise no indication that the existing level has been scaled back.

When most people think of Manuel Noriega, they recall the U.S. invasion of Panama and the capture of the odious dictator. One declared purpose of the December, 1989, U.S. military operation in Panama was to apprehend Noriega and bring him to Florida for trial on narcotics trafficking charges.

That was hardly the beginning of the relationship between the U.S. and Noriega, though. In the years before the 1989 invasion, Washington's relationship with him had been of a very different nature. For years, there had been close cooperation as the Panamanian strongman assisted Washington in its drive to undermine the leftist Sandinista regime in Nicaragua and prop up the right-wing government of El Salvador against Marxist rebels. Noriega had also received praise from the DEA for his cooperation in helping to stanch the flow of narcotics through his country. The latter was no small consideration, since Panama was a major transit point in the illegal drug trade.

Washington's enthusiasm for Noriega's apparent dedication to the drug war began as early as 1978 when DEA administrator Peter Bensinger thanked him for his support in the fight against drugs. Eight years later, one of Bensinger's successors, John Lawn, sent Noriega an effusive thank you letter. "I would like to take this opportunity to reiterate my deep appreciation for the vigorous anti-drug trafficking policy that you have adopted, which is reflected in the numerous expulsions from Panama of accused traffickers," Lawn wrote. In May, 1987, Lawn praised the Panamanian leader for his "personal commitment" to one important drug investigation: "I look forward to our continued efforts together. Drug traffickers around the world are now on notice that the proceeds and profits of their illegal ventures are not welcome in Panama." The following year, DEA spokesman Cornelius Dougherty conceded that there had been many such letters of praise over the years. "The bottom line is that he was helpful and cooperative," Dougherty maintained.

Yet, throughout the 1980s, Noriega systematically undermined democratic rule—typically by rigging elections to ensure the victory of compliant civilian front men while he held the real reins of power as the head of Panama's armed forces. Noriega was also not above harassing, jailing, and torturing political opponents. Indeed, he was apparently not above murdering them.

Noriega's domestic political troubles first became acute in late 1987 when Roberto Diaz, a retired high-ranking Panamanian military officer and former Noriega confidant, made a series of explosive accusations. Most notably, Diaz presented evidence that the general had set up the 1984 murder of a leading opposition politician who had spoken out against Noriega's alleged involvement in drug trafficking.

Until these high-profile allegations, Washington seemed impervious to evidence that Noriega was perverting Panama's political system and brutalizing political opponents. In that respect, the actions of American officials were consistent with an increasingly familiar pattern. As long as the ruler in question seemed cooperative on the drug war, U.S. leaders were willing to look the other way regarding his conduct, however repugnant. What is perhaps more surprising is that U.S. officials seemed impervious to evidence that Noriega himself was involved in the drug trade.

Ironically, throughout the period when Noriega was winning praise for his antidrug measures, there were mounting indications of his corruption. He had been cited by at least one source as the person at the center of Panama's drug trafficking network a decade before his indictment and the subsequent U.S. invasion. As *Wall Street Journal* correspondent Frederick Kempe noted, "Noriega had been arresting many drug traffickers and extraditing some of them to the United States, but just as often he extorted traffickers before they could gain their release." In essence, while appearing to help the Americans fight the drug trade, "he was only turning in his competition, as he skimmed off the profits from a multibillion-dollar industry," Kempe pointed out.

Noriega was engaged in a delicate balancing act, protecting the interests of the Colombian cartels while retaining the support of U.S. officials. "It was a tricky game," Kempe indicates, "but American agents in Panama were particularly easy to con," and it worked for many years. "With each major drug bust that Noriega assisted, and with each fugitive that he helped to extradite, Noriega grew in the DEA's esteem, at the same time that he was expanding business with the cartel. It was a remarkable balancing act that can only be explained one way: Noriega was using the DEA as his own private enforcer." The invasion of Panama and the arrest of Noriega were a dramatic admission of just how misguided previous U.S. policy had been.

Anyone who might have assumed that the Noriega experience had taught U.S. officials a sobering lesson about cooperating with corrupt dictators in the name of waging the war on drugs soon received evidence to the contrary. The most-graphic example was the increasingly cozy relationship between Washington and the government of Peru's autocratic president, Alberto Fujimori, in the 1990s.

The trend toward democracy in Latin America experienced a major blow in April, 1992, when Fujimori declared to the nation that he had assumed exclusive control of the government in an *autogolpe* ("self-coup") with the support of the military. His revamped regime moved quickly to shut down all independent branches of the government. He dissolved the Peruvian congress and eviscerated the judicial system by summarily dismissing 13 supreme court justices as well as all the judges on the Tribunal of Constitutional Guarantees. During the early years of his authoritarian rule, the U.S. State and Justice departments frequently condemned the regime's human rights abuses. As the Fujimori government pressed its campaign against the Maoist Sendero Luminoso (Shining Path) guerrillas, there was an abundance of such abuses.

Fujimori's offensive against the Shining Path affected many of the peasants in the Upper Huallaga Valley and other remote locales, who grew much of the coca crop and at least countenanced, if not actively supported, the guerrillas. As the effort to stamp out the Shining Path gained momentum in the mid and late 1990s, Washington began to look on the autocratic regime in Lima with greater tolerance. Indeed, from the standpoint of U.S. officials, Fujimori's decision to unleash the military offered the promise of a dual benefit. Not only did it promise to weaken a dangerous radical-left political force, it seemed to be disrupting the source of the bulk of the cocaine flowing from the Andean region.

Between 1995 and 1998, the acreage under coca cultivation in Peru dropped 40%. By 1999, the decline reached 56%. U.S. officials used terms such as "amazing" and "astonishing" and were quick to credit the Peruvian government. In truth, however, the principal reason for the decline was a fungus that swept through the Peruvian coca crop during those years.

During the 1990s, the U.S. military assisted the Peruvian government in interdicting planes carrying drugs out of Peru to processing facilities in Colombia. American radar monitoring of suspect flights was crucial to that operation. By 1998, Washington was significantly expanding its drug war financial aid to the Peruvian government in other ways. Under one program, a five-year, $60,000,000 effort, the U.S. sought to expand Peru's force of river patrol boats greatly to combat the drug trade in the Amazon basin. At that time, the Peruvian military had just 16 such boats. The U.S. aid would provide another 54, as well as funds to train the additional military personnel needed to man them.

The Fujimori government's prosecution of the drug war was more apparent than real, though. As far as the Peruvian military was concerned, the principal offense of the peasants engaged in growing coca was not that they were involved in the drug trade, but that they helped fund the Shining Path. A cynic might even argue that the military's real complaint was that too many peasants paid off the Shining Path instead of the military.

Throughout the 1990s, allegations surfaced repeatedly that Vladimiro Montesinos, the head of the National Intelligence Service, used his office to shield friendly drug traffickers, even as the military used force against drug-crop peasants who were deemed enemies of the regime. After Fujimori fell from power and fled the country in late 2000, those allegations soared in number. Evidence surfaced that Montesinos may have received as much as $1,000,000 from a leading Mexican drug cartel. At the same time, he and his intelligence apparatus were apparently receiving up to $1,000,000 a year from the CIA.

Despite the unsavory nature of the Fujimori-Montesinos regime, U.S. praise for Peru's antidrug efforts increased steadily during the 1990s. Between 1995 and 1998, coca production in Peru supposedly declined by 40% and the price of coca leaves fell by half. That result drew praise from U.S. Ambassador Dennis Jett. Peru had "demonstrated that the battle can be won against an enemy that doesn't respect frontiers or laws," he stated. It didn't seem to bother Washington unduly that it was cooperating with a regime that had used the military to undermine democracy in Peru.

Learning From the Past

The willingness of U.S. administrations to collaborate with the most-odious dictatorships in the war on drugs is long-standing and continuing. It is more than a little distressing to see the U.S. government betray America's values in that fashion. Moreover, it has been a myopic, utterly futile policy. In case after case, Washington's ostensible partners in the antidrug crusade have themselves been extensively involved in trafficking. The fiascos with Noriega and Afghanistan's Taliban government were just the most-notorious examples.

One might well speculate about why a succession of administrations, Republican and Democrat, conservative and liberal, would engage in such conduct. The core reason is probably continued frustration at the lack of lasting, meaningful results in the international phase of the war on drugs. Over the last three decades, the U.S. has made a concerted effort to cut off, or at least significantly reduce, the flow of drugs into the country from Latin America, Central Asia, and Southeast Asia. Despite that effort, more illegal drugs enter the U.S. from those sources today than did when the "supply-side" campaign began.

Instead of facing the reality that a prohibitionist strategy is doomed to fail, that it merely creates a lucrative black-market premium that attracts new producers, U.S. officials are willing to make common cause with any regime that promises to combat the scourge of narcotics, even when the regime in question is thoroughly repressive.

The folly of collaborating with unsavory partners in the international war on drugs may be of more than historical interest. Bush Administration officials and Congressional drug warriors alike are fairly gushing with enthusiasm over the election of Alvaro Uribe as Colombia's new president. Uribe campaigned on a platform advocating vigorous resistance to Colombia's leftist insurgents and an intensified effort to eradicate the country's lucrative drug trade. Perhaps Uribe is a sincere and honorable man who is merely mistaken in his belief that pursuing a prohibitionist strategy toward drugs can ever be effective.

Nevertheless, there are troubling signs that he may be from the same mold as some of Washington's repugnant partners in the drug war. One disturbing indicator was that members of the principal right-wing paramilitary organization, the United Self-Defense Forces of Colombia (AUC), openly backed Uribe's candidacy. The AUC is on the State Department's list of terrorist organizations, and Colombia's outgoing president, Andres Pastrana, has accused it of being responsible for at least 70% of the atrocities committed in his country's complex civil war.

In addition to the unsettling reality of the AUC's enthusiasm for Uribe, one of the new president's closest associates has been accused of involvement in the drug trade. Perhaps these factors will prove to be nothing more than ephemeral dark clouds, but it is also possible that Washington is acquiring another unsavory associate in the war on drugs.

POSTSCRIPT

Should the United States Put More Emphasis on Stopping the Importation of Drugs?

The drug trade spawns violence; people die from using drugs or by dealing with people in the drug trade; families are ruined by the effects of drugs on family members; prisons are filled with tens of thousands of people who were and probably still are involved with illegal drugs; and drugs can devastate aspirations and careers. The adverse consequences of drugs can be seen everywhere in society. Would more people be helped by reducing the availability of drugs, or would more people benefit if they could be persuaded that drugs are harmful to them?

Two paths that are traditionally followed involve reducing either the supply of or the demand for drugs. Four major agencies involved in the fight against drugs in the United States—the Drug Enforcement Administration (DEA), the Federal Bureau of Investigation (FBI), the U.S. Customs Service, and the U.S. Coast Guard—have seized thousands of pounds of marijuana, cocaine, and heroin during the past few years. Drug interdiction appears to be reducing the availability of drugs. But what effect does drug availability have on use? If a particular drug were not available, would other drugs be used in its place? Would the cost of drugs increase if there were a shortage of drugs? If costs increase, will drug-related violence go up as well?

Annual surveys of 8th-, 10th-, and 12th-grade students indicate that availability is not a major factor in drug use. Throughout the 1980s drug use declined dramatically even though marijuana and cocaine could be obtained easily. According to the surveys, the perceived harm of these drugs, not their availability, is what affects students' drug use. As individuals' perceptions of drugs as harmful increase, usage decreases; as perceptions of harm decrease, usage increases.

Efforts to prevent drug use may prove fruitless if people have a natural desire to alter their consciousness. In his 1989 book *Intoxication: Life in the Pursuit of Artificial Paradise* (E. P. Dutton), Ronald Siegel contends that the urge to alter consciousness is as universal as the craving for food and sex.

Articles that examine international efforts to deal with the issue of drugs include "U.S. Versus Them: Challenging America's War on Drugs—U.S. Policy," by Susan Taylor Martin, *The St. Petersburg Times* (July 29, 2001); "Narcoterrorism as a Threat to International Security," by Stephen Blank, *The World & I* (December 2001); and "Addicted to the Drug War," by Kenneth Sharp, *The Chronicle of Higher Education* (October 6, 2000). Finally, Philippe Bordes, in "Drugs: Surveillance or Punishment?" *UNESCO Courier* (October 1998), looks at the drug problem from an international perspective.

ISSUE 3

Will a Lower Blood Alcohol Level for Drunk Driving Reduce Automobile Accidents?

YES: Thomas S. Dee, from "Does Setting Limits Save Lives: The Case of 0.08 BAC Laws," *Journal of Policy Analysis and Management* (vol. 20, no. 1, 2001)

NO: General Accounting Office, from "How Effective Are '.08' Drunk-Driving Laws?" *Consumers' Research Magazine* (August 1999)

ISSUE SUMMARY

YES: Professor of economics Thomas S. Dee supports a .08 blood alcohol concentration (BAC) level for drunk driving. He maintains that alcohol-related fatalities are lower in those states that have adopted a .08 BAC. Dee concludes that an estimated 1,200 fewer deaths would result from the adoption of such a limit.

NO: The General Accounting Office (GAO) states that the evidence supporting the beneficial effects of establishing a lower blood alcohol level for drunk driving is inconclusive. The GAO maintains that the government's methods for determining the effectiveness of a lower blood alcohol level are faulty and that rates for drunk driving have declined regardless of changes in BAC legal limits.

When discussions of drinking and driving arise, many people justifiably express concern. Too many people die needlessly because of others' poor judgment regarding whether or not they can safely operate a motor vehicle after consuming alcohol. However, the news is not all bad. In the last 20 years, the number of alcohol-related driving fatalities in the United States has decreased significantly. In the early 1980s about 26,000 people died each year because of drivers under the influence of alcohol. In 1998 the number of people killed in automobile accidents on American highways because of drunk drivers was around 17,000. This represents a 30 percent decline. Despite this significant reduction, few would argue against further improvement.

The figure of 17,000 alcohol-related automobile fatalities represents the number of people who were killed by a driver who was legally intoxicated at the time of the accident. Missing from this figure is the number of people who were killed by drivers who may have been drinking but who were not legally drunk. However, one does not need to be drunk to be impaired. A number of studies have demonstrated that driving ability is impaired with a blood alcohol concentration (BAC) level as low as .04.

The BAC is the amount of alcohol that is in a person's body as measured by the weight of the alcohol in a certain volume of blood. A person's BAC can be measured by testing the blood, breath, urine, or saliva. The U.S. Senate approved a national blood alcohol level standard of .08 in March 1998. States refusing to adopt this standard risk losing federal funding for highways. The Senate debated whether or not the federal government should interfere in what many senators see as a state's option. Research indicates that lowering the BAC limit from .10 or higher to .08 reduces the number of people who get behind the wheel of a car after drinking. However, the senators are not debating whether or not a lower standard like .08 is desirable; they are arguing what the role of the federal government should be in this matter.

The precedent for penalizing states who refuse to adopt the .08 blood alcohol level standard was set in the early 1980s when President Ronald Reagan threatened to withdraw highway funds from states that did not raise the drinking age to 21. That situation, like the current issue, raises a fundamental question: Should the federal government have the right to dictate to individual states what is an acceptable BAC standard? Is the role of government to conduct research in order to allow states to make informed decisions? If, as Senator Jack Reed (D-Rhode Island) has indicated, a .08 BAC saves between 500 and 600 lives a year, shouldn't the federal government take a more strident stand? Yet is the research cited by these senators accurate? Should government impose laws when the supporting research is suspect?

In the following selections, Thomas S. Dee argues that the need to lower the acceptable BAC for drunk driving is clear. The federal government should enact a national BAC standard of .08 for driving while intoxicated in order to save lives and to prevent serious injuries. The General Accounting Office does not dispute the fact that automobile accidents have declined over the past two decades, but it questions the validity of studies that provide evidence that it is the lowering of blood alcohol levels that caused the decline. The GAO asserts that the decline in automobile accidents may have occurred anyway, regardless of changes in the law.

Thomas S. Dee

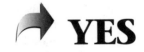 **YES**

Does Setting Limits Save Lives?
The Case of 0.08 BAC Laws

Abstract

Nineteen states have established laws that make it illegal per se to drive with a blood alcohol concentration (BAC) of 0.08. The controversy over extending this stricter definition throughout the nation has focused largely on whether the state laws have been effective at saving lives. Prior evidence on this question has been mixed as well as criticized on several methodological grounds. This study presents novel, panel-based evaluations of 0.08 BAC laws, which address the potential methodological limitations of previous studies. The results of this study indicate that 0.08 BAC laws have been effective in reducing the number of traffic fatalities, particularly among younger adults. These estimates suggest that the nationwide adoption of 0.08 BAC laws would generate substantial gains, reducing the annual count of traffic fatalities by at least 1200.

Introduction

Over the last 25 years, almost every state has adopted a law that makes it illegal per se to drive with certain blood alcohol concentrations (BAC).[1] Most states initially established this limit at a BAC of 0.10 or higher. However, by the end of 1998, 14 states had established an illegal per se limit at a BAC of 0.08 (Table 1).[2] The continued expansion of this stricter standard has been strongly advocated by law enforcement groups, insurance industry advocates, and traffic safety organizations like Mothers Against Drunk Driving (MADD) who claim that these regulations can save lives by reducing the prevalence of drunk driving. However, these claims have also been contested aggressively by the alcohol and restaurant industries, which argue that this regulation merely punishes responsible social drinkers who pose no threat to others. Over the last several years, much of this debate has focused on possible actions by the federal government to compel all states to adopt this stricter BAC standard. In particular, in March of 1998, the Senate approved by a vote of 62 to 32 a transportation appropriations bill that would withhold federal highway funds from states that do not adopt an

From Thomas S. Dee, "Does Setting Limits Save Lives? The Case of 0.08 BAC Laws," *Journal of Policy Analysis and Management,* vol. 20, no. 1 (2001). Copyright © 2001 by The Association for Public Policy Analysis and Management. Reprinted by permission of John Wiley & Sons, Inc.

Table 1

Effective Dates of 0.08 BAC Laws and Administrative License Revocations, 1982–1998

State	Effective Dates	
	Illegal Per Se at 0.08 BAC	Administrative License Revocation
Alabama	August 1995	August 1996
California	January 1990	July 1990
Florida	January 1994	October 1990
Idaho	July 1997	July 1994
Illinois	July 1997	January 1986
Kansas	July 1993	July 1988
Maine	August 1988	January 1986
New Hampshire	January 1994	July 1992
New Mexico	January 1994	July 1984
North Carolina	October 1993	October 1983
Oregon	October 1983	July 1984
Utah	August 1983	August 1983
Vermont	July 1991	December 1989
Virginia	July 1994	January 1995

Note: Hawaii, Washington, Texas, Kentucky, and Rhode Island also adopted 0.08 BAC laws in 1995, 1999, 1999, 2000, and 2000, respectively.

illegal per se limit of 0.08. The Clinton administration also endorsed this legislation. However, there was less support for this measure among Republican leaders in the House. After a period of intense lobbying, the Senate's initial decision was reversed: the final legislation did not withhold highway funds from states without a 0.08 BAC standard. And there was no threat of a presidential veto in response to this change (Pianin, 1998).[3] Commentators attributed the demise of this drunk-driving legislation in part to aggressive lobbying by the alcohol and restaurant industries as well as to a propensity among many legislators to allow states to make these decisions for themselves (Weisman, 1998). However, unclear statistical evidence on the effects of previous state-level 0.08 BAC laws was also cited as an important part of the public debate. The final legislation acknowledged this concern by directing the General Accounting Office (GAO) to evaluate the existing studies of the efficacy of state 0.08 BAC laws. In their subsequent report, the GAO (1999) cited several methodological concerns with this research in concluding that available evidence had not clearly established that the state-level 0.08 BAC laws actually reduced alcohol-related traffic fatalities.[4]

These concerns about the uncertain effects of state-level experiences with 0.08 BAC laws are likely to surface again: in its most recent transportation appropriations bill, the Senate has again approved the withholding of highway funds from states that do not have a 0.08 BAC standard. This study addresses these issues by presenting new empirical evidence on how state-level 0.08 BAC laws influenced traffic fatalities. These evaluations are based on data and empirical specifications that address the potential methodological limitations of the prior research reviewed in GAO (1999). For example, these evaluations are based on a relatively long (1982–1998) panel of annual state-level data on traffic fatality rates, instead of data on alcohol involvement in fatal crashes.[5] Furthermore, the specifications adopted here improve upon much of the previous literature partly by introducing a broader set of controls for potentially confounding and omitted determinants of traffic safety. These include explicit regressors that control for several of the key traffic-related policies that were also being introduced within states over this period (for example, other drunk-driving policies, seat-belt laws, speed limits). New state regulations that allow licensing authorities to revoke the driver's license of allegedly drunk drivers before any court action (administrative license revocations) are of particular concern in this context. More specifically, several of the states that introduced 0.08 BAC laws introduced administrative license revocations almost simultaneously (Table 1). Some studies have been criticized for failing to control for the possibly confounding influence of this contemporaneous drunk-driving policy (GAO, 1999).

Furthermore, several traffic safety studies have recognized that other important and unobserved determinants of traffic safety may vary substantially from one geographic area to another as well as over time periods (for example, state-specific or year-specific cultural sentiment toward drunk driving). As in these studies (for example, Benson, Rasmussen, and Mast, 1999; Cook and Tauchen, 1984; Dee, 1999; Evans and Graham, 1988; Evans, Neville, and Graham, 1991; Mast, Benson, and Rasmussen, 1999; Ruhm, 1996; Young and Likens, 2000), the results presented here control for the influence of these unobserved and potentially confounding omitted variables through the use of state and year fixed effects. This study also presents some counterfactual evaluations that validate this study's key inferences by exploiting the patterns in the timing of alcohol involvement in fatal traffic accidents. It is well known that traffic fatalities that occur on weekends and at night are substantially more likely to involve drunk driving than those that occur during the day or on weekdays. This pattern presents a compelling opportunity to evaluate the reliability of the inferences presented here. More specifically, if the fixed effects specifications were generating reliable inferences, life-saving benefits of introducing drunk-driving policies like 0.08 BAC laws would be expected to be relatively concentrated in observed reductions of weekend and nighttime traffic fatalities. If, in contrast, these models suggest that such policies are more effective in reducing daytime and weekday traffic fatalities, it would point to the possible existence of confounding specification errors.

The results of these evaluations clearly indicate that the adoption of state-level 0.08 BAC laws generated large and statistically significant reductions in the prevalence of traffic fatalities. Furthermore, these results suggest that the law-driven reductions in traffic fatalities were particularly large among teenagers and young adults. However, it is important to note that 0.08 BAC laws were almost never in effect without administrative license revocations

(Table 1). This implies that the "direct" effects of 0.08 standards cannot be effectively distinguished from its potentially interactive effects with administrative license revocations. However, from a policy perspective, this caveat is not particularly constraining given that most states already have administrative license revocations in place. In particular, even under the conservative assumption that 0.08 BAC laws would only save lives when combined with administrative license revocations already in effect, the results presented here suggest that the nationwide adoption of this policy would reduce traffic fatalities by roughly 1200 annually.

Evaluating 0.08 BAC Laws

According to the National Highway Traffic Safety Administration (NHTSA), an average 170-pound man would reach a BAC of 0.08 by consuming his fifth 12-ounce beer (4.5 percent alcohol by volume) within a two-hour period (GAO, 1999). An average 120-pound woman would have a BAC of 0.08 after consuming three beers over the same period.[6] Varied evidence suggests that driving at such levels of intoxication is associated with increased traffic fatality risk (Levitt and Porter, 1999; Zador, 1991; Zador, Krawchuk, and Voas, 2000). For example, Zador, Krawchuk, and Voas (2000) found that the fatality risk for drivers with blood alcohol concentrations between 0.08 and 0.10 was at least six times higher than for sober drivers and that the increased risk was particularly high among young males. Similarly, NHTSA claims that impairment of visual function, reaction time, steering, and emergency responsiveness is substantial among drivers with a 0.08 BAC (GAO, 1999). However, alcohol industry associations have disputed this evidence and suggested that a nationwide 0.08 BAC law would only punish "responsible social drinking."[7]

More direct evidence on the potential efficacy of 0.08 BAC laws has been based on reduced-form evaluations of the available state-level experiences with such regulations. More specifically, seven studies have evaluated how the adoption of 0.08 BAC laws may have influenced the proportion of alcohol involvement in fatal crashes and the number of alcohol-related fatalities (GAO, 1999). Two studies focused on the effects of California's 0.08 BAC law, which was adopted at the beginning of 1990 (NHTSA, 1991; OTS, 1995). The first of these studies reported a 12 percent decline in alcohol-related fatalities after the adoption of the 0.08 BAC law. However, the GAO criticized this study in part because the post-law period was so short and because just six months into this post-law period, California introduced administrative license revocations for drunk drivers (Table 1). The second California study, which was based on four years of data, reported mixed results regarding the 0.08 BAC law. NHTSA (1994) examined data from five states that adopted 0.08 BAC laws (California, Maine, Oregon, Utah, and Vermont). This study considered how six measures of alcohol involvement (driver involvement in fatal crashes by certain BAC levels, nighttime involvement) changed after the adoption of 0.08 BAC laws in these five states. They reported significant decreases in nine of the 30 measures. Hingson, Heeren, and Winter (1996) also evaluated the changed rates of alcohol involvement in fatal crashes for these five states. However, this study compared the changes in these states with those in nearby comparison states to provide potential controls for the shared but unobserved time-series determinants of alcohol involvement.[8] Nonetheless, both of these studies have been reasonably criticized for failing to control for other important time-varying determinants. In particular, as Hingson, Heeren, and Winter (1996) recognized, three of the five states in these studies also adopted administrative license revocations within only 10 months of their 0.08 BAC law (Table 1). The study by Hingson, Heeren, and Winter (1996) has also been criticized for the potentially problematic nature of the comparison states.[9]

NHTSA released three other studies on 0.08 BAC laws in April of 1999. One of these studies (Foss, Stewart, and Reinfurt, 1998) focused on North Carolina and concluded that the 0.08 BAC law had no clear effect and that reductions in alcohol-related traffic fatalities appeared to be part of a long-term trend that began before the adoption of a 0.08 BAC law. Apsler et al. (1999) presented time-series evaluations for the 11 states that had a 0.08 BAC law by the end of 1994. They found that 0.08 BAC laws significantly reduced alcohol involvement in only two to five of these 11 states. Voas, Tippetts, and Fell (2000) conducted an evaluation of 0.08 BAC laws by estimating regression models based on quarterly data from all 50 states and the District of Columbia from 1982 through 1997. These regression models included controls for other determinants of alcohol involvement such as administrative license revocations, vehicle miles traveled, urbanicity, shared trends, and fixed state-level variables for whether each state had adopted certain traffic safety policies at any time over this period.[10] They found that 0.08 BAC laws reduced the involvement of drinking drivers relative to sober drivers. GAO (1999) criticizes this study in part for excluding young drivers, noting that many young drivers have been prosecuted under the 0.08 BAC law in California.

In reviewing the mixed evidence from these seven state-level studies, GAO (1999) concluded that they fell short of clearly establishing the efficacy of 0.08 BAC laws. This study presents novel evaluations of the effect of 0.08 BAC laws, which address the potential methodological limitations of these previous studies. One class of innovations in this study simply involves the nature of the data being analyzed. The evaluations presented here are based on annual state-level panel data on traffic fatality rates from 1982 to 1998. These data are sufficiently recent to provide observations well after most states enacted 0.08 BAC laws (Table 1). Furthermore, these data reflect total fatalities including those among young adults who were excluded from some prior studies (for example, NHTSA, 1994; Voas, Tippetts, and Fell, 2000).[11] And some of the evaluations presented here focus specifically on traffic fatality rates among younger adults. However, another potentially important distinction in the data set under study here is simply that the key outcomes are traffic fatality rates. Most studies have instead examined how 0.08 BAC laws influenced rates of alcohol involvement in fatal crashes. The rate of alcohol involvement in crashes is undoubtedly a policy-relevant outcome as it is strongly associated with fatality risk. However, tests for alcohol involvement are not actually conducted and recorded for all fatal crashes. Therefore, NHTSA has simply imputed much of the available data on alcohol involvement. In contrast, the actual number of traffic fatalities, which are ultimately the outcome of interest, is essentially observed without error in each state and year.[12] Similarly, other key attributes of fatal crashes known to be associated with alcohol use (time of accident, age of victims) are also recorded for nearly all accidents and allow construction of alcohol-sensitive measures of traffic fatalities.

A second class of innovations in this study involves the research design employed to identify the effects of 0.08 BAC laws. The most recent studies on 0.08 BAC laws have employed multiple regression techniques to purge the potentially confounding influence of other observed and unobserved determinants of traffic safety (Apsler et al., 1999; Voas, Tippetts, and Fell, 2000). However, the number of controls included in previous studies may be too limited. The period over which 0.08 BAC laws were adopted was characterized by considerable within-state variation in other important policies related to traffic safety (other drunk-driving measures, seat-belt laws, speed limits, etc.). Furthermore, other less tangible attributes that influence traffic safety may also vary substantially from one geographic area to another and over periods of time (for example, state-specific or period-specific cultural sentiment toward drunk driving). By definition, such unobserved determinants are inherently difficult to measure. However, omitting controls for these determinants could easily bias statistical inferences regarding traffic safety measures as well as attenuate the precision of those inferences. Several empirical studies of traffic safety have controlled for such omitted variable biases by introducing state and year fixed effects, which unambiguously purge the influence of unobserved state-specific determinants as well as shared, year-specific determinants.[13] This study presents multiple regression results based on such two-way fixed effects models. As noted earlier, the method adopted by Hingson, Heeren, and Winter (1996) is conceptually consistent with this approach because it relies on comparing the within-state changes in 0.08 BAC states with the contemporaneous changes in states that did not adopt 0.08 BAC laws. However, the two-way fixed effects models presented here generalize this approach in at least two important ways. One is that the effective "comparison" states are less selective because they are drawn from the entire nation. The second is that it allows for other important robustness checks because other variables reflecting important state policy changes over this period can easily be included as controls.

Nonetheless, even the use of fixed effects and an expanded set of control variables does not obviate all reasonable concerns about the possibly confounding influence of omitted variables or other specification errors. As an additional check on these results, this study presents evidence from counterfactual estimations that attempt to exploit the patterns in the timing of alcohol-related accidents. It is well established that the rates of alcohol involvement in fatal crashes are substantially larger during weekends and at nighttime.[14] For example, NHTSA (1999) reports that, in 1988, 49 percent of the drivers killed during weekends were in accidents involving someone who was intoxicated (that is, a BAC of at least 0.10). In contrast, only 29 percent of the drivers killed during weekdays in 1988 were in accidents involving someone who was intoxicated. Similarly, the rate of alcohol involvement for driver fatalities in 1988 was 56 percent at night and 16 percent during the day.[15] Because of these patterns, several empirical studies of alcohol policies (including this one) have focused on these alcohol-sensitive weekend or nighttime outcomes. However, the much lower rates of alcohol involvement in weekday and daytime fatalities also present a compelling opportunity. More specifically, if the conventional regression models were generating reliable inferences about the effects of 0.08 BAC laws, one would reasonably expect these effects to be smaller in similarly specified models of weekday or daytime traffic fatalities. However, if 0.08 BAC laws appeared to have relatively large and statistically significant effects in such models, it would suggest a confounding specification error. This study presents such counterfactual evidence by comparing the results from similarly specified models of weekend, weekday, nighttime, and daytime traffic fatality rates. These ad hoc comparisons are particularly useful in this context because they provide a compelling way of validating the inferences from these models without simply introducing additional controls that exhaust the already limited sample variation in 0.08 BAC laws and traffic fatalities. However, the power of these simple comparisons as a specification test should not be overstated. Comparisons of evaluation results for models of daytime, nighttime, weekend, and weekday traffic fatalities may yield a plausible heterogeneity even in the presence of some specification error. Furthermore, drunk-driving measures such as 0.08 BAC laws may actually have no detectable effects on daytime and weekday traffic fatalities if efforts at enforcement are substantially lower during these periods. Alternatively, 0.08 BAC standards may have larger effects on weekday and daytime fatalities if those at risk for driving drunk during these periods are more responsive to illegal per se laws. Nonetheless, the patterns of response heterogeneity across these types of traffic fatalities can provide a useful additional commentary on this study's main results. . . .

Conclusions

Over the last 20 years, an extensive array of legislative initiatives has attempted to reduce the prevalence of drunk driving. Although, by most accounts, these efforts have been successful, drunk driving continues to exact a heavy toll. In 1998, 38 percent of the 41,471 traffic fatalities in the United States were classified as alcohol-involved (NHTSA, 1999). Such disturbing facts motivate the continued legislative efforts to discourage risky drunk driving. The focus of the most recent activity has largely been on state laws that establish an explicit blood alcohol concentration (BAC) at which it is illegal per se to drive. In most states, this standard has been set at a BAC of 0.10. However, to date, 19 states have adopted a stricter BAC standard of 0.08. Further expansion of this stricter drunk-driving standard has been under consideration in most states as well as at the federal level. The nationwide adoption of 0.08 BAC laws has been strongly supported by traffic safety advocates who argue that these regulations save lives by reducing driving at unsafe BAC levels. However, these claims have also been aggressively contested by the alcohol and restaurant industries, which argue that these regulations merely punish responsible social drinking. In 1998, a federal proposal sought to withhold highway funds from states that do not adopt a 0.08 BAC standard. Congressional negotiators ultimately rejected that proposal after a period of intense lobbying that one official characterized as "deep emotions versus deep pockets" (Dao, 1998).

However, much of the controversy over extending the 0.08 BAC standard has also focused on arguably legitimate concerns about the mixed empirical evidence on the efficacy of the earliest state laws. In particular, evaluations of 0.08 BAC laws have been explicitly criticized on a variety of methodological grounds (GAO, 1999). This study presents novel evaluations of state-level 0.08 BAC laws that address the criticisms raised in the GAO report as well as several specification issues that are not. The regression models presented here examine these potential shortcomings through the analysis of a relatively long and recent panel data set on traffic fatalities and through the inclusion of additional controls for other contemporaneous and potentially confounding determinants of traffic safety. The results suggest that methodological criticisms, like those raised in GAO (1999), are indeed valid. In particular, these evaluations indicated that the failure to control for the influence of other traffic safety policies could lead to highly inflated estimates of the life-saving benefits of 0.08 BAC laws.

Nonetheless, the results of these evaluations also demonstrated that state-level 0.08 BAC laws have generated statistically significant reductions in traffic fatality rates. The preferred specification indicate that this stricter BAC standard reduced fatality rates by 7.2 percent. This evidence appears to be quite robust and was validated, in part, by the results of counterfactual estimations that exploited the timing of alcohol involvement in fatal traffic accidents. Interestingly, these results also indicate that these policy-induced reductions in traffic fatalities were particularly large among younger drivers. One relevant caveat to these results is that the direct effects of 0.08 BAC laws cannot be clearly distinguished from their potentially interactive effects with administrative license revocations because states that adopted the 0.08 BAC standard almost always had administrative license revocations in effect (Table 1). However, this qualification is not particularly constraining with respect to the policy relevance of these results in light of the fact that most states have already adopted administrative license revocations. For example, the U.S. Congress is currently reconsidering withholding highway funds from any state without a 0.08 BAC standard. This study's results suggest that federal actions that led to the nationwide expansion of 0.08 BAC laws would generate a considerable reduction in the number of annual traffic fatalities. More specifically, this study's results can be used to estimate the number of lives that would be saved annually by expanding the 0.08 BAC standard under the conservative assumption that this policy would only be effective in states that already have administrative license revocations. Twenty-three states (excluding Alaska) currently have administrative license revocations but have not yet adopted 0.08 BAC laws. In these states, during 1998, there were roughly 90.1 million people and the total traffic fatality rate averaged 18.7 per 100,000 in the population. A 7.2 percent reduction in traffic fatality rates in these states would imply roughly 1200 lives saved annually. . . . [T]hese saved lives would be disproportionately young. In considering the policy implications of such simulations and the future of BAC standards in the United States, it should also be noted that other types of evidence point to the likely efficacy of 0.08 BAC laws. Medical evidence suggests that driver ability is significantly impaired at this BAC level. Studies based on actual crash data (Levitt and Porter 1999; Zador, Krawchuk, and Voas, 2000) also demonstrate a sharply increased risk associated with driving at relatively modest BAC levels, which may not be conventionally associated with drunk driving.

Notes

1. Only Massachusetts and South Carolina have no established BAC at which it is illegal per se to drive. BAC is measured as the weight of alcohol in a certain volume of blood and can be determined through the analysis of blood, urine, breath and saliva.

2. Since then, five other states (Hawaii, Washington, Texas, Kentucky, and Rhode Island) have also adopted 0.08 BAC laws. Several other industrialized nations also define drunk-driving at a BAC of 0.08 or lower.

3. However, as part of the compromise, the legislation allocated $500 million for incentive grants to states that adopted the 0.08 BAC standard.

4. However, GAO (1999) noted that there were "strong indications" that the interaction of these laws with other drunk-driving measures may be effective. The GAO study also suggested that direct medical evidence of driver impairment at such BAC levels should be considered.

5. One criticism of some previous studies has been that they have had too little data after the adoption of 0.08 BAC laws. Another potential shortcoming in prior studies of 0.08 BAC laws has been the focus on rates of alcohol involvement in fatal crashes. Since alcohol involvement in fatal crashes is not always determined, much of the available data are actually imputed. In contrast, the prevalence of traffic fatalities, which are arguably the true outcome of interest, is essentially observed in every state and year without error.

6. Such calculations vary because the absorption of alcohol into the bloodstream depends on a number of individual characteristics, such as age.

7. Public rhetoric on how many drinks it actually takes to reach a 0.08 BAC (and, by implication, what may constitute responsible social drinking) has often been based on misleadingly varied choices of weight, gender, and drink type for a representative person (Gawande, 1998).

8. This approach is analogous to a basic "difference-in-differences" estimator, since it compares changes in the "treatment" state to contemporaneous changes in the "control" states. The preferred regression specifications adopted here, which include state and year fixed effects, provide a more general and flexible variation on this basic identification strategy.

9. For example, California was paired with Texas. GAO (1999) suggests that, in this context, it is better to compare "treatment" states to several states or the rest of the nation. The two-way fixed effects specifications employed here effectively adopt this approach and allow the introduction of other potentially relevant controls that vary within states over time.

10. However, these specifications included trend variables instead of year fixed effects. They also omitted unrestrictive state fixed effects, including instead time-invariant dummy variables for states that had certain traffic safety policies any time over the study period. Their specifications also excluded variables representing other potentially important policies that varied within states over this period (speed limits and other drunk-driving policies).

11. GAO (1999) noted that in 1997, more under-21 California drivers were convicted under the state's 0.08 BAC law than under the "zero tolerance" law.

12. Since 1975, NHTSA has obtained data on all traffic-related fatalities through its Fatal Accident Reporting System (FARS). The economic literature on traffic safety has focused almost exclusively on fatalities as the key dependent variable (for example, Chaloupka, Saffer, and Grossman, 1993; Cook and Tauchen, 1984; Dee, 1999; Evans and Graham, 1988; Evans, Neville, and Graham, 1991; Mast, Benson, and Rasmussen, 1999; Ruhm, 1996; Young and Likens, 2000).

13. Ruhm (1996) addressed this issue directly and finds that the omission of such controls can lead to confounded inferences about alcohol-related traffic safety policies.

14. NHTSA (1999) defines the weekend as the period from 6:00 PM on Friday to 5:59 AM on Monday and defines nighttime as the period from 6:00 PM to 5:59 AM. These definitions are also adopted here.

15. These patterns of alcohol involvement are typical even though they are partly based on imputed data and are only for 1988 drivers. According to the author's calculations with the 1982–1998 FARS data on all traffic fatalities, the patterns of police-reported rates of alcohol involvement are quite similar.

References

Apsler, R., Char, A.R., Harding, W.M., & Klein, T.M. (1999). The effects of 0.08 BAC laws. Washington, DC: National Highway Traffic Safety Administration.

Benson, B.L., Rasmussen, D.W, & Mast, B.D. (1999). Deterring drunk driving fatalities: An economics of crime perspective. International Review of Law and Economics, 19(2), 205–225.

Chaloupka, F.J., Saffer, H., & Grossman, M. (1993). Alcohol-control policies and motor-vehicle fatalities. Journal of Legal Studies, 22(1), 161–186.

Cook, P.J. & Tauchen, G. (1984). The effect of minimum drinking age legislation on youthful auto fatalities, 1970–1977. Journal of Legal Studies, 13, 169–190.

Dao, J. (1998). Highway bill accord rejects tougher standard on alcohol. The New York Times, A1.

Dee, T.S. (1999). State alcohol policies, teen drinking and traffic fatalities. Journal of Public Economics, 72(2), 289–315.

Evans, W.N. & Graham, J.D. (1988). Traffic safety and the business cycle. Alcohol, Drugs and Driving, 4(1), 31–38.

Evans, W.N., Neville, D., & Graham, J.D. (1991). General deterrence of drunk driving: Evaluation of recent American policies. Risk Analysis, 11(2), 279–289.

Foss, R.D., Stewart, J.R., & Reinfurt, D.W. (1998). Evaluation of the effects of North Carolina's 0.08% BAC law. Washington, DC: National Highway Traffic Safety Administration.

GAO [U.S. General Accounting Office] (1999). Highway Safety: Effectiveness of State .08 Blood Alcohol laws. Washington, DC: GAO.

Gawande, A. (1998). One for my baby, but 0.08 for the road. Slate Magazine. (http://slate.msn.com/MedicalExaminer/98-02-26/MedicalExaminer.asp).

Hingson, R., Heeren, T., & Winter, M. (1996). Lowering state legal blood alcohol limits to 0.08%: The effect on fatal motor vehicle crashes. American Journal of Public Health, 86(9), 1297–1299.

Levitt, S.D. & Porter, J. (1999). Estimating the effect of alcohol on driver risk using only fatal accident statistics. Working Paper 6944. Cambridge, MA: National Bureau of Economic Research.

Mast, B.D., Benson, B.L., & Rasmussen, D.W. (1999). Beer taxation and alcohol-related traffic fatalities. Southern Economic Journal, 66(2), 214–249.

NHTSA [National Highway Traffic Safety Administration]. (1991). The effects following the implementation of .08 BAC limit and an administrative per se Law in California. Washington, DC: NHTSA.

NHTSA [National Highway Traffic Safety Administration]. (1994). A preliminary assessment of the impact of lowering the illegal BAC per se limit to 0.08 in five states. Washington, DC: NHTSA.

NHTSA [National Highway Traffic Safety Administration]. (1999). Traffic safety facts 1998—alcohol. Washington, DC: U.S. Department of Transportation.

OTS [Office of Traffic Safety]. (1995). The general deterrent impact of California's .08% blood alcohol concentration limit and administrative per se license suspension laws. Office of Traffic Safety, State of California.

Pianin, E. (1998). How pressure politics bottled up a tougher drunk-driving rule. The Washington Post. Washington, DC: A20.

Ruhm, C.J. (1996). Alcohol policies and highway vehicle fatalities. Journal of Health Economics, 14(5), 583–603.

Voas, R.B., Tippetts, A.S., & Fell, J. (2000). The relationship of alcohol safety laws to drinking drivers in fatal crashes. Accident Analysis and Prevention, 32, 483–492.

Weisman, J. (1998). Industry may kill alcohol measure. The Baltimore Sun. Baltimore, MD: 1A.

Young, D. & Likens, T. (2000). Alcohol regulation and auto fatalities. International Review of Law and Economics, 20(1), 107–126.

Zador P.L. (1991). Alcohol-related relative risk of fatal driver injuries in relation to driver age and sex. Journal of Studies on Alcohol, 52(4), 302–310.

Zador, P.L., Krawchuk, S.A., & Voas, R.B. (2000). Alcohol-related relative risk of driver fatalities and driver involvement in fatal crashes in relation to driver age and sex: An update using 1996 data. Journal of Studies on Alcohol, 61(3), 387–395.

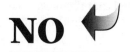
How Effective Are ".08" Drunk-Driving Laws?

Inconclusive Results

State efforts to combat drunk driving have, by all accounts, worked to good effect. Alcohol-related fatalities have declined sharply over the past 15 years. Currently, it is illegal in every state to drive while under the influence of alcohol. In addition, all but two have blood alcohol "per se" laws—laws that make it unlawful for a person to drive with a specific amount of alcohol in his blood. How low this amount should be has drawn controversy. Thirty-two states have set this limit at .10 BAC (blood alcohol content). In 16 states, however, the per se limit is 20% lower, or .08 BAC, and the Clinton Administration has pushed to extend this limit to other states, raising concerns that drivers who pose little threat on the highways will be unfairly penalized. As the following excerpts from a recent General Accounting Office report reveal, the effectiveness of these '.08' limits has not been sufficiently supported by the safety data, despite official assertions to the contrary.—Ed.

Since 1970, the National Highway Traffic Safety Administration (NHTSA) has espoused a "systems approach" to reducing drunk driving, including enforcement, judicial, legislative, licensing, and public information components. In 1997, NHTSA published an action plan developed with other participants to reduce alcohol-related driving fatalities to 11,000 by the year 2005. This plan recommended that all states pass a wide range of laws, including ones establishing .08 BAC limits, license revocation laws—under which a person deemed to be driving under the influence has his or her driving privileges suspended or revoked—comprehensive screening and treatment programs for alcohol offenders, vehicle impoundment, "zero tolerance" BAC and other laws for youth, and primary enforcement laws for safety belts. The plan also called for increased public awareness campaigns, with an emphasis on target populations such as young people and repeat offenders.

The value of public education and enforcement has been demonstrated in a number of studies. A recent NHTSA evaluation of a sobriety checkpoint program in Tennessee, a state with a .10 BAC limit, concluded that the program and its attendant publicity reduced alcohol-related fatal accidents in that state by 20.4%.

•◦•

One of NHTSA's principal arguments for nationwide adoption of .08 BAC laws is that the medical evidence of drivers' impairment at that level is substantial and conclusive. According to NHTSA, reaction time, tracking and steering, and emergency responses are impaired at even low levels, and substantially impaired at .08 BAC. As a result, the risk of being in a motor vehicle crash increases when alcohol is involved, and increases dramatically at .08 BAC and higher levels. In contrast to NHTSA's position, industry associations critical of .08 BAC laws contend that .08 BAC is an acceptable level of impairment for driving a motor vehicle and that these laws penalize "responsible social drinking."

These associations also believe that .08 BAC laws do not address the problem of drunk driving because many more drivers using alcohol are reported at the "high" BAC levels (above .10 BAC) than at the lower BAC levels. Because we were directed to review the impact of .08 BAC laws on the number and severity of crashes involving alcohol, we did not review the medical evidence on impairment or other arguments in favor of or in opposition to .08 BAC laws.

NHTSA also believes that lowering the BAC limit to .08 is a proven effective measure that will reduce the number of crashes and save lives. For example, in a December 1997 publication, NHTSA stated that "recent research . . . has been quite conclusive in showing the impaired driving reductions already attributable to .08, as well as the potential for saving additional lives if all states adopted .08 BAC laws." In May 1998, the NHTSA Administrator stated, "The traffic safety administration is aware of four published studies, . . . [and] each study has shown that lowering the illegal blood alcohol limit to .08 is associated with significant reductions in alcohol-related fatal crashes." In a fact sheet distributed to state legislatures considering these laws, NHTSA stated that the agency's "analysis of five states that lowered the BAC limit to .08 showed that significant decreases in alcohol-related fatal crashes occurred in four out of the five states as a result of the legislation." NHTSA used these study results to encourage states to enact .08 BAC laws, testifying in one instance before a state legislature: "We conservatively project a 10% reduction in alcohol-related crashes, deaths, and injuries" in the state.

Seven studies have been published assessing the effect of .08 BAC laws on motor vehicle crashes and fatalities in the United States. Four studies published between 1991 and 1996 assessed the effectiveness of .08 BAC laws in the five states that enacted them between 1983 and 1991. On April 28, 1999, NHTSA released three additional studies.

Early studies had limitations and raised methodological concerns   Although NHTSA characterized the first four studies on the effectiveness of .08 BAC laws as conclusively establishing that .08 BAC laws resulted in substantial reductions in fatalities involving alcohol, we found that three of the four studies had limitations and raised methodological concerns that called their conclusions into question. For example, while a NHTSA-endorsed Boston University study concluded that 500 to 600 fewer fatal crashes would occur each year if all states adopted .08 BAC laws, this study has been criticized for, among other reasons, its method of comparing states; and a recent NHTSA study characterized the earlier study's conclusion as "unwarranted." The fourth study reported mixed results. Therefore, these studies did not provide conclusive evidence that .08 BAC laws by themselves have resulted in reductions in drunk driving crashes and fatalities. A task force of the New Jersey State Senate examined this evidence and, in a report issued in December 1998, reached a similar conclusion.

⋆◈⋆

Recent studies are more comprehensive, but results are mixed   On April 28, 1999, NHTSA released three studies that it sponsored. These studies are more comprehensive than the earlier studies and show many positive results but fall short of conclusively establishing that .08 BAC laws by themselves have resulted in reductions in alcohol-related fatalities. For example, during the early 1990s, when the involvement of alcohol in traffic fatalities declined from around 50% to nearly 40%—a trend in states with both .08 BAC and .10 BAC laws—eight states' .08 BAC laws became effective, and the recent studies disagree on the degree to which .08 BAC laws played a role. Two of the studies reached different conclusions about the effect of one state's .08 BAC law; one concluded that the law brought about reductions in drunk driving deaths in North Carolina, while another concluded that the state's reductions occurred as the result of a long-term trend that began before the law was enacted.

In a statement releasing the three studies, NHTSA credited the nation's progress in reducing drunk driving to a combination of strict state laws and tougher enforcement, and stated that "these three studies provide additional support for the premise that .08 BAC laws help to reduce alcohol-related fatalities, particularly when they are implemented in conjunction with other impaired driving laws and programs."

Eleven-state study   An April 1999 NHTSA study of 11 states with .08 BAC laws assessed whether the states experienced statistically significant reductions in three measures of alcohol involvement in crashes after the law took effect: (1) the number of fatalities in crashes in which any alcohol was involved, (2) the number of fatalities in crashes where drivers had a BAC of .10 or greater ("high BAC"), and (3) the proportion of fatalities involving "high BAC" drivers to fatalities involving sober drivers. The study performed a similar analysis for license revocation laws and also modeled and controlled for any pre-existing long-term declining trends these states may have been experiencing when their .08 BAC laws went into effect. The study found that five of the 11 states had reductions in at least one measure and that two of the 11 states had reductions in all three measures.

The study was careful not to draw a causal relationship between the reductions it found and the passage of .08 BAC laws by themselves. Rather, it concluded that .08 BAC laws added to the impact that enforcement, public information, and legislative activities, particularly license revocation laws, were having. In addition to the two states where .08 BAC and license revocation laws were found to be effective in combination, the study noted that the five states with .08 BAC laws that showed reductions already had license revocation laws in place. One of the authors told us that this suggested the .08 BAC laws had the effect of expanding the scope of the license revocation laws to a new portion of the driving public.

University of North Carolina study   A NHTSA-sponsored study by the University of North Carolina concluded, in contrast to the 11-state study, that the .08 BAC law in North Carolina had little clear effect. The study examined alcohol-related crashes and crashes involving drivers with BACs greater than .10 from 1991 through 1995; compared fatalities among drivers with BACs greater than .10 in North Carolina with such fatalities in 11 other states; and compared six measures of alcohol involvement in North Carolina and 37 states that did not have .08 BAC laws at that time. The study controlled for and commented on external factors that could confound the results, such as the state's sobriety checkpoints, enforcement, and media coverage. The study found the following:

- No statistically significant decrease in alcohol-related crashes after passage of North Carolina's .08 BAC law in three direct and two "proxy" measures.
- A continual decline in the proportion of fatally injured drivers with BACs equal to or greater than .10 but no abrupt change in fatalities that could be attributed to the .08 BAC law.
- Decreases in alcohol-related crashes in North Carolina and in the 11 other states studied. While North Carolina's decreases were greater, the study concluded that no specific effects could be attributed to the .08 BAC law.
- No statistically significant difference between North Carolina and 37 states without .08 BAC laws in four of the six measures. While reductions in police-reported and estimated instances of alcohol involvement were found to be statistically significant, these reductions happened 18 months before North Carolina lowered its BAC limit. The authors attributed these decreases, in part, to increased enforcement.

The study concluded that the .08 BAC law had little clear effect on alcohol-related fatalities in North Carolina, that a downward trend was already occurring before North Carolina enacted its .08 BAC law, and that this trend was not affected by the law. The authors offered several possible explanations, including (1) the effects of the .08 BAC laws were obscured by a broader change in drinking-driving behavior that was already occurring; (2) North Carolina had made substantial progress combating drunk driving and that the remaining drinking and driving population in North Carolina was simply not responsive to the lower BAC law; and (3) .08 BAC laws are not effective in measurably affecting the behavior of drinking drivers.

50-state study   The third April 1999 NHTSA study evaluated .08 BAC laws by comparing two groups—states with .08 BAC laws with states with .10 BAC laws, before and after the laws were passed. This study concluded that states that enacted .08 BAC laws experienced an 8% reduction in the involvement of drivers with both high and low BACs when compared with the involvement of sober drivers. The study estimated that 274 lives have been saved in the states that enacted .08 BAC laws and that 590 lives could be saved annually if all states enacted .08 BAC laws.

While more comprehensive than other studies, the study used a method to calculate the 8% reduction that is different from, and thus not directly comparable, to those for fatality estimates reported in other studies and publications. In particular, this method can produce a numerical effect that is larger than other methods.

⁓⊙⁓

Another reason why this study's results cannot be directly compared to other studies' is because it did not include data for drivers under 21. In 1997, drivers under 21 accounted for around 14% of the drivers in fatal crashes and about 12% of the drivers in fatal crashes involving alcohol.

Including persons under 21 years old would have changed these study results. In particular, the study would have found no statistically significant reductions associated with .08 BAC laws for drivers at low BAC levels. The findings regarding drivers at high BAC levels—a group that contains over three times as many drivers—would have remained substantially unchanged.

The study warns that "it is important to interpret estimates of lives saved due to any single law with considerable caution." In particular, as the study notes, factors such as public education, enforcement, and changes in societal norms and attitudes toward alcohol have produced long-term reductions in drunk driving deaths over many years. This study did more to control for extraneous factors than any of the other multi-state studies, but this is inherently difficult to do, and in this case the authors estimate that 50% to 60% of the reductions in alcohol-related fatalities are explained by the laws it reviewed and the other factors it considered, a moderate level for statistical analyses of this type. Because of the uncertainties, the study's estimate of lives saved is also expressed as a range—and the number of lives saved in states with .08 BAC laws could have been as few as 88 or as many as 472.

While the study reported results for the three laws it reviewed, including .08 BAC laws, the study also concluded that "the attribution of savings to any single law should be made with caution since each new law builds to some extent on existing legislation and on other ongoing trends and activities."

While indications are that .08 BAC laws in combination with other drunk-driving laws, as well as sustained public education and information efforts and strong enforcement, can be effective, the evidence does not conclusively establish that .08 BAC laws by themselves result in reductions in the number and severity of crashes involving alcohol. Until recently, limited published evidence existed on the effectiveness of .08 BAC laws, and NHTSA's position—that this evidence was conclusive—was overstated. In 1999, more comprehensive studies have been published that show many positive results, and NHTSA's characterization of the results has been more balanced. Nevertheless, these studies fall short of providing conclusive evidence that .08 BAC laws by themselves have been responsible for reductions in fatal crashes.

Because a state enacting a .08 BAC law may or may not see a decline in alcohol-related fatalities, it is difficult to predict accurately how many lives would be saved if all states passed .08 BAC laws. The effect of a .08 BAC law depends on a number of factors, including the degree to which the law is publicized; how well it is enforced; other drunk driving laws in effect; and the unique culture of each state, particularly public attitudes concerning alcohol.

As drunk driving continues to claim the lives of thousands of Americans each year, governments at all levels seek solutions. Many states are considering enacting .08 BAC laws, and the Congress is considering requiring all states to enact these laws. Although a strong causal link between .08 BAC laws by themselves and reductions in traffic fatalities is absent, other evidence, including medical evidence on impairment, should be considered when evaluating the effectiveness of .08 BAC laws. A .08 BAC law can be an important component of a state's overall highway safety program, but a .08 BAC law alone is not a "silver bullet." Highway safety research shows that the best countermeasure against drunk driving is a combination of laws, sustained public education, and vigorous enforcement.

Five Bottles of Beer

On average, according to NHTSA, a 170-pound man reaches .08 BAC after consuming five 12-ounce beers (4.5% alcohol by volume) over a two-hour period. A 120-pound woman reaches the same level after consuming three beers over the same period. NHTSA publishes a BAC estimator that computes the level of alcohol in a person's blood on the basis of the person's weight and gender and the amount of alcohol consumed over a specified period of time.

This estimator assumes average physical attributes in the population; in reality, alcohol affects individuals differently, and this guide cannot precisely predict its effect on everyone. For example, younger people have higher concentrations of body water than older people; therefore, after consuming the same amount of alcohol, a 170-pound 20-year-old man attains a lower BAC level on average than a 170-pound 50-year-old man.

NHTSA's estimator shows that the difference between the .08 BAC and .10 BAC levels for a 170-pound man is one beer over two hours. The difference between the .08 BAC and .10 BAC levels for a 120-pound woman is one-half a beer over the same time period.

Alcohol use is a significant factor in fatal motor vehicle crashes. In 1997, the most recent year for which data are available, there were 16,189 alcohol-related fatalities, representing 38.6% of the nearly 42,000 people killed in fatal crashes that year. In the states with .08 BAC laws, alcohol was involved in 36% of all traffic fatalities, lower than the national average and the 39.5% rate of alcohol involvement in the rest of the states. Utah had the lowest level at 20.6%; the District of Columbia had the highest at 58.5%. Among the 10 states with the lowest levels of alcohol-related fatalities, three were states with .08 BAC laws and seven were states with .10 BAC laws. Among the 10 states with the highest levels of alcohol-related fatalities, two were states with .08 BAC laws, seven were states with .10 BAC laws, and one had no BAC per se law.

Although alcohol use remains a significant factor in fatal crashes, fatalities involving alcohol have declined sharply over the past 15 years. In 1982, 25,165 people died in crashes involving alcohol, 57.3% of the nearly 44,000 traffic fatalities that year. The proportion of fatal crashes that involved alcohol declined during the 1980s, falling below 50% for the first time in 1989. The involvement of alcohol in fatal crashes declined markedly in the early 1990s, from about 50% of the fatal crashes in 1990 to nearly 40% in 1994. During this time, the number of people killed in crashes involving alcohol declined by around 25%. The proportion of fatalities involving alcohol rose slightly in the next two years before falling, in 1997, to its lowest level since 1982.

POSTSCRIPT

Will a Lower Blood Alcohol Level for Drunk Driving Reduce Automobile Accidents?

An important follow-up question to the discussion of whether or not a national BAC standard of .08 for driving while intoxicated would reduce the number of alcohol-related accidents is, Is the federal government unreasonably imposing laws concerning blood alcohol levels when the evidence for those laws can be seen as questionable? Is the federal government being presumptuous in trying to implement a policy that it feels is best for its citizens? On the other hand, if it has been shown that a .08 BAC limit lowers the rate of alcohol-related accidents, doesn't the federal government have a moral and ethical obligation to prevent these accidents?

Alcohol abuse is a serious problem. Although restricting a person from drinking and driving may not reduce the incidence of alcohol abuse, it may reduce other problems. Driving a motor vehicle after drinking alcohol is clearly dangerous. Not only are the drinker and the drinker's passengers endangered, but anyone else who may be driving a car in the vicinity of the intoxicated driver is at risk. Thousands of people, including pedestrians, are killed or maimed each year by drunk drivers. Lowering the blood alcohol limit to .08 may not reduce alcohol abuse, but will it reduce the risks faced by others?

Balancing the rights of individual states to establish their own laws against the need of the federal government to implement a policy that it believes is right is a recurring issue. There is a lack of consistency in the matter of federal and state laws. During the oil crisis of the 1970s, for example, the federal government required states to have speed limits no higher than 55 miles per hour. Yet each state has its own laws regarding the sale of alcohol. There is little debate that reducing the number of alcohol-related accidents is a high priority. However, how far should the federal government go to ensure that this occurs? Should the federal government *dictate* how we should act, or should it *recommend* how we should act? In addition, is the evidence clear that a lower BAC would result in fewer automobile accidents?

The National Safety Council and the National Highway Traffic Safety Administration's publication *Setting Limits, Saving Lives* (2000) addresses the effects of a .08 blood alcohol level on automobile accidents. Other publications are "Drinking and Driving: Factors Influencing Accident Risk," by the National Institute on Alcohol Abuse and Alcoholism, *Alcohol Alert No. 31* (January 1996); the National Highway Traffic Safety Administration report "Zero-Tolerance Laws to Reduce Alcohol-Impaired Driving by Youth" (January 1998); and "Preventing Impaired Driving," by Ralph W. Hingson, Timothy Heeren, and Michael R. Winter, *Alcohol Research & Health* (Winter 1999).

ISSUE 4

Should We Be Concerned About "Club Drugs"?

YES: Eric Sigel, from "Club Drugs: Nothing to Rave About," *Contemporary Pediatrics* (October 2002)

NO: Jacob Sullum, from "Sex, Drugs and Techno Music," *Reason* (January 2002)

ISSUE SUMMARY

YES: Assistant professor of pediatrics Eric Sigel argues that club drugs such as Ecstasy, GHB, Rohypnol, and Special K are dangerous. Their use, especially at rave parties, allows participants to overlook social barriers and helps individuals to relate better to others. Sigel cautions that some drugs that are taken at rave parties, especially GHB, have led to date rape.

NO: Jacob Sullum, a senior editor at *Reason* magazine, contends that the effects of drugs such as Ecstasy, particularly with regard to sexual behavior, are exaggerated. He refers to the history of marijuana and how it too was deemed a drug that would make people engage in behaviors in which they would not typically engage. Sullum maintains that the public's reaction to club drugs is unjustified.

According to national surveys of secondary school students in the United States, the use of club drugs, especially Ecstasy (MDMA), has risen significantly. In the most recent survey, over 8 percent of high school seniors had used Ecstasy in the previous 12 months. Not surprisingly, the number of people admitted to emergency rooms due to adverse reactions to Ecstasy and other club drugs has also increased. In the year 2000 almost 5,000 people were admitted to emergency rooms due to GHB (gamma-hydroxybutyrate), over 4,500 emergency room visits can be attributed to Ecstasy, and over 700 people were admitted to emergency rooms due to either Ketamine (Special K) or Rohypnol (Roofies). Emergency room visits due to Ecstasy and GHB jumped significantly between 1999 and 2000.

The taking of GHB, Ecstasy, Rohypnol, and Ketamine is not limited to rave parties. A *Time* magazine article indicates that these drugs are showing up at hip-hop parties, on Bourbon Street in New Orleans, and in many other places. However, their use at rave parties is not unusual. Many people agree that making rave parties illegal will not stop the use of these drugs, but it would remove one venue where their use occurs. Also, drug use is deeply embedded in the culture of rave parties. This raises the question, Is making rave parties illegal an effective strategy for reducing the use of club drugs? Further, would people who attend rave parties but who do not use drugs be unfairly penalized if such parties were outlawed?

Attempts to make rave parties and similar activities illegal are being made on the national level as well as on the local level. A bipartisan bill was introduced into the Senate recently "to prohibit an individual from knowingly opening, maintaining, managing, controlling, renting, leasing, making available for use, or profiting from any place for the purpose of manufacturing, distributing, or using any controlled substance, and for other purposes." This act is referred to as the Reducing Americans' Vulnerability to Ecstasy Act of 2002, or the RAVE Act. Penalties could include 20 years in prison or a fine of $250,000 or twice the gross receipts derived from each violation, whichever is more.

One reason for the RAVE Act is that raves have become a way to exploit American youth. These parties are said to be manipulating young people as a means of making money. There is concern that drug use at these parties leads to adverse physical reactions as well as reckless behavior. For example, one consequence of Ecstasy use is dehydration. To capitalize on this effect, some club owners charge excessive amounts of money for water. Others have "chilling rooms" one can go into—for a price. Those who object to rave parties point to these examples as proof that club owners are engaging in exploitation. One potential problem with the bill is that its language is broad enough to close down any business or establishment where any drug use or transaction occurs; in fact, in Chicago the city council passed an ordinance to put building owners or managers in jail if they allow raves to be held on their property.

One of the problems associated with buying illegal drugs is that they are not always what they are purported to be. One cannot be sure of the authenticity of the drug being purchased. Moreover, if one is sold a bogus drug, one has no legal recourse. One group that attends rave parties is DanceSafe. This group tests pills for purity. Therefore, someone who purchases an Ecstasy pill can have it tested to determine whether or not it is indeed Ecstasy. DanceSafe attempts to reduce the harm associated with misidentified drugs. Does DanceSafe give the impression that rave patrons can safely use Ecstasy?

The following selections ask whether or not we should be concerned about club drugs. The effects of club drugs represent a serious threat to the physical and emotional well-being of young people, according to Eric Sigel. Because of the drugs' presence at rave parties, Sigel contends that raves should be illegal. Jacob Sullum acknowledges that drugs like Ecstasy have the potential to cause harm. He notes that many drugs sold as Ecstasy are something else entirely. However, he maintains that warnings associated with these drugs are blown out of proportion and that rave parties should not be closed down.

Eric Sigel

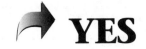 **YES**

Club Drugs: Nothing to Rave About

Ecstasy and other so-called club drugs have caught on with many teens and young adults as a way to enhance the fun of rave parties. Here's what you need to know to counsel your patients about the dangers—including date rape—of this risky kind of recreation.

Club drugs, considered novel in the early 1990s have become mainstream. (1) In particular, we have witnessed a striking rise in the use of Ecstasy since the mid-1990s. The use of club drugs has its roots in the club and rave scene, which originated in the late 1980s and has, like the drugs associated with it, moved from the margins toward the mainstream of teenage culture. It is essential for any health-care practitioner who cares for youth to understand the epidemiology, biology, and psychological impact of club drugs on teenagers and young adults.

Raves: Cradle of Club Drugs

Recognizing the nature of raves is important to understanding the evolution of club drugs into popular culture. (2) Raves are all-night dance parties that began underground, hidden from the law and mainstream culture. Originally, they represented an alternative to mainstream socialization, an outlet for teens and young adults who did not identify with the popular peer groups. Because of the desire to stay separate from the mainstream and the law, rave organizers would send out notices at the last minute letting concertgoers know where the upcoming event was to be held—usually an abandoned warehouse or remote area of the countryside.

Rave music was initially noncommercial and computer generated, reflecting the so-called techno age. It has been described as repetitive, remorseless, loud, and fast, surging past the listener in mind-numbing waves. Over the last 10 to 15 years, rave music has evolved into a new genre, appealing to a wide range of teenagers and adults. Some of the different types of music within this genre are referred to as techno, house, and trance.

Raves also have become increasingly popular. It is easy to log on to the World Wide Web and find out where a rave is being held on any given night.

(3,4) Concert promoters sponsor raves (legally) at prominent venues in most major cities.

The link between raves and drugs derives in part from the nature of raves. Raves typically last all night. Drug use helps participants stay up all night and then come down when dawn arrives. The drugs also enable participants to dismiss classic social barriers and connect to peers, regardless of sex, ethnic background, or social class.

In general, adolescent substance use in the United States reached a peak in the mid-1990s; the use of some substances has leveled off since then and the use of others has declined slightly. (5) Ecstasy is the one drug whose use has increased dramatically over the last five years, though the rate of increase slowed somewhat for the first time in 2001. (6) Nearly 12% of high school seniors have tried Ecstasy at least once.

When interpreting statistics concerning club drug use, physicians must apply the numbers to clinical situations to get an accurate picture. We tend not to attach great significance to drugs that "only 1% to 2%" of a population are using, as is the case with some club drugs. Consider, however, that if 2% of high school students are using Gamma-hydroxybutyrate (GHB), for example, and you are working in a clinic that sees 50 adolescents a week, you will likely see one GHB user weekly, which is significant.

Ecstasy: Euphoria at a Price

MDMA (3-4-methylenedioxymethamphetamine), or "Ecstasy," is an amphetamine that has hallucinogenic properties similar to mescaline. (7,8) Street names include, in addition to Ecstasy, Adam, Bean, E, M, Roll, X, XTC, and Lovers Speed. In the 1970s, psychiatrists used Ecstasy to decrease patients' inhibitions, allowing them to talk freely and openly. In 1985, once the physical dangers of the drug were recognized, the US Drug Enforcement Agency reclassified MDMA as a schedule I drug, and it became a banned substance. Media attention has focused increasingly on Ecstasy in recent years, both because of the rapid rise in its use and much-publicized deaths connected with the drug.

Ecstasy is readily available; more than 50% of high school students say they can obtain it easily. Forty-one percent of tenth graders and 61% of 12th graders say that Ecstasy is "fairly easy" or "very easy" to get. (5) It comes in the form of tablets, often with names such as Playboy bunnies or Nike swoosh CK. Each "brand" of tablet is thought to have a slightly different effect. The drug can be made in home labs but is most often imported from Europe.

Studies have shown different tablets to contain anywhere from 0 mg to 140 mg of MDMA. The average dose is 100 mg. A point to stress when talking to patients about Ecstasy is that the user has no way to know what is actually in the tablet; it may be cut with any one of a number of undesirable drugs, such as ephedrine, dextromethorphan, or amphetamine.

Effects   Onset of action occurs 20 minutes after ingestion of the drug and can last up to six hours. Ecstasy increases sensory input. Users report that they feel extremely happy, peaceful, and euphoric with enhanced sensation from touch and other sensory systems. Social inhibitions disappear, sexual sensation increases, and people feel close, or connected, to others.

MDMA is metabolized by the liver and excreted by the kidney. It produces its effects by indirect sympathetic activation, releasing norepinephrine, dopamine, and serotonin from terminals in the central and autonomic nervous systems. It can inhibit monoamine oxidase. Alcohol potentiates toxicity.

Ecstasy produces multiple physiologic effects. (9) Short-term cardiac effects include tachycardia, vasoconstriction, unpredictable blood pressure changes, arrhythmias, hypertension, and paradoxical hypotension (with depletion of catecholamines). (10) Users may develop myocardial ischemia or infarction, as well as coronary artery spasm. Longer term cardiac effects include irreversible cardiomyopathy, noncardiogenic pulmonary edema, and pulmonary hypertension.

Other medical consequences of Ecstasy use include increased muscle tension, involuntary teeth clenching, malignant hyperthermia, blurred vision, syncope, chills, sweating, dehydration, and seizures. Users may develop hepatitis, which is thought to result from hepatic cell damage related to metabolism of MDMA by the liver. The effects are usually similar to viral hepatitis, with elevated liver enzymes that return to normal after weeks or months. One study found Ecstasy to be the second leading cause of liver damage in people under 25 years of age. (11) In rare cases, the damage can lead to liver failure.

Neurologic effects of MDMA result primarily from its action on the serotonin system. Ecstasy releases serotonin, reducing levels of serotonin (5-hydroxytriptamine [5-HT]) and its metabolite 5HIAA as well as 5-HT transporter. This effect has been demonstrated in several species, including primates. (12) Increasing doses of MDMA lead to degeneration of serotenergic axon terminals throughout the entire brain.

Brain changes in the axonal terminals are detectable seven years after recreational Ecstasy use. Positron emission tomography scans . . . have shown decreased brain 5-HT transporter binding that correlates with the extent of prior use. (13) In addition, Ecstasy produces a demonstrated up-regulation of postsynaptic 5-[HT.sub.2] receptors, which may put users at risk for microvascular changes in the brain and subsequent cerebrovascular accidents. (14)

Persons who have used Ecstasy recreationally show impaired cognitive function affecting performance in complex tasks requiring attention, memory, and learning, and tasks that reflect general intelligence. (15) Performance deteriorates with heavier use of the drug.

Short-term psychological difficulties associated with Ecstasy use include confusion, depression, sleep problems, drug craving, severe anxiety, and paranoia while and sometimes weeks after taking MDMA. Other psychological effects include increased somatization, obsessionality, and hostility. (16)

Deaths from Ecstasy have been attributed to a wide range of medical complications, including rhabdomyolysis, hyperpyrexia, intravascular coagulopathy, hepatic necrosis, cardiac arrhythmias, cerebrovascular accidents, and suicide.

Treatment   Acute MDMA intoxication can be treated initially by administering activated charcoal within the first hour after ingestion to decrease absorption of the drug. General treatment is supportive. In cases of severe intoxication, monitor serum electrolytes, renal and liver function tests, creatine phosphokinase, complete blood count, and coagulation studies. Anxiety and agitation should be treated with a benzodiazepine. Seizures and hypertension should be treated appropriately. (17) No indication exists at present to evaluate brain function or learning ability specifically, although such an assessment should be considered if unusual or specific deficits are observed.

Because Ecstasy has so much appeal, counseling is important, especially in the early teen years. Healthcare professionals need to be aware of several myths about MDMA use that they may encounter among their patients. Many users of MDMA believe that using the drug "the right way" prevents sequelae. The "right way" includes drinking appropriate fluids, avoiding getting overheated, and having enough energy in one's system. As with any drug, users believe they cannot get addicted to MDMA, which is false.

In some countries, such as Canada, raves have health stations and tools to help attendees determine the purity of their Ecstasy. If the content of a pill is determined to be less than 90% MDMA, users usually will not take it. If "ravers" develop acute medical symptoms, the medical team can intervene and send patients to emergency rooms if necessary. Ethical questions have been raised as to whether providing health stations condones the use of Ecstasy and other drugs.

GHB: Date Rape Drug of Choice

Gamma-hydroxybutyrate is a sedative and amnestic that is often used at the end of a rave to help people come down from their Ecstasy high. Street names include Liquid Ecstasy, Soap, Easy Lay, and Georgia Home Boy.

GHB has been used clinically outside the US to treat narcolepsy and opiate and ethanol withdrawal. It has also been used as an anesthetic (for single-agent intravenous anesthesia for emergency procedures and anesthesia for cataract surgery and labor, for example), although other, more effective agents have largely supplanted it.

Since about 1990, GHB has been abused in the US for its euphoric, sedative, and anabolic (bodybuilding) effects. (18) It was widely available over the counter in health food stores from the 1980s until 1992 and was purchased mostly by body builders to aid fat reduction and muscle building. Ingredients in GHB, gamma-butyrolactone (GBL) and 1,4-butanediol, can be converted by the body into GHB. These ingredients are still found in a number of dietary supplements available in health food stores and gymnasiums to induce sleep, build muscles, and enhance sexual performance despite warnings about GBL-related products issued by the Food and Drug Administration in 1997 and 1999. (19) GHB is now more often used as a club drug than a dietary supplement and, because of its amnestic properties, is one of the most commonly used "date rape" drugs. Around 1.6% of high school seniors report having used GHB in the last year. (5)

GHB can be produced in clear liquid, white powder, tablet, and capsule forms and is tasteless if mixed in drinks. (20) Like many other club drugs, it can be made in home laboratories.

Because of GHB's toxicity, overdoses have increased dramatically—from 55 in 1994 to 2,973 in 1999. (21) In 1999, GHB accounted for 32% of illicit-drug-related calls to poison centers in Boston. (21)

Effects   Onset of action occurs 10 to 20 minutes after the drug is taken. Effects can last up to four hours, depending on the dosage. Alcohol potentiates the effects. At lower doses, GHB can relieve anxiety and produce relaxation. As the dose increases, however, the sedative effects may result in sleep and eventual coma or death.

GHB is a naturally occurring metabolite of the inhibitory neurotransmitter gamma-aminobutyric acid and also functions as a neurotransmitter on its own. It binds to receptors in the hippocampus, cortex, midbrain, basal ganglia, and substantia nigra. GHB mediates sleep cycles, temperature regulation, cerebral glucose metabolism and blood flow, memory, and emotional control. (22) In low doses, it inhibits dopamine release, but at high doses it stimulates dopamine release.

The neurologic effects are primary, leading to central nervous system depression with sedation, confusion, amnesia, and coma. It can decrease the seizure threshold and intracranial pressure and cause nystagmus, dizziness, and ataxia.

Other effects include decreased heart rate and blood pressure (at low doses), nausea, and respiratory depression and apnea, which can lead to hypoxia and respiratory failure.

Treatment is generally supportive. If the patient is unconscious, aspiration precautions should be taken. Pulse oximetry should be initiated, and the patient should be observed for respiratory depression and bradycardia. Bradycardia can be treated with epinephrine or, if the rhythm disturbance is getting worse, with atropine. (23) Patients typically return to consciousness two to six hours after ingestion.

Ketamine: Not for Dogs Only

Ketamine is an injectable anesthetic that has been approved for both human and animal use in medical settings since 1970. (24) About 90% of the ketamine sold legally today is intended for veterinary use. Street names include Special K, K, Vitamin K, Cat Valium.

Ketamine became popular as a drug of abuse in the 1980s, when it was realized that a large dose causes a dream-like state and hallucinations similar to those associated with phencyclidine (PCP). Around 1.3% of eighth graders and 2.5% of 12th graders report using ketamine in the past year. (5)

Ketamine is produced in liquid form or as a white powder that is often snorted or smoked with marijuana or tobacco. Recently, intramuscular injection of the drug has been reported.

Effects   Ketamine has receptors in the hippocampus and cerebral cortex. It is a noncompetitive N-methyl-D-aspartate (NMDA) receptor antagonist that prevents excretion of excitatory neurotransmitters. It produces a dissociative state characterized by profound analgesia and amnesia without loss of consciousness. (25) Drug abusers seek the delusional effects of ketamine.

Neurologic effects include sedation, anxiety, agitation, slurred speech, dilated pupils, and psychotic symptoms such as delusions and hallucinations. Low-dose intoxication impairs attention, learning ability, and memory. Systemic effects resulting from an increase in catecholamines include increased heart rate and blood pressure, palpitations, chest pain, and tachypnea. A high dose can lead to respiratory depression.

Treatment is supportive. For acute anxiety reactions, a benzodiazepine may be indicated.

Rohypnol: Forget About It!

Rohypnol (flunitrazepam) is a benzodiazepine that is not approved for prescribing in the US. It is approved in Europe and is used in more than 60 countries as a treatment for insomnia, a sedative, and a presurgical anesthetic. It is produced in tablet form and smuggled into the US from Latin America and Europe. Street names include Roofies, Rophies, Roche, and Forget-me Pill.

Relatively few adolescents admit to using Rohypnol—around 1.7% of high school seniors say they have used it during their lifetime. Fewer than 1% of eighth and 12th graders say they have used Rohypnol in the last year. (5)

Effects   Rohypnol causes profound "anterograde amnesia." (26) Users may not remember events they experienced while under the influence of the drug but do not necessarily lose consciousness. Rohypnol's amnestic effect—along with the fact that it is tasteless and odorless and dissolves easily in carbonated beverages—makes it attractive as a date rape drug. Concurrent use of alcohol aggravates the sedative and toxic effects of Rohypnol. Even without alcohol, a dose of Rohypnol as small as 1 mg can cause impairment for eight to 12 hours. It has been used to enhance highs produced by heroin and to ease the negative effects of cocaine.

Rohypnol is a central nervous system depressant. Users become drowsy and may lose consciousness. Other side effects include decreased blood pressure, respiratory depression, visual disturbances, dizziness, confusion, nausea, vomiting, and urinary retention.

Treatment for Rohypnol intoxication is supportive and, except in an acute overdose with respiratory depression or hypotension, medical intervention is unnecessary. (27) Exploring with the patient's peers what may have occurred under the influence is important, because it may reveal other medical concerns that need to be evaluated, such as sexual assault.

Methamphetamine: The Downside of Uppers

Methamphetamine is an addictive stimulant drug that causes the body to release norepinephrine, dopamine, and serotonin in the central and autonomic nervous system. (28) It is a crystal-like powdered substance—usually white or slightly yellow, depending on purity—that sometimes comes in large rock-like chunks. When the powder flakes off the rock, the shards look like glass, which is a nickname for the drug. Other street names include Chalk, Crank, Croak, Crypto, Crystal, Fire, Meth, Speed, and White Cross. (29) Methamphetamine can be taken orally, injected, snorted, or smoked.

Methamphetamine can be made easily using a combination of over-the-counter products including cold preparations containing pseudophedrine. The drug has received much media attention because police raids of methamphetamine labs have increased substantially, consuming significant resources of local drug agencies.

About 2.2% of eighth graders and 6% of high school seniors report using methamphetamine within the last year; 10% of high school seniors report having used the drug over their lifetimes. (5)

Methamphetamine overdoses treated in emergency rooms increased 30% nationwide between 1999 and 2000. (30)

Effects   Immediately after smoking or intravenously injecting methamphetamine, the user experiences an intense sensation, called a "rush" or "flash," caused by the catecholamine release. The sensation lasts only a few minutes and is described as extremely pleasurable. Oral or intranasal use produces euphoria—a high, but not a rush. Other short-term effects include irritability and aggression, anxiety, nervousness, convulsions, and insomnia.

Generally, methamphetamine has similar sympathomimetic side effects to those caused by Ecstasy. Short-term effects include tachycardia, hypertension, hyperthermia, mydriasis, and diaphoresis. Cardiac arrhythmia can lead to stroke or myocardial infarctions. (28) Necrotizing vasculitis involving medium and small arteries in most organs can lead to widespread ischemia and intracranial hemorrhage. Alcohol can potentiate toxicity.

Methamphetamine is neurotoxic. Abusers may have significant reductions in dopamine transporters. Research shows that users risk long-term damage to their brain cells similar to that caused by a stroke or Alzheimer's disease. (31) Irreversible cardiomyopathy also has been noted. Psychological symptoms of prolonged use include paranoia, hallucinations, repetitive behavior patterns, and delusions of parasites or insects under the skin. Users often obsessively scratch their skin to get rid of the imagined insects.

As noted, methamphetamine is addictive, and users can develop a tolerance quickly, needing higher doses to get high and going on longer binges to achieve the desired effect. Some users avoid sleep for three to 15 days while on a binge.

Treatment   Emergent treatment targets the symptoms of overdose—hyperthermia, tachycardia, and hypertension. (32) Hyperthermia above 40[degrees]

C requires cooling measures, such as cooling blankets. Seizures can be controlled with a benzodiazepine. Unless hypertension is life-threatening and requires aggressive treatment, monitoring vital signs until they stabilize is appropriate. Activated charcoal, administered within one hour of ingestion, can help decrease absorption of methamphetamine.

Symptomatic patients require monitoring of electrolytes, renal and hepatic function, creatine phosphokinase, and the electrocardiogram. A specific urine test—a semiquantitative homogeneous enzyme-multiplied immunoassay test (EMIT)—can detect the class of amphetamine that was used.

Methamphetamine addiction is generally treated with cognitive-behavioral therapy. Support groups can also help addicts.

LSD: Still a Bad Trip

Lysergic acid diethylamide (LSD) is a hallucinogen. It alters cognitive and perceptual states, leading to auditory and visual hallucinations. Street names include Acid, Boomers, and Yellow Sunshines.

LSD is manufactured from lysergic acid, which is found in ergot, a fungus that grows on rye and other grains. (33) It is sold in tablet, capsule, and liquid forms as well as on pieces of blotter paper impregnated with the drug. It is typically taken by mouth. Around 3.4% of eighth graders and 10.9% of 12th graders have used LSD in their lifetime; 6.6% of 12th graders have used the drug in the past year. (5)

Effects   LSD is a potent $5\text{-}[HT.sub.1]$ (serotonin) agonist. Its effects are unpredictable and depend on the amount taken, the surroundings in which the drug is used, and the user's personality, mood, and expectations. Typically the user feels the effects of the drug 30 to 90 minutes after taking it. Initial physical effects include dilated pupils, hyperthermia, tachycardia, hypertension, diaphoresis, lightheadedness, and tremors. In the next phase of intoxication, the visual, auditory, and sensory alterations develop; they can last several hours. The user's sense of time and self changes. Sensations may seem to "cross over," giving the user the feeling of hearing colors and seeing sounds. These changes can be frightening and cause panic.

The late phase of intoxication produces euphoria, mood swings, and depression. Tension and anxiety may develop, leading to panic attacks. Sensations and feelings change much more dramatically than the physical signs. The user may feel several different emotions at once or swing rapidly from one emotion to another.

A high dose of LSD can lead to hyperventilation, and severe toxicity can cause apnea, seizures, coma, and respiratory arrest. Other life-threatening sequelae include neuroleptic malignant syndrome, characterized by hyperthermia, muscle rigidity, rhabdomyolysis, and stupor, which may progress to coma and death.

Two long-term disorders are associated with LSD use: persistent psychosis and posthallucinogen perception disorder, a condition marked by visual disturbances, such as trails of light. LSD users may experience acute psychotic reactions and paranoia, which can develop in persons without a history of schizophrenia.

Flashbacks occur in 15% to 77% of LSD users, often weeks or years after taking LSD. (43) They are generally related to the chronicity of LSD use, but can happen to anyone who has used LSD.

Although users do not become physically addicted to LSD, they often need to increase the dose to achieve similar effects. This results in increased risk of medical side effects.

Treatment   General treatment IS supportive. Activated charcoal administered within one hour of ingestion can help decrease absorption, but is not typically recommended for recreational LSD use. A benzodiazepine can benefit those who are significantly agitated. For those undergoing a so-called bad trip, talking them down in a quiet, dimly lit room can be helpful. For acute psychosis, haloperidol can be effective. Hospital admission may be warranted for prolonged psychosis. (35)

Screening and Counseling

In-depth assessment of drug use is beyond the scope of this article. Primary care health providers should recognize that any adolescent who demonstrates "at-risk behavior" is more likely than other youth to use club drugs. Early onset of any drug use, younger age of sexual debut, and academic difficulties are just a few of the risk factors. High-functioning teenagers are not immune to risk, however, as they may experiment out of boredom or curiosity.

Adolescents and young adults should be asked about the availability of MDMA and other club drugs, what their philosophy is on using these drugs—especially Ecstasy because of its popularity—and whether they have experimented. Counseling college-bound youth about what they may be exposed to on campus and their responsibilities regarding drug use is an additional avenue to pursue.

Counseling about side effects and risks associated with acute toxicity is essential. Use of any amphetamine puts the user at risk of death the next time he or she uses it because of the idiosyncratic cardiovascular effects of these drugs. Some practitioners believe use of club drugs is reason to bring parents into the discussion, breaking confidentiality if a patient is in imminent danger. . . .

Evaluating youth for depression or other mental health disorders is vital and can help determine the appropriate course of intervention. If the patient seems addicted, referral to a drug treatment program is indicated. If the patient has been experimenting and appears to have a comorbid psychiatric condition such as depression, treating the condition with counseling and medication is appropriate.

Although most drugs are metabolized within a few days, performing random Monday urine screening can be used to monitor drug use as an adjunct to treatment. Some club drugs—including MDMA, methamphetamine, and

Rohypnol (as a benzodiazepine)—can be detected on comprehensive drug screens. Specific screens must be ordered for other drugs, such as LSD and ketamine. The physician needs to know what is available from the lab he or she uses and customize drug testing accordingly.

So that adolescents can make responsible, informed decisions, they need to be made aware that club drugs have potentially high morbidity and mortality. In counseling adolescents and young adults, it is essential to remind them always to be on the lookout for themselves and each other, especially at parties or in bars where they do not know everyone. Because it is easy to dope drinks in these situations, youth need to know exactly where a drink came from and who made it.

The availability and properties of date rape drugs may make the idea of sexually victimizing peers more enticing, so a serious conversation with males about the morality and legal aspects of date rape is worth pursuing. Young women need to be aware of how date rape may be perpetrated and how they can team up with peers to prevent it. Encouraging young women to buddy-up at parties and in bars and check in with each other consistently during the evening is one way to prevent such consequences as sexual assault.

Physicians should familiarize themselves with drug treatment resources in the community. Schools often offer mini-courses on drug use. Most cities have drug treatment facilities that can help assess the extent of an adolescent's drug use and determine whether significant intervention, such as residential treatment or day treatment, is indicated. Adolescent specialists can help the primary care practitioner work through complicated situations.

References

1. National Institute on Drug Abuse: Club drugs. Community Drug Alert Bulletin, December 1999. http://www.nida.nih.gov/ClubAlert/ClubDrugAlert.html
2. Weir E: Raves: A review of the culture, the drugs, and the prevention of harm. CMAJ 2000; 162(13):1843
3. http://www.come.to/DenverRaves
4. http://www.ravehousetech.about.com/mbody.htm
5. The Monitoring the Future Study: Trends in the use of various drugs. 2001 data from in-school surveys of 6th, 10th, and 12th grade students. Ann Arbor, Mich., University of Michigan News and Information Services, December 2001. www.monitoringthefuture.org
6. Johnson LD, O'Malley PM, Bachman JG: Rise in ecstasy use among American teens begins to slow. Ann Arbor, Mich., University of Michigan News and Information Services, December 19, 2001. www.monitoringthefuture.org
7. Schwartz R, Miller N: MDMA (Ecstasy) and the rave: A review. Pediatrics 1997; 100:705
8. National Institute on Drug Abuse: Ecstasy. 2001. http://www.nida.nih.gov/Infofax/Clubdrugs.html
9. Kalant H: The pharmacology and toxicology of "Ecstasy" (MDMA) and related drugs. CMAJ 2001; 165(7):917
10. Lester SJ, Baggott M, Welm S, et al: Cardiovascular effects of 3,4-methylenedioxymethamphetamine: A double-blind, placebo-controlled trial. Ann Intern Med 2000; 133:969

11. Andreu V: Ecstasy: A common cause of severe acute hepatotoxicity. J Hepatol 1998; 29:94

12. Ricaurte GA, Yuan J, McCann UD: 3,4 Methylenedioxymethamphetamine ("Ecstasy")-induced serotonin neurotoxicity: Studies in animals. Neuropsychobiology 2000; 42:5

13. McCann UD, Szabo S, Scheffel U, et al: Positron emission tomographic evidence of toxic effect of MDMA ("Ecstasy") on brain serotonin neurons in human beings. Lancet 1998; 352:1433

14. Reneman L, Habraken J: MDMA (Ecstasy) and its association with cerebrovascular accidents: Preliminary findings. Am J Neuroradiol 2000; 21:1001

15. Gouzoulis-May F: Impaired cognitive performance in drug-free use of recreational Ecstasy. J Neurol Neuorosurg Psychiatry 2000; 68:719

16. Parrot AC, Sisk E, Turner JJD: Psychobiologic problems in heavy "Ecstasy" (MDMA) polydrug users. Drug and Alcohol Dependence 2000; 60:105

17. Hallucinogenic amphetamines. Poisindex, Micromedex Inc, vol 113

18. O'Connell T, Kaye L, Plosay J: Gamma-hydroxybutyrate (GHB): A newer drug of abuse. Am Fam Physician 2000; 62:2478

19. US Department of Health and Human Services, Food and Drug Administration: FDA warns about GBL-related products. January 21, 1999. www.cfsan.fda.gov

20. National Institute on Drug Abuse: GHB. 2001. http://www.nida.nih.gov/Infofax/Clubdrugs.html

21. Substance Abuse and Mental Health Services Administration (SAMHSA): The DAWN Report, December 2000. www.samhsa.org

22. U J, Stokes SA, Woeckener A: A tale of novel intoxication: A review of the effects of gamma-hydroxybutyric acid with recommendations for management. Ann Emerg Med 1998; 31(6):739

23. GHB. Poisindex, Micromedex Inc, vol 113

24. National Institute on Drug Abuse: Ketamine. 2001. http://www.nida.nih.gov/Infofax/Clubdrugs.html

25. Kohrs R, Duriex M: Ketamine: Teaching an old drug new tricks. Anesth Analg 1998; 87:1186

26. National Institute on Drug Abuse: Rohypnol. 2001. http://www.nida.nih.gov/Infofax/Clubdrugs.html

27. Rohypnol. Poisindex, Micromedex Inc, vol 113

28. Ghuran A, Nolan J: Recreational drug misuse: Issues for the cardiologist. Heart 2000; 83:627

29. National Institute on Drug Abuse: Methamphetamine. 2001. http://www.nida.nih.gov/Infofax/Clubdrugs.html

30. Drug Abuse Warning Network (DAWN Report): Year-end 2000 emergency department data, www.whitehousedrugpolicy.gov/news/yearend2000

31. National Institute on Drug Abuse: Methamphetamine: Abuse and addiction. Research Report series, 1998. http://www.nida.nih.gov/ResearchReports/methamph/Methamph.html

32. Amphetamines and related drugs. Poisindex, Micromedex Inc, vol 113

33. National Institute on Drug Abuse: LSD. 2001. http://www.nida.nih.gov/infofax/lsd.html

34. Haddad LM, Shannon MW, Winchester JF: Clinical Management of Poisoning and Drug Overdose, ed 3. Philadelphia, WB Saunders, 1998

35. LSD. Poisindex, Micromedex Inc, vol 113

NO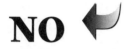

Jacob Sullum

Sex, Drugs, and Techno Music

[In 2001], the Chicago City Council decided "to crack down on wild rave parties that lure youngsters into environments loaded with dangerous club drugs, underage drinking and sometimes predatory sexual behavior," as the *Chicago Tribune* put it. The newspaper described raves as "one-night-only parties . . . often held in warehouses or secret locations where people pay to dance, do drugs, play loud music, and engage in random sex acts." Taking a dim view of such goings-on, the city council passed an ordinance threatening to jail building owners or managers who allowed raves to be held on their property. Mayor Richard Daley took the occasion to "lash out at the people who produce the huge rogue dance parties where Ecstasy and other designer drugs are widely used." In Daley's view, rave promoters were deliberately seducing the innocent. "They are after all of our children," he warned. "Parents should be outraged by this."

The reaction against raves reflects familiar anxieties about what the kids are up to, especially when it comes to sex. As the chemical symbol of raves, MDMA—a.k.a. Ecstasy—has come to represent sexual abandon and, partly through association with other "club drugs," sexual assault. These are not the only fears raised by MDMA. The drug, whose full name is methylenedioxymethamphetamine, has also been accused of causing brain damage and of leading people astray with ersatz feelings of empathy and euphoria (concerns discussed later in this article). But the sexual angle is interesting because it has little to do with the drug's actual properties, a situation for which there is considerable precedent in the history of reputed aphrodisiacs.

A relative of both amphetamine and mescaline, MDMA is often described as a stimulant with psychedelic qualities. But its effects are primarily emotional, without the perceptual changes caused by LSD. Although MDMA was first synthesized by the German drug company Merck in 1912, it did not gain a following until the 1970s, when the psychonautical chemist Alexander Shulgin, a Dow researcher turned independent consultant, tried some at the suggestion of a graduate student he was helping a friend supervise. "It was not a psychedelic in the visual or interpretive sense," he later wrote, "but the lightness and warmth of the psychedelic was present and quite remarkable." MDMA created a "window," he decided. "It enabled me to see out, and to see my own insides, without distortions or reservations."

From Jacob Sullum, "Sex, Drugs and Techno Music," *Reason*, vol. 33, no. 8 (January 2002). Copyright © 2002 by The Reason Foundation, 3415 S. Sepulveda Blvd., Suite 400, Los Angeles, CA 90034. http://www.reason.com. Reprinted by permission.

After observing some striking examples of people who claimed to have overcome serious personal problems (including a severe stutter and oppressive guilt) with the help of MDMA, Shulgin introduced the drug to a psychologist he knew who had already used psychedelics as an aid to therapy. "Adam," the pseudonym that Shulgin gave him (also a nickname for the drug), was on the verge of retiring, but was so impressed by MDMA's effects that he decided to continue working. He shared his techniques with other psychologists and psychiatrists, and under his influence thousands of people reportedly used the drug to enhance communication and self-insight. "It seemed to dissolve fear for a few hours," says a psychiatrist who tried MDMA in the early '80s. "I thought it would have been very useful for working with people with trauma disorders." Shulgin concedes that there was "a hint of snake-oil" in MDMA's reputed versatility, but he himself considered it "an incredible tool." He quotes one psychiatrist as saying, "MDMA is penicillin for the soul, and you don't give up penicillin, once you've seen what it can do."

Shulgin did not see MDMA exclusively as a psychotherapeutic tool. He also referred to it as "my low-calorie martini," a way of loosening up and relating more easily to others at social gatherings. This aspect of the drug came to the fore in the '80s, when MDMA became popular among nightclubbers in Texas, where it was marketed as a party drug under the name *Ecstasy*. The open recreational use of Ecstasy at clubs in Dallas and Austin brought down the wrath of the Drug Enforcement Administration [DEA], which decided to put MDMA in the same legal category as heroin. Researchers who emphasized the drug's psychotherapeutic potential opposed the ban. "We had no idea psychiatrists were using it," a DEA pharmacologist told *Newsweek* in 1985. Nor did they care: Despite an administrative law judge's recommendation that doctors be allowed to prescribe the drug, the ban on MDMA took effect the following year.

Thus MDMA followed the same pattern as LSD, moving from discreet psychotherapeutic use to the sort of conspicuous consumption that was bound to provoke a government reaction. Like LSD, it became illegal because too many people started to enjoy it. Although the DEA probably would have sought to ban any newly popular intoxicant, the name change certainly didn't help. In *Ecstasy: The MDMA Story*, Bruce Eisner quotes a distributor who claimed to have originated the name *Ecstasy*. He said he picked it "because it would sell better than calling it 'Empathy.' 'Empathy' would be more appropriate, but how many people know what it means?" In its traditional sense, *ecstasy* has a spiritual connotation, but in common usage it simply means intense pleasure—often the kind associated with sex. As David Smith, director of the Haight-Ashbury Free Clinic, observed, the name "suggested that it made sex better." Some marketers have been more explicit: A 1999 article in the *Journal of Toxicology* (headlined "SEX on the Streets of Cincinnati") reported an analysis of "unknown tablets imprinted with 'SEX'" that turned out to contain MDMA.

Hyperbolic comments by some users have reinforced Ecstasy's sexual connotations. "One enthusiast described the feeling as a six-hour orgasm!" exclaimed the author of a 2000 op-ed piece in Malaysia's *New Straits Times*, picking up a phrase quoted in *Time* a couple of months before. A column in *The*

Toronto Sun, meanwhile, stated matter-of-factly that MDMA "can even make you feel like a six-hour orgasm." If simply taking MDMA makes you feel that way, readers might reasonably conclude, MDMA-enhanced sex must be indescribably good.

Another reason MDMA came to be associated with sex is its reputation as a "hug drug" that breaks down emotional barriers and brings out feelings of affection. The warmth and candor of people who've taken MDMA may be interpreted as flirtatiousness. More generally, MDMA is said to remove fear, which is one reason psychotherapists have found it so useful. The same effect could also be described as a loss of inhibitions, often a precursor to sexual liaisons. Finally, users report enhanced pleasure from physical sensations, especially the sense of touch. They often trade hugs, caresses, and back rubs.

Yet the consensus among users seems to be that MDMA's effects are more sensual than sexual. According to a therapist quoted by Jerome Beck and Marsha Rosenbaum in their book *Pursuit of Ecstasy*, "MDMA and sex do not go very well together. For most people, MDMA turns off the ability to function as a lover, to put it indelicately. It's called the love drug because it opens up the capacity to feel loving and affectionate and trusting." At the same time, however, it makes the "focusing of the body and the psychic energy necessary to achieve orgasm . . . very difficult. And most men find it impossible. . . . So it is a love drug but not a sex drug for most people."

Although this distinction is widely reported by users, press coverage has tended to perpetuate the connection between MDMA and sex. In 1985 *Newsweek* said the drug "is considered an aphrodisiac," while *Maclean's* played up one user's claim of "very good sexual possibilities." *Life* also cited "the drug's reputation for good sex," even while noting that it "blocks male ejaculation." More recently, a 2000 story about MDMA in *Time* began by describing "a classic Southeast Asian den of iniquity" where prostitutes used Ecstasy so they could be "friendly and outgoing." It warned that "because users feel empathetic, ecstasy can lower sexual inhibitions. Men generally cannot get erections when high on e, but they are often ferociously randy when its effects begin to fade." The story cited a correlation between MDMA use and "unprotected sex." A cautionary article in *Cosmopolitan* began with the account of "a 28-year-old lawyer from Los Angeles" who brought home a man with whom she felt "deeply connected" under the influence of MDMA. "We would have had sex, but he couldn't get an erection," she reported. "The next day, I was horrified that I had let a guy I couldn't even stand into my bed!"

Rape Drugs

MDMA has been linked not just to regrettable sexual encounters but to rapes in which drugs are used as weapons. The connection is usually made indirectly, by way of other drugs whose effects are quite different but which are also popular at raves and dance clubs. In particular, the depressants GHB and Rohypnol have acquired reputations as "date rape drugs," used to incapacitate victims to whom they are given surreptitiously. Needless to say, this is not the main use for these substances, which people generally take on purpose because they like their effects. It's not clear exactly how often rapists use GHB or Rohypnol, but such cases are surely much rarer than the hysterical reaction from the press and Congress (which passed a Date Rape Drug Prohibition Act [in 2001]) would lead one to believe. The public has nonetheless come to view these intoxicants primarily as instruments of assault, an impression that has affected the image of other "club drugs," especially MDMA.

Grouping MDMA with GHB and Rohypnol, a 2000 Knight Ridder story warned that the dangers of "club drugs" include "vulnerability to sexual assault." Similarly, the *Chicago Tribune* cited Ecstasy as the most popular "club drug" before referring to "women who suspect they were raped after they used or were slipped a club drug." In a *Columbus Dispatch* op-ed piece, pediatrician Peter D. Rogers further obscured the distinction between MDMA and the so-called rape drugs by saying that "Ecstasy . . . comes in three forms," including "GHB, also called liquid Ecstasy," and "Herbal Ecstasy, also known as ma huang or ephedra" (a legal stimulant), as well as "MDMA, or chemical Ecstasy." He asserted, without citing a source, that "so-called Ecstasy"—it's not clear which one he meant—"has been implicated nationally in the sexual assaults of approximately 5,000 teen-age and young adult women." Rogers described a 16-year-old patient who "took Ecstasy and was raped twice. She told me that she remembers the rapes but, high on the drug, was powerless to stop them. She couldn't even scream, let alone fight back." If Rogers, identified as a member of the American Academy of Pediatrics' Committee on Substance Abuse, had trouble keeping the "club drugs" straight, it's not surprising that the general public saw little difference between giving a date MDMA and slipping her a mickey.

As the alleged connections between MDMA and sex illustrate, the concept of an aphrodisiac is complex and ambiguous. A drug could be considered an aphrodisiac because it reduces resistance, because it increases interest, because it improves ability, or because it enhances enjoyment. A particular drug could be effective for one or two of these purposes but useless (or worse) for the others. Shakespeare observed that alcohol "provokes the desire, but it takes away the performance." Something similar seems to be true of MDMA, except that the desire is more emotional than sexual, a sense of closeness that may find expression in sex that is apt to be aborted because of difficulty in getting an erection or reaching orgasm. Also like alcohol, MDMA is blamed for causing people to act against their considered judgment. The concern is not just that people might have casual sex but that they might regret it afterward.

Surely this concern is not entirely misplaced. As the old saw has it, "Candy is dandy, but liquor is quicker." When drinking precedes sex, there may be a fine line between seducing someone and taking advantage, between lowering inhibitions and impairing judgment. But the possibility of crossing that line does not mean that alcohol is nothing but a trick employed by cads. Nor does the possibility of using alcohol to render someone incapable of resistance condemn it as a tool of rapists.

The closest thing we have to a genuine aphrodisiac—increasing interest, ability, and enjoyment—is Viagra, the avowed purpose of which is to enable people to have more and better sex. Instead of being deplored as an aid to hedonism, it is widely praised for increasing the net sum of human happiness. Instead of being sold on the sly in dark nightclubs, it's pitched on television by a former Senate majority leader. The difference seems to be that Viagra is viewed as a legitimate medicine, approved by the government and prescribed by doctors.

But as Joann Ellison Rodgers, author of *Drugs and Sexual Behavior*, observes, "there is great unease with the idea of encouraging sexual prowess. . . . At the very least, drugs in the service of sex do seem to subvert or at least trivialize important aspects of sexual experiences, such as love, romance, commitment, trust and health." If we've managed to accept Viagra and (to a lesser extent) alcohol as aphrodisiacs, it may be only because we've projected their darker possibilities onto other substances, of which the "club drugs" are just the latest examples.

Signal of Misunderstanding

The current worries about raves in some ways resemble the fears once symbolized by the opium den. The country's first anti-opium laws, passed by Western states in the late 19th century, were motivated largely by hostility toward the low-cost Chinese laborers who competed for work with native whites. Supporters of such legislation, together with a sensationalist press, popularized the image of the sinister Chinaman who lured white women into his opium den, turning them into concubines, prostitutes, or sex slaves. Although users generally find that opiates dampen their sex drive, "it was commonly reported that opium smoking aroused sexual desire," writes historian David Courtwright, "and that some shameless smokers persuaded 'innocent girls to smoke in order to excite their passions and effect their ruin.'" San Francisco authorities lamented that the police "have found white women and Chinamen side by side under the effects of this drug—a humiliating sight to anyone who has anything left of manhood." In 1910 Hamilton Wright, a U.S. diplomat who was a key player in the passage of federal anti-drug legislation, told Congress that "one of the most unfortunate phases of the habit of smoking opium in this country" was "the large number of women who [had] become involved and were living as common-law wives or cohabiting with Chinese in the Chinatowns of our various cities."

Fears of miscegenation also played a role in popular outrage about cocaine, which was said to make blacks uppity and prone to violence against whites, especially sexual assault. In 1910 Christopher Koch, a member of the Pennsylvania Pharmacy Board who pushed for a federal ban on cocaine, informed Congress that "the colored people seem to have a weakness for it. . . . They would just as leave rape a woman as anything else, and a great many of the southern rape cases have been traced to cocaine." Describing cocaine's effect on "hitherto inoffensive, law abiding negroes" in the *Medical Record*, Edward Huntington Williams warned that "sexual desires are increased and perverted."

Marijuana, another drug that was believed to cause violence, was also linked to sex crimes and, like opium, seduction. Under marijuana's influence, according to a widely cited 1932 report in *The Journal of Criminal Law and Criminology*, "sexual desires are stimulated and may lead to unnatural acts, such as indecent exposure and rape." The authors quoted an informant who "reported several instances of which he claimed to have positive knowledge, where boys had induced girls to use the weed for the purpose of seducing them." The federal Bureau of Narcotics, which collected anecdotes about marijuana's baneful effects to support a national ban on the drug, cited "colored students at the Univ. of Minn. partying with female students (white) smoking [marijuana] and getting their sympathy with stories of racial persecution. Result pregnancy." The bureau also described a case in which "two Negroes took a girl fourteen years old and kept her for two days in a hut under the influence of marijuana. Upon recovery she was found to be suffering from syphilis."

Drug-related horror stories nowadays are rarely so explicitly racist. A notable and surprising exception appears in the 2000 film *Traffic*, which is critical of the war on drugs but nevertheless represents the utter degradation of an upper-middle-class white teenager who gets hooked on crack by showing her having sex with a black man. Whether related to race or not, parental anxieties about sexual activity among teenagers have not gone away, and drugs are a convenient scapegoat when kids seem to be growing up too fast.

The link between drugs and sex was reinforced by the free-love ethos of the '60s counterculture that embraced marijuana and LSD. In the public mind, pot smoking, acid dropping, and promiscuous sex were all part of the same lifestyle; a chaste hippie chick was a contradiction in terms. When Timothy Leary extolled LSD's sex-enhancing qualities in a 1966 interview with *Playboy*, he fueled the fears of parents who worried that their daughters would be seduced into a decadent world of sex, drugs, and rock 'n' roll. The Charles Manson case added a sinister twist to this scenario, raising the possibility of losing one's daughter to an evil cult leader who uses LSD to brainwash his followers, in much the same way as Chinese men were once imagined to enthrall formerly respectable white girls with opium.

The alarm about the sexual repercussions of "club drugs," then, has to be understood in the context of warnings about other alleged aphrodisiacs, often identified with particular groups perceived as inferior, threatening, or both. The fear of uncontrolled sexual impulses, of the chaos that would result if we let our basic instincts run wild, is projected onto these groups and, by extension, their intoxicants. In the case of "club drugs," adolescents are both victims and perpetrators. Parents fear for their children, but they also fear them. When Mayor Daley warned that "they are after all of our children," he may have been imagining predators in the mold of Fu Manchu or Charles Manson. But the reality is that raves—which grew out of the British "acid house" movement, itself reminiscent of the psychedelic dance scene that emerged in San Francisco during the late '60s—are overwhelmingly a youth phenomenon.

The experience of moving all night to a throbbing beat amid flickering light has been likened to tribal dancing around a fire. But for most people over 30, the appeal of dancing for hours on end to the fast, repetitive rhythm of techno music is hard to fathom. "The sensationalist reaction that greets every mention of the word *Ecstasy* in this country is part of a wider, almost unconscious fear of young people," writes Jonathan Keane in the British *New Statesman*, and the observation applies equally to the United States. For "middle-aged and middle-class opinion leaders . . . E is a symbol of a youth culture they don't understand."

This is not to say that no one ever felt horny after taking MDMA. Individual reactions to drugs are highly variable, and one could probably find anecdotes suggesting aphrodisiac properties for almost any psychoactive substance. And it is no doubt true that some MDMA users, like the woman quoted in *Cosmo*, have paired up with sexual partners they found less attractive the morning after. But once MDMA is stripped of its symbolism, these issues are no different from those raised by alcohol. In fact, since MDMA users tend to be more lucid than drinkers, the chances that they will do something regrettable are probably lower.

I Love You Guys

Another alcohol-related hazard, one that seems to be more characteristic of MDMA than the risk of casual sex or rape, is the possibility of inappropriate emotional intimacy. The maudlin drunk who proclaims his affection for everyone and reveals secrets he might later wish he had kept is a widely recognized character, either comical or pathetic depending upon one's point of view. Given MDMA's reputation as a "love drug," it's natural to wonder whether it fosters the same sort of embarrassing behavior.

Tom Cowan, a systems analyst in his 30s, has used MDMA a few times, and he doesn't think it revealed any deep emotional truths. (All names of drug users in this story are pseudonyms.) "For me," he says, "it was almost too much of a fake. . . . It was too artificial for me. . . . I felt warm. I felt loved. All of those sensations came upon me. . . . I had all these feelings, but I knew that deep down I didn't feel that, so at the same time there was that inner struggle as far as just letting loose and just being. . . . That was difficult because of the fakeness about it for me." More typically, MDMA users perceive the warm feelings as real, both at the time and in retrospect. Some emphasize an enhanced connection to friends, while others report a feeling of benevolence toward people in general.

"I was very alert but very relaxed at the same time," says Alison Witt, a software engineer in her 20s. "I didn't love everybody. . . . It's a very social drug, and you do feel connected to other people, but I think it's more because it creates a sense of relaxation and pleasure with people you're familiar with." Walter Stevenson, a neuroscientist in his late 20s, gives a similar account: "I felt really happy to have my friends around me. I just enjoyed sitting there and spending time with them, not necessarily talking about anything, but not to the degree that I felt particularly attracted or warm to people I didn't know. I was very friendly and open to meeting people, but there wasn't anything inappropriate about the feeling."

Adam Newman, an Internet specialist in his 20s, believes his MDMA use has helped improve his social life. "It kind of catapulted me past a bunch of shyness and other mental and emotional blocks," he says. Even when he wasn't using MDMA, "I felt a lot better than I had in social interactions before." Bruce Rogers, a horticulturist in his 40s, says one thing he likes about MDMA is that "you can find something good in somebody that you dislike." He thinks "it would make the world a better place if everybody did it just once."

That's the kind of assertion, reminiscent of claims about LSD's earthshaking potential, that tends to elicit skeptical smiles. But the important point is that many MDMA users believe the drug has lasting psychological benefits, even when it's taken in a recreational context—the sort of thing you don't often hear about alcohol.

Not surprisingly, people who use MDMA in clubs and at raves emphasize its sensual and stimulant properties, the way it enhances music and dancing. But they also talk about a sense of connectedness, especially at raves. Jasmine Menendez, a public relations director in her early 20s who has used MDMA both at raves and with small groups of friends, says it provides "a great body high. I lose all sense of inhibition and my full potential is released. . . . It allows me to get closer to people and to myself."

Too Much Fun

Euphoria is a commonly reported effect of MDMA, which raises the usual concerns about the lure of artificial pleasure. "It was an incredible feeling of being tremendously happy where I was and being content in a basic way," Stevenson recalls of the first time he felt MDMA's effects. He used it several more times after that, but it never became a regular habit.

Menendez, on the other hand, found MDMA "easy to become addicted to" because "you see the full potential in yourself and others; you feel like you won the lottery." She began chasing that feeling one weekend after another, often taking several pills in one night. "Doing e as much as I did affected my relationship with my mother," she says. "I would come home cracked out from a night of partying and sleep the whole day. She couldn't invite anyone over because I was always sleeping. She said that my party habits were out of control. We fought constantly. I would also go to work high from the party, if I had to work weekends. The comedown was horrible because I wanted to sleep and instead I had to be running around doing errands."

Menendez decided to cut back on her MDMA consumption, and recently she has been using it only on special occasions. "I think I've outgrown it finally," she says. "I used e to do some serious soul-searching and to come out of my shell, learning all I could about who I really am. I'm grateful that I had the experiences that I did and wouldn't change it for the world. But now, being 23, I'm ready to embrace mental clarity fully. Ecstasy is definitely a constructive tool and if used correctly can benefit the user. It changed my life for the better, and because of what I learned about myself, I'm ready to start a new life without it."

Sustained heavy use of MDMA is rare, partly because it's impractical. MDMA works mainly by stimulating the release of the neurotransmitter serotonin. Taking it depletes the brain's supply, which may not return to normal levels for a week or more. Some users report a hangover period of melancholy and woolly-headedness that can last a few days. As frequency of use increases, MDMA's euphoric and empathetic effects diminish and its unpleasant side effects, including jitteriness and hangovers, intensify. Like LSD, it has a self-limiting quality, which is reflected in patterns of use. In a 2000 survey, 8.2 percent of high school seniors reported trying MDMA in the previous year. Less than half of them (3.6 percent) had used it in the previous month, and virtually none reported "daily" use (defined as use on 20 or more occasions in the previous 30 days). To parents, of course, any use of MDMA is alarming, and the share of seniors who said they'd ever tried the drug nearly doubled between 1996 and 2000, when it reached 11 percent.

Parental fears have been stoked by reports of sudden fatalities among MDMA users. Given the millions of doses consumed each year, such cases are remarkably rare: The Drug Abuse Warning Network counted nine MDMA-related deaths in 1998. The most common cause of death is dehydration and overheating. MDMA impairs body temperature regulation and accelerates fluid loss, which can be especially dangerous for people dancing vigorously in crowded, poorly ventilated spaces for hours at a time. The solution to this problem, well-known to experienced ravers, is pretty straightforward: avoid clubs and parties where conditions are stifling, take frequent rests, abstain from alcohol (which compounds dehydration), and drink plenty of water. MDMA also interacts dangerously with some prescription drugs (including monoamine oxidase inhibitors, a class of antidepressants), and it raises heart rate and blood pressure, of special concern for people with cardiovascular conditions.

Another hazard is a product of the black market created by prohibition: Tablets or capsules sold as Ecstasy may in fact contain other, possibly more dangerous drugs. In tests by private U.S. laboratories, more than one-third of "Ecstasy" pills turned out to be bogus. (The samples were not necessarily representative, and the results may be on the high side, since the drugs were submitted voluntarily for testing, perhaps by buyers who had reason to be suspicious.) Most of the MDMA substitutes, which included caffeine, ephedrine, and aspirin, were relatively harmless, but one of them, the cough suppressant dextromethorphan (DXM), has disturbing psychoactive effects in high doses, impedes the metabolism of MDMA, and blocks perspiration, raising the risk of overheating. Another drug that has been passed off as MDMA is paramethoxyamphetamine (PMA), which is potentially lethal in doses over 50 milligrams, especially when combined with other drugs. In 2000 the DEA reported 10 deaths tied to PMA. Wary Ecstasy users can buy test kits or have pills analyzed by organizations such as DanceSafe, which sets up booths at raves and nightclubs.

Nervous Breakdown

Generally speaking, a careful user can avoid the short-term dangers of MDMA. Of more concern is the possibility of long-term brain damage. In animal studies, high or repeated doses of MDMA cause degeneration of serotonin nerve receptors, and some of the changes appear to be permanent. The relevance of these studies to human use of MDMA is unclear because we don't know whether the same changes occur in people or, if they do, at what doses and with what practical consequences. Studies of human users, which often have serious methodological shortcomings, so far have been inconclusive.

Still, the possibility of lasting damage to memory should not be lightly dismissed. There's enough reason for concern that MDMA should no longer be treated as casually as "a low-calorie martini." If the fears of neurotoxicity prove to be well-founded and a safe dose cannot be estimated with any confidence, a prudent person would need a good reason—probably better than a fun night out—to take the risk. On the other hand, the animal research suggests that it may be possible to avoid neural damage by preventing hyperthermia or by taking certain drugs (for example, Prozac) in conjunction with MDMA. In that case, such precautions would be a requirement of responsible use.

However the debate about MDMA's long-term effects turns out, we should be wary of claims that it (or any drug) makes people "engage in random sex acts." Like the idea that certain intoxicants make people lazy, crazy, or violent, it vastly oversimplifies a complex interaction between the drug, the user, and the context. As MDMA's versatility demonstrates, the same drug can be different things to different people. Michael Buchanan, a retired professor in his early 70s, has used MDMA several times with one or two other people. "It's just wonderful," he says, "to bring closeness, intimacy—not erotic intimacy at all, but a kind of spiritual intimacy, a loving relationship, an openness to dialogue that nothing else can quite match." When I mention MDMA use at raves, he says, "I don't understand how the kids can use it that way."

POSTSCRIPT

Should We Be Concerned About "Club Drugs"?

There is little argument that mind-altering drugs can cause physical and emotional havoc for the user. On drugs, people might become less inhibited and engage in behaviors they would not typically exhibit. However, if one attends a rave party, is one more likely to use drugs? Are individuals who go to raves the types of people who would use drugs regardless? If going to raves increases the likelihood of drug use, is that a valid argument for making raves illegal?

Sigel contends that club drugs are readily available at rave parties. Furthermore, the clandestine nature of rave parties offers some degree of obscurity from law enforcement officials. Earmarking raves as places where drugs may be used might increase the probability that drug use will occur. One might think that it is appropriate, perhaps expected, to engage in drug use at a rave party.

Sullum argues that history shows that bringing attention to certain drugs results in their increased use. Young people would not know to alter their consciousness with certain drugs unless they were alerted to their effects. However, if young people participate in an activity that is potentially harmful to them, one could argue that it is the government's responsibility to step in. At what point is too much information counterproductive? How should we balance the right to know about certain drugs with the publicity generated by informing the public about these drugs?

There are many interesting questions associated with the issue of whether or not we should be concerned about club drugs. For example, when is a drug a club drug? Can people just get together to enjoy music and to socialize without being looked upon suspiciously? If a club brings in a musical group that plays techno music, does the club become a front for a rave? If patrons at a club use illegal drugs, is that the responsibility of the club owner or manager?

There are a number of articles that look at the issue of club drugs and rave parties. One good article is "As Raves Go Uptown, Cities Take Aim at Drugs, Noise," by Donna Leinwand, *USA Today* (November 12, 2002). Other informative articles are "Ecstasy and Its Agony," by Peter Jensen, *The Baltimore Sun* (January 28, 2001); "The Lure of Ecstasy," by John Cloud, *Time* (June 5, 2000); and "Ecstasy Use Among Club Rave Attendees," by Amelia Arria et al., *Archives of Pediatrics and Adolescent Medicine* (March 2002). One group that sponsors research into the therapeutic benefits of Ecstasy and other drugs is the Multidisciplinary Association for Psychedelic Studies (MAPS), located online at http://www.maps.org.

ISSUE 5

Should Pregnant Drug Users Be Prosecuted?

YES: Paul A. Logli, from "Drugs in the Womb: The Newest Battlefield in the War on Drugs," *Criminal Justice Ethics* (Winter/Spring 1990)

NO: Drew Humphries, from *Crack Mothers: Pregnancy, Drugs, and the Media* (Ohio State University Press, 1999)

ISSUE SUMMARY

YES: Paul A. Logli, an Illinois prosecuting attorney, argues that it is the government's duty to enforce every child's right to begin life with a healthy, drug-free mind and body. Logli maintains that pregnant women who use drugs should be prosecuted because they may harm the life of their unborn children. He feels it is the state's responsibility to ensure that every baby is born as healthy as possible.

NO: Researcher Drew Humphries argues that the prosecution of women who use drugs while pregnant has resulted from overzealous efforts on the part of a handful of state prosecutors. Humphries asserts that the prosecution of pregnant drug users is unfair because poor women are more likely to be the targets of such prosecution and that these cases do not hold up to legal standards.

The effects that drugs have on a fetus can be mild and temporary or severe and permanent, depending on the extent of drug use by the mother, the type of substance used, and the stage of fetal development at the time the drug crosses the placental barrier and enters the bloodstream of the fetus. Both illegal and legal drugs, such as cocaine, crack, marijuana, alcohol, and nicotine, are increasingly found to be responsible for incidents of premature births, congenital abnormalities, fetal alcohol syndrome, mental retardation, and other serious birth defects. The exposure of the fetus to these substances and the long-term involuntary physical, intellectual, and emotional effects are disturbing. In addition, the medical, social, and economic costs to treat and care for babies who are exposed to or become addicted to drugs while in utero (in the uterus) warrant serious concern.

An important consideration regarding the prosecution of pregnant drug users is whether this is a legal problem or a medical problem. In recent years, attempts have been made to establish laws that would allow the incarceration of drug-using pregnant women on the basis of "fetal abuse." Some cases have been successfully prosecuted: mothers have been denied custody of their infants until they enter appropriate treatment programs, and criminal charges have been brought against mothers whose children were born with drug-related complications. The underlying presumption is that the unborn fetus should be afforded protection against the harmful actions of another person, specifically the use of harmful drugs by the mother.

Those who profess that prosecuting pregnant women who use drugs is necessary insist that the health and welfare of the unborn child is the highest priority. They contend that the possibility that these women will avoid obtaining health care for themselves or their babies because they fear punishment does not absolve the state from the responsibility of protecting the babies. They also argue that criminalizing these acts is imperative to protect fetuses and newborns that cannot protect themselves. It is the duty of the legal system to deter pregnant women from engaging in future criminal drug use and to protect the best interests of infants.

Others maintain that drug use and dependency by pregnant women is a medical problem, not a criminal one. Many pregnant women seek treatment, but they often find that rehabilitation programs are limited or unavailable. Shortages of openings in chemical dependency programs may keep a prospective client waiting for months, during which time she will most likely continue to use the drugs to which she is addicted and prolong her fetus's drug exposure. Many low-income women do not receive drug treatment and adequate prenatal care due to financial constraints. Women who fear criminal prosecution because of their drug use might simply avoid prenatal care altogether.

Some suggest that medical intervention, drug prevention, and education—not prosecution—are needed for pregnant drug users. Prosecution, they contend, drives women who need medical attention away from the very help they and their babies need. Others respond that prosecuting pregnant women who use drugs will help identify those who need attention, at which point adequate medical and social welfare services can be provided to treat and protect the mother and child.

In the following selections, Paul A. Logli, arguing for the prosecution of pregnant drug users, contends that it is the state's responsibility to protect the unborn and the newborn because they are least able to protect themselves. He charges that it is the prosecutor's responsibility to deter future criminal drug use by mothers who he feels violate the rights of their potential newborns to have an opportunity for a healthy and normal life. Drew Humphries contends that many of the pregnant women who are prosecuted are minorities and that there is therefore a racist element to such prosecution. She asserts that prosecuting pregnant drug users may be counterproductive to improving the quality of infant and maternal health. The threat of arrest and incarceration may decrease the likelihood that pregnant drug users will seek out adequate prenatal care.

Paul A. Logli

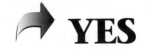 **YES**

Drugs in the Womb: The Newest Battlefield in the War on Drugs

Introduction

The reported incidence of drug-related births has risen dramatically over the last several years. The legal system and, in particular, local prosecutors have attempted to properly respond to the suffering, death, and economic costs which result from a pregnant woman's use of drugs. The ensuing debate has raised serious constitutional and practical issues which are far from resolution.

Prosecutors have achieved mixed results in using current criminal and juvenile statutes as a basis for legal action intended to prosecute mothers and protect children. As a result, state and federal legislators have begun the difficult task of drafting appropriate laws to deal with the problem, while at the same time acknowledging the concerns of medical authorities, child protection groups, and advocates for individual rights.

The Problem

The plight of "cocaine babies," children addicted at birth to narcotic substances or otherwise affected by maternal drug use during pregnancy, has prompted prosecutors in some jurisdictions to bring criminal charges against drug-abusing mothers. Not only have these prosecutions generated heated debates both inside and outside of the nation's courtrooms, but they have also expanded the war on drugs to a controversial new battlefield—the mother's womb.

A 1988 survey of hospitals conducted by Dr. Ira Chasnoff, Associate Professor of Northwestern University Medical School and President of the National Association for Perinatal Addiction Research and Education (NAPARE) indicated that as many as 375,000 infants may be affected by maternal cocaine use during pregnancy each year. Chasnoff's survey included 36 hospitals across the country and showed incidence rates ranging from 1 percent to 27 percent. It also indicated that the problem was not restricted to urban populations or particular racial or socio-economic groups. More recently a study at Hutzel Hospital in Detroit's inner city found that 42.7 percent of its newborn babies were exposed to drugs while in their mothers' wombs.

From Paul A. Logli, "Drugs in the Womb: The Newest Battlefield in the War on Drugs," *Criminal Justice Ethics*, vol. 9, no. 1 (Winter/Spring 1990), pp. 23–29. Copyright © 1990 by *Criminal Justice Ethics*. Reprinted by permission of The Institute for Criminal Justice Ethics, 555 West 57th Street, Suite 601, New York, NY

The effects of maternal use of cocaine and other drugs during pregnancy on the mother and her newborn child have by now been well-documented and will not be repeated here. The effects are severe and can cause numerous threats to the short-term health of the child. In a few cases it can even result in death.

Medical authorities have just begun to evaluate the long-term effects of cocaine exposure on children as they grow older. Early findings show that many of these infants show serious difficulties in relating and reacting to adults and environments, as well as in organizing creative play, and they appear similar to mildly autistic or personality-disordered children.

The human costs related to the pain, suffering, and deaths resulting from maternal cocaine use during pregnancy are simply incalculable. In economic terms, the typical intensive-care costs for treating babies exposed to drugs range from $7,500 to $31,000. In some cases medical bills go as high as $150,000.

The costs grow enormously as more and more hospitals encounter the problem of "boarder babies"—those children literally abandoned at the hospital by an addicted mother, and left to be cared for by the nursing staff. Future costs to society for simply educating a generation of drug-affected children can only be the object of speculation. It is clear, however, that besides pain, suffering, and death the economic costs to society of drug use by pregnant women is presently enormous and is certainly growing larger.

The Prosecutor's Response

It is against this backdrop and fueled by the evergrowing emphasis on an aggressively waged war on drugs that prosecutors have begun a number of actions against women who have given birth to drug-affected children. A review of at least two cases will illustrate the potential success or failure of attempts to use existing statutes.

People v. Melanie Green   On February 4, 1989, at a Rockford, Illinois hospital, two-day-old Bianca Green lost her brief struggle for life. At the time of Bianca's birth both she and her mother, twenty-four-year-old Melanie Green, tested positive for the presence of cocaine in their systems.

Pathologists in Rockford and Madison, Wisconsin, indicated that the death of the baby was the result of a prenatal injury related to cocaine used by the mother during the pregnancy. They asserted that maternal cocaine use had caused the placenta to prematurely rupture, which deprived the fetus of oxygen before and during delivery. As a result of oxygen deprivation, the child's brain began to swell and she eventually died.

After an investigation by the Rockford Police Department and the State of Illinois Department of Children and Family Services, prosecutors allowed a criminal complaint to be filed on May 9, 1989, charging Melanie Green with the offenses of Involuntary Manslaughter and Delivery of a Controlled Substance.

On May 25, 1989, testimony was presented to the Winnebago County Grand Jury by prosecutors seeking a formal indictment. The Grand Jury, however, declined to indict Green on either charge. Since Grand Jury proceedings in the State of Illinois are secret, as are the jurors' deliberations and votes, the reason for the decision of the Grand Jury in this case is determined more by conjecture than any direct knowledge. Prosecutors involved in the presentation observed that the jurors exhibited a certain amount of sympathy for the young woman who had been brought before the Grand Jury at the jurors' request. It is also likely that the jurors were uncomfortable with the use of statutes that were not intended to be used in these circumstances.

It would also be difficult to disregard the fact that, after the criminal complaints were announced on May 9th and prior to the Grand Jury deliberations of May 25th, a national debate had ensued revolving around the charges brought in Rockford, Illinois, and their implications for the ever-increasing problem of women who use drugs during pregnancy.

People v. Jennifer Clarise Johnson   On July 13, 1989, a Seminole County, Florida judge found Jennifer Johnson guilty of delivery of a controlled substance to a child. The judge found that delivery, for purposes of the statute, occurred through the umbilical cord after the birth of the child and before the cord was severed. Jeff Deen, the Assistant State's Attorney who prosecuted the case, has since pointed out that Johnson, age 23, had previously given birth to three other cocaine-affected babies, and in this case was arrested at a crack house. "We needed to make sure this woman does not give birth to another cocaine baby."

Johnson was sentenced to fifteen years of probation including strict supervision, drug treatment, random drug testing, educational and vocational training, and an intensive prenatal care program if she ever became pregnant again.

Support for the Prosecution of Maternal Drug Abuse

Both cases reported above relied on a single important fact as a basis for the prosecution of the drug-abusing mother: that the child was born alive and exhibited the consequences of prenatal injury.

In the Melanie Green case, Illinois prosecutors relied on the "born alive" rule set out earlier in *People v. Bolar.* In *Bolar* the defendant was convicted of the offense of reckless homicide. The case involved an accident between a car driven by the defendant, who was found to be drunk, and another automobile containing a pregnant woman. As a result, the woman delivered her baby by emergency caesarean section within hours of the collision. Although the newborn child exhibited only a few heart beats and lived for approximately two minutes, the court found that the child was born alive and was therefore a person for purposes of the criminal statutes of the State of Illinois.

The Florida prosecution relied on a live birth in an entirely different fashion. The prosecutor argued in that case that the delivery of the controlled substance occurred after the live birth via the umbilical cord and prior to the cutting of the cord. Thus, it was argued, that the delivery of the controlled substance occurred not to a fetus but to a person who enjoyed the protection of the criminal code of the State of Florida.

Further support for the State's role in protecting the health of newborns even against prenatal injury is found in the statutes which provide protection for the fetus. These statutes proscribe actions by a person, usually other than the mother, which either intentionally or recklessly harm or kill a fetus. In other words, even in the absence of a live birth, most states afford protection to the unborn fetus against the harmful actions of another person. Arguably, the same protection should be afforded the infant against intentional harmful actions by a drug-abusing mother.

The state also receives support for a position in favor of the protection of the health of a newborn from a number of non-criminal cases. A line of civil cases in several states would appear to stand for the principle that a child has a right to begin life with a sound mind and body, and a person who interferes with that right may be subject to civil liability. In two cases decided within months of each other, the Supreme Court of Michigan upheld two actions for recovery of damages that were caused by the infliction of prenatal injury. In *Womack v. Buckhorn* the court upheld an action on behalf of an eight-year-old surviving child for prenatal brain injuries apparently suffered during the fourth month of the pregnancy in an automobile accident. The court adopted with approval the reasoning of a New Jersey Supreme Court decision and "recognized that a child has a legal right to begin life with a sound mind and body." Similarly, in *O'Neill v. Morse* the court found that a cause of action was allowed for prenatal injuries that caused the death of an eight-month-old viable fetus.

Illinois courts have allowed civil recovery on behalf of an infant for a negligently administered blood transfusion given to the mother prior to conception which resulted in damage to the child at birth. However, the same Illinois court would not extend a similar cause of action for prebirth injuries as between a child and its own mother. The court, however, went on to say that a right to such a cause of action could be statutorily enacted by the Legislature.

Additional support for the state's role in protecting the health of newborns is found in the principles annunciated in recent decisions of the United States Supreme Court. The often cited case of *Roe v. Wade* set out that although a woman's right of privacy is broad enough to cover the abortion decision, the right is not absolute and is subject to limitations, "and that at some point the state's interest as to protection of health, medical standards and prenatal life, becomes dominant."

More recently, in the case of *Webster v. Reproductive Health Services,* the court expanded the state's interest in protecting potential human life by setting aside viability as a rigid line that had previously allowed state regulation only after viability had been shown but prohibited it before viability. The court goes on to say that the "fundamental right" to abortion as described in *Roe* is now accorded the lesser status of a "liberty interest." Such language surely supports a prosecutor's argument that the state's compelling interest in potential human life would allow the criminalization of acts which if committed by a pregnant woman can damage not just a viable fetus but eventually a born-alive infant. It follows that, once a pregnant woman has abandoned her right to abort and has decided to carry the fetus to term, society can well impose a duty on the mother to insure that the fetus is born as healthy as possible.

A further argument in support of the state's interest in prosecuting women who engage in conduct which is damaging to the health of a newborn child is especially compelling in regard to maternal drug use during pregnancy. Simply put, there is no fundamental right or even a liberty interest in the use of psycho-active drugs. A perceived right of privacy has never formed an absolute barrier against state prosecutions of those who use or possess narcotics. Certainly no exception can be made simply because the person using drugs happens to be pregnant.

Critics of the prosecutor's role argue that any statute that would punish mothers who create a substantial risk of harm to their fetus will run afoul of constitutional requirements, including prohibitions on vagueness, guarantees of liberty and privacy, and rights of due process and equal protection. . . .

In spite of such criticism, the state's role in protecting those citizens who are least able to protect themselves, namely the newborn, mandates an aggressive posture. Much of the criticism of prosecutorial efforts is based on speculation as to the consequences of prosecution and ignores the basic tenet of criminal law that prosecutions deter the prosecuted and others from committing additional crimes. To assume that it will only drive persons further underground is to somehow argue that certain prosecutions of crime will only force perpetrators to make even more aggressive efforts to escape apprehension, thus making arrest and prosecution unadvisable. Neither could this be accepted as an argument justifying even the weakening of criminal sanctions. . . .

The concern that pregnant addicts will avoid obtaining health care for themselves or their infants because of the fear of prosecution cannot justify the absence of state action to protect the newborn. If the state were to accept such reasoning, then existing child abuse laws would have to be reconsidered since they might deter parents from obtaining medical care for physically or sexually abused children. That argument has not been accepted as a valid reason for abolishing child abuse laws or for not prosecuting child abusers. . . .

The far better policy is for the state to acknowledge its responsibility not only to provide a deterrant to criminal and destructive behavior by pregnant addicts but also to provide adequate opportunities for those who might seek help to discontinue their addiction. Prosecution has a role in its ability to deter future criminal behavior and to protect the best interests of the child. The medical and social welfare establishment must assume an even greater responsibility to encourage legislators to provide adequate funding and facilities so that no pregnant woman who is addicted to drugs will be denied the opportunity to seek appropriate prenatal care and treatment for her addiction.

One State's Response

The Legislature of the State of Illinois at the urging of local prosecutors moved quickly to amend its juvenile court act in order to provide protection to those children born drug-affected. Previously, Illinois law provided that a court could assume jurisdiction over addicted minors or a minor who is generally declared neglected or abused.

Effective January 1, 1990, the juvenile court act was amended to expand the definition of a neglected or abused minor. . . .

> those who are neglected include . . . any newborn infant whose blood or urine contains any amount of a controlled substance. . . .

The purpose of the new statute is to make it easier for the court to assert jurisdiction over a newborn infant born drug-affected. The state is not required to show either the addiction of the child or harmful effects on the child in order to remove the child from a drug-abusing mother. Used in this context, prosecutors can work with the mother in a rather coercive atmosphere to encourage her to enter into drug rehabilitation and, upon the successful completion of the program, be reunited with her child.

Additional legislation before the Illinois Legislature is House Bill 2835 sponsored by Representatives John Hallock (R-Rockford) and Edolo "Zeke" Giorgi (D-Rockford). This bill represents the first attempt to specifically address the prosecution of drug-abusing pregnant women. . . .

The statute provides for a class 4 felony disposition upon conviction. A class 4 felony is a probationable felony which can also result in a term of imprisonment from one to three years.

Subsequent paragraphs set out certain defenses available to the accused.

> It shall not be a violation of this section if a woman knowingly or intentionally uses a narcotic or dangerous drug in the first twelve weeks of pregnancy and: 1. She has no knowledge that she is pregnant; or 2. Subsequently, within the first twelve weeks of pregnancy, undergoes medical treatment for substance abuse or treatment or rehabilitation in a program or facility approved by the Illinois Department of Alcoholism and Substance Abuse, and thereafter discontinues any further use of drugs or narcotics as previously set forth.

. . . A woman, under this statute, could not be prosecuted for self-reporting her addiction in the early stages of the pregnancy. Nor could she be prosecuted under this statute if, even during the subsequent stages of the pregnancy, she discontinued her drug use to the extent that no drugs were present in her system or the baby's system at the time of birth. The statute, as drafted, is clearly intended to allow prosecutors to invoke the criminal statutes in the most serious of cases.

Conclusion

Local prosecutors have a legitimate role in responding to the increasing problem of drug-abusing pregnant women and their drug-affected children. Eliminating the pain, suffering and death resulting from drug exposure in newborns must be a prosecutor's priority. However, the use of existing statutes to address the problem may meet with limited success since they are burdened with numerous constitutional problems dealing with original intent, notice, vagueness, and due process.

The juvenile courts may offer perhaps the best initial response in working to protect the interests of a surviving child. However, in order to address more serious cases, legislative efforts may be required to provide new statutes that will specifically address the problem and hopefully deter future criminal conduct which deprives children of their important right to a healthy and normal birth.

The long-term solution does not rest with the prosecutor alone. Society, including the medical and social welfare establishment, must be more responsive in providing readily accessible prenatal care and treatment alternatives for pregnant addicts. In the short term however, prosecutors must be prepared to play a vital role in protecting children and deterring women from engaging in conduct which will harm the newborn child. If prosecutors fail to respond, then they are simply closing the doors of the criminal justice system to those persons, the newborn, who are least able to open the doors for themselves.

NO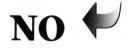

Drew Humphries

The Point of Moral Panic

In any moral panic the decisive moment arrives when moral entrepreneurs—experts, spokespeople, officials—determine that disapproved conduct exceeds the boundaries of permissible behavior. In this case, too many cocaine mothers had harmed their babies, or a few cocaine mothers had inflicted too great a harm on their babies. However overstated such claims might be, the point is that moral entrepreneurs came to believe that existing systems of social control no longer sufficed. Pregnant drug users were perceived as ignoring medical warnings, physician advice, and referrals to drug treatment or prenatal care. Termination of parental rights, a sanction available through social services, was not seen as a severe enough penalty to force drug users to halt maternal cocaine use. Firmer action was required.

Reacting to these perceptions, a handful of county prosecutors took the step that triggered the panic: treating cocaine mothers as criminals. Across the nation prosecutors brought over 160 criminal cases against women who used crack or cocaine during pregnancy. Although most cases were dismissed or overturned on appeal, the county prosecutors profiled in this [selection] pursued the high-publicity cases that defined the issues and turned the crack mothers episode into a classic case of moral panic.

Consider what the prosecutions were not. They did not arise in America's big cities, nor did they necessarily reflect local epidemics of crack babies. The communities that generated them were like many other small- and medium-sized towns and cities. They ran the gamut from wealthy suburb to worn-out industrial center. They were overwhelmingly white; minority populations did not exceed the national average. So, many of the explanations developing from the symbolic implications of the prosecutions are ill suited to actual circumstances. The prosecutions did not arise in communities where affluent white groups felt threatened by unemployment, poverty, or minorities.

The prosecutions were localized responses to national priorities. Crack was the drug targeted by federal authorities. Any politically astute, ambitious, or ideologically inclined prosecutor understood that crack was also the target drug at the local level. At this level crack was a powerful symbol. It epitomized all the ills associated with America's urban centers. County prosecutors—white professionals occupying positions of power and privilege in small cities and medium-sized towns—labored to keep crack and big cities' problems out. As the suburbs turned against the big cities, prosecutors turned against cocaine mothers. The highly publicized cases that resulted galvanized hostility, directing it against some of the most vulnerable women in America.

It can be said that county prosecutors brought the cases in part because they could. Prosecutors have far-reaching latitude in how they conduct the business of prosecution (Jacoby, 1979): County prosecutors decide whether to prosecute a case. They make decisions that affect who is prosecuted, the charges that are to be filed, and the kinds of plea bargains that are struck. They decide which cases are to be pursued more aggressively than others. In this [selection], we will see how reports of crack mothers reached prosecutors, and we will examine some of the factors that influenced the decision to prosecute in the first place, to charge at the high end of the penalty spectrum, and to prosecute aggressively. The kind of power held over defendants, even before a judge gets involved, reflects the unparalleled role prosecutors play in the criminal justice system.

Across the country most prosecutors declined to prosecute women who had used drugs during pregnancy. States like Florida and California limited or declined to authorize criminal prosecution in cases of cocaine-exposed infants under the child abuse and neglect laws (Spitzer, 1987; Gomez, 1997). Alternatives existed. The statutes on possession and distribution of drugs applied to women, pregnant or not. Child protective services investigated cocaine-exposed newborns and, where warranted, brought abusive or negligent parents into family or juvenile court to terminate parental rights. And the federal Ad Hoc Drug Policy Group had by 1991 recommended prevention and treatment for the mothers as well as shifts in the mission of child welfare services to cope with maternal drug use and drug-exposed children. The group's recommendations reflected a broader, but less visible, consensus about the efficacy of services over prosecution (U.S. Department of Health and Human Services, 1992).

Legal precedents made it unlikely that any attempt to criminally prosecute cocaine mothers would be successful. A fetus is not, legally speaking, a person. The state may act to protect fetal life, and often it imposes criminal sanctions for intentionally harming a fetus—but typically only someone else's fetus. In *Roe v. Wade* (1973) and later in *Webster v. Reproductive Health Services* (1989), the Supreme Court left no doubt that the state's interest in protecting fetal life is outweighed by a woman's interest in controlling her own reproductive life. Thus, a woman's fetus may be protected from other people, but not really from herself.

The fetal-rights advocates have never accepted this, asking, if a third party can be punished for harming a fetus, why can't the mother be punished, too? For years they have pushed at the limits of *Roe v. Wade* (1973), trying to read much into the "important and legitimate interest" the Supreme Court Justices said the state may have in a first- or second-trimester fetus. Knowing a declaration that legal life begins at conception is beyond them, right-to-life jurists have tried to work around the edges, using related issues like maternal drug use to advance their cause.

In no state was there a criminal statute in place applying to the specific circumstances of cocaine-exposed newborns. This meant that prosecutors drew from the statutes available, stretching the meaning of their provisions beyond the legislature's original intentions (Maschke, 1995). A 1986 case in San Diego shows the lengths to which prosecutors went in finding applicable statutes (Moss, 1988). Pamela Rae Stewart was charged with child abuse for failing to provide "medical attendance" for her unborn child. Stewart had disregarded doctor's instructions to avoid cocaine and other illicit drugs and to avoid sexual intercourse. And she delayed getting help when she started to hemorrhage. When she reached the hospital, the infant she delivered tested positive for cocaine, and it died of brain damage. The statute used to charge Stewart had been designed to force fathers to provide for the women they had impregnated. It had been amended, however, to require mothers to support their children as well. The prosecutors seized on this later provision to charge Stewart, but because the legislature had not intended it to penalize conduct during pregnancy, the case was dismissed.

A few years later, riding a wave of anti-drug hysteria, county prosecutors in a handful of other states acted. Karen Maschke suggests that these prosecutors had a "conviction psychology" (1995). Some had prosecuted child abuse cases; others were strong advocates of victims' rights. They all believed that babies had a right to be born free of defect—a variant of the defeated fetal-rights argument. They all believed that the mothers should be held responsible.

But the county prosecutors who tried the cocaine mother cases shared other things as well. As elected officials, they identified voters as their primary constituency (Jacoby, 1979), and their need to remain visible led them to make politically popular decisions. The early Stewart case had set off a national controversy without settling the issues; other statutes remained to be tested. Publicity earned by prosecuting a high-profile case had carryover value in winning higher office or attracting the attention of national decision makers. Indeed, their need to remain visible led prosecutors to legally questionable decisions. Paul Logli, the state's attorney from Rockford, Illinois, said the plight of cocaine-exposed babies was so severe in Winnebago County that one could do no less than to exploit all avenues of the law. Other prosecutors were every bit as adamant and inventive. Using manslaughter, drug-trafficking, and child-abuse statutes, they applied existing laws to a situation never envisaged by the legislature: a mother and her cocaine-exposed newborn.

Irrespective of how individual prosecutors justified their action, the decision to prosecute reflects the isolation of public prosecutors as a group of privileged white professionals. Dwight Greene, who wrote about Tony Tague, the Michigan county prosecutor discussed below, calls this isolation "pluralistic ignorance" (Greene, 1991). Tague made his decisions about the case, said Greene, on the basis of "false knowledge"—misconceptions about women, race, and poverty that he shared with other attorneys. It's hard to know whether any of the prosecutors reviewed in this chapter saw the women they prosecuted as real people; they apparently saw them as symbolic targets in a battle to save children. What they did not see or would not admit were the increasing depth of urban poverty, the desperation of the people burdened by it, and the impact of crack on the lives of people, especially of young women. Prosecutors instead saw women who had refused to help themselves, who had used up all their chances, and who required the full impact of the criminal sanction to get them to carry out their duties as mothers.

Here, then, are the highly publicized cases that signaled the moral panic. The defendants were for the most part poor, single mothers who had succumbed to crack because it defined the social worlds in which they lived. Two defendants were white. The case against Lynn Bremer, a white attorney, helped county prosecutor Tony Tague fend off accusations of racism for having charged Kimberly Hardy, a black single mother whose baby tested positive for cocaine. Josephine Pelligrini, the other white defendant, came from a middle-class family in Brockton, Massachusetts, but the father of her infant was black. The remaining defendants were poor, black, single mothers: Melanie Green in Illinois, Jennifer Johnson in Florida, and Kimberly Hardy in Michigan. Several additional cases grew out of a program in Charleston, South Carolina; defendants in these cases were almost all black, too. Charges filed against these women included involuntary manslaughter, delivery of a controlled substance to a minor, and child abuse or neglect. The cases were filed in Illinois, Florida, Michigan, Massachusetts, and South Carolina. Paul Logli, state's attorney for Winnebago County; Jeffrey Deen, assistant state attorney in Seminole County; Anthony Tague, county attorney for Muskegon County; William O'Malley, district attorney in Plymouth County; and Charles M. Condon, ninth circuit solicitor in Charleston prosecuted the cases.

Melanie Green and Involuntary Manslaughter

Melanie Green, 24, was the first cocaine mother in the country to be charged with manslaughter in the death of her baby. She was as unlikely as any other poor, single mother to find herself at the center of a national debate about women's rights and drug abuse. Raised in a large working-class black family in Rockford, Illinois, she had dropped out of high school before drifting into drug use. When she was 17, she pleaded guilty to shoplifting charges; later she attributed her problems to having got involved with the wrong people. She gave birth to her son, Damen, in 1983.

Green was pregnant with her second child in September of 1988. Back in Illinois from an extended stay in Iowa, she was on welfare and had sought help for a drug problem, but the waiting list was too long, so she tried on her own to cut back. Six months later, Green gave birth to a daughter, Bianca, and both tested positive for cocaine. Bianca was underweight, had suffered brain damage, and she died within days of her birth. Later Melanie described the loss of her daughter as the most difficult days of her life. When another close family member died in April, Melanie Green was emotionally less prepared than ever for what was to come. Three months after the death of her daughter, she was arrested at her home as she waited for her son Damen to return from school.

The state's attorney for Winnebago County, Paul Logli, had in the meantime been pondering the legal situation presented by the death of Bianca Green. "It was a living, breathing baby that died, for no other reason, we believe, than that cocaine was ingested by the mother," Logli said. "To ignore that is unconscionable. It borders on barbarism" (Stein, 1989). His frustrations were with the law. If a living infant was prenatally exposed to cocaine, an Illinois prosecutor can bring the mother before the juvenile court for a hearing to determine custody. If, on the other hand, the cocaine-exposed infant dies, the Illinois law provides no remedy. "The statutes of this state," Logli said in a published interview, "specifically exempt mothers from the aggravated battery or manslaughter of a fetus." He went on to explain, "That's so prosecutors like me can't use that to get around the [U.S. Supreme Court abortion] decision [in *Roe v. Wade*]" (Reardon, 1989, May 14).

Logli disputed suggestions that his Roman Catholic background—he attended Catholic high school and a Catholic-affiliated college—had any bearing on his decision in the Green case (Stein, 1989). As the legal test that he proposed and later wrote about, Logli reported finding precedent for filing criminal charges against Melanie Green in a 1982 Illinois reckless homicide case (Logli, 1992). The facts were straightforward: a car driven by the drunken defendant collided with another car in which a pregnant woman rode as a passenger. Within hours of the collision, the woman delivered a baby who died a few minutes later. The injury to the baby was prenatal. But because the baby was born alive—like Bianca Green—Logli hoped this could be the precedent for holding Melanie Green responsible for her own child's death. Thus, the Rockford office of the state's attorney presented to the grand jury one charge of involuntary manslaughter in the death of Green's daughter and one count of delivering drugs to a minor.

The obstacles to the involuntary manslaughter charge were serious (Reardon, 1989, May 28). The American Civil Liberties Union (ACLU) had entered the case, pointing out that the injury was prenatal. In attempting to hold a mother criminally responsible for prenatal injury to her own child, the ACLU argued, Logli ran afoul of the U.S. Supreme Court ruling in *Roe v. Wade*: the fetus is not a person with protectable rights (Kreiter, 1989, May 10). Prosecuting a woman for acts to her own body is an unconstitutional intrusion into the right to privacy (Kreiter, 1989, May 27). Harvey Grossman, legal director of the ACLU in Chicago, defended Melanie Green and said of the case, "It's a question of how society related to women, period. She is not simply a vessel for carrying a fetus. She doesn't lose her rights to personal autonomy because of pregnancy" (Parson, 1993).

The eight women and four men on the grand jury agreed and chose not to indict Green on either the manslaughter or the drug delivery charge. Bowing to defeat, Logli admitted that manslaughter may not have been the best mechanism for charging women who used drugs during pregnancy (Lamb, 1989). Questions asked by the grand jurors, he conceded, showed that they had concerns about Green's right to privacy, that is, her right to make decisions about her body free from government interference. There were also some risks, Logli admitted, in criminalizing the behavior in question (Reardon, 1989, May 28).

From where did this high-profile prosecution come? Logli cited the local epidemic of crack babies, although Winnebago County, Illinois, was not the most likely place for a prosecutorial campaign (Logli, 1990). While 27 babies born to women allegedly using cocaine had been identified in the hospitals between the summer of 1988 and May of 1989, this figure is small in contrast with the much larger estimates from urban centers like New York City or Los Angeles (Stein, 1989).

Logli may have been more concerned with keeping big-city problems, including crack babies, from taking hold in the smaller community of Rockford. And Logli was frustrated with the war on drugs (Logli, 1990). "We undertook this prosecution in an effort to find one more way to fight a cocaine war that all society is presently losing," Logli wrote in a 1990 law journal article (Logli, 1990). "Concerned citizens and child welfare authorities" who wanted to remedy the problem of substance-abused infants had asked him to step in, he said (Logli, 1992). Criminal sanctions, Logli maintained, remained an effective remedy. They "raised the consequences of maternal drug use to a tough enough position that these persons . . . might be encouraged to seek the treatment, the help they need" (Primetime Live, 1989).

The Green case gave Paul Logli national exposure. On the day he filed charges against Green, he flew to New York City to appear on two national television shows (Reardon, 1989, May 11), and television talk show hosts continued to provide a forum for him to express his prosecutorial views. Reports circulating in the late 1980s had it that Paul Logli was considering a run for Congress, but he remained state's attorney for Winnebago County well into the 1990s (Stein, 1989). He became president of the Illinois State's Attorney Association in 1996.

Melanie Green, on the other hand, tried to escape the publicity that surrounded her case. Even though she was unavailable for interviews, the troubles she experienced in 1989 were played out on national television. As she mourned the death of her daughter and an aunt, she faced very serious criminal charges: the drug distribution charge carried a sentence of 15 years in prison, the manslaughter charge, of 5. And had Logli tacked on the drug possession charge he threatened to file after the grand jury dismissed the others, Green would have faced 3 years in prison. After the grand jury dismissed charges against her, Green left Rockford to enter a three-week day-treatment program. To avoid the permanent stigma of being Rockford's most infamous crack mother, she announced plans to relocate. . . .

Crack Mothers in Charleston, South Carolina

Charles Malony Condon, South Carolina's ninth circuit solicitor from 1980 to 1991, served both Charleston and Berkeley Counties. One of the things that attracted Condon to the job of solicitor was its promise of autonomy and discretion. In an article profiling his career, he told interviewers that the job allowed him to pick his cases, discarding bad ones to concentrate on good ones: "I think the prosecutor should always wear the white hat. And if you don't wear the white hat, you're not doing your job" (MacDougall, 1991).

In the late 1990s, now state attorney general for South Carolina, Charles Condon looks back on a career that includes developing the program he says reduced the number of cocaine-addicted babies in Charleston (MacDougall,

1991). Hospital officials from the Medical University of South Carolina (MUSC) had originally called in the Circuit Solicitor's Office when nurses and doctors began seeing five or six pregnant women a week who had used cocaine or crack, some with hemorrhaging or other complications related to pregnancy (Lewin, 1990). Physicians linked the symptoms to cocaine, and because they felt they were witnessing a crime, went to the circuit solicitor (Siegel, 1994).

Condon had already enlisted in the war on drugs, and with a politician's eye to a winning issue, agreed that the hospital had an obligation to report such cases (Siegel, 1994). In a *Los Angeles Times* article, Condon is reported to have admonished hospital officials, "It's nice you came in . . . But the fact is, you have to come in. There's no patient-doctor privilege on this. If you don't report it, it's a crime" (Siegel, 1994). In response, Dr. Edgar Horger and nurse Shirley Brown, both from MUSC, joined Condon in developing a program for drug-using pregnant women that sent a deterrent message: Seek drug treatment or face arrest and jail time (Condon, 1995).

The program developed in three stages. From October 1988 to September 1989, during clinic visits urine drug tests were administered to pregnant women suspected of using cocaine or other illicit drugs. The testing program identified 119 cases of cocaine use among pregnant women. For most, the drug test coincided with the delivery of their babies. Referrals for drug rehabilitation were made for 15 women tested for drugs early in their pregnancies, but their babies tested positive for cocaine when they returned to the hospital for delivery.

In the program's shock stage, arrests were made. In October, November, and December 1989, patients were arrested if they or their newborns tested positive for cocaine. Ten women were arrested, their babies turned over to foster care. In a final stage, beginning in January 1990, the program modified its procedures so that patients could avoid arrest by successfully completing drug counseling. The threat of arrest, made real by the program's shock period, was thereafter used to "leverage" women into treatment. Over the program's five-year life, 42 women were arrested, some of whom avoided charges by agreeing to drug treatment (Associated Press, 1994).

Following an investigation in January 1990, the ACLU and the Center for Reproductive Law and Policy pointed to serious deficiencies in the MUSC program (Goetz, Fox, and Bates, 1990). Screening procedures were discriminatory. Doctors began by screening patients on a discretionary basis, but implementation of a nine-point protocol intended to reduce bias still permitted selective drug screening. Combined with the fact that MUSC served poor patients, this meant that poor women, the majority of whom were black, were singled out as drug-abusing mothers.

The MUSC program was also punitive. Once the hospital identified drug-using women, the circuit solicitor recommended against releasing them on their own recognizance, insisting instead on bail. The judge set bail, which had the effect of keeping cash-strapped, postpartum women in jail and away from adequate medical attention or drug treatment. The MUSC program purported to give mothers a choice between treatment and jail, but treatment was either nonexistent or inappropriate. Initially, the hospital had not developed treatment options for women, but when it did, the program did not work well for most. This population needed day treatment, child care, and transportation, or residential facilities with accommodations for children—none of which existed in Charleston.

Still, Condon defended the program as effective in reducing the number of cocaine babies (MacDougall, 1991). The program's evaluation reportedly showed that MUSC had reduced the number of drug-using women coming to the hospital for delivery, but a flawed methodology made it a poor demonstration of effectiveness (Horger, Brown, and Condon, 1990). Nonetheless, in a 1990 interview on *Nightline*, Condon summed up the MUSC experience: "We have been able to demonstrate quite clearly that with an effective prosecution program available as a last resort and the women knowing that something will in fact happen to them eventually, they [the women] have simply stopped using cocaine" (1990). And because there had been growing criticism that prosecutions like those in South Carolina frightened women away from needed prenatal care, he added, "And there's absolutely no evidence here locally that the women are not seeking prenatal care. . . . They go to the same hospitals as before."

His experience in South Carolina, Condon said, showed that without the threat of prosecution, women who used cocaine during pregnancy would do nothing to help themselves or their future children: "When the women have been coming into the hospital and have been told simply and educated simply that cocaine use is bad, it can hurt you or your fetus and can cause great damage, many women continue to use cocaine" (Nightline, 1990). In a different context, Condon predicted, "Until they [cocaine mothers] suffer sanctions, . . . you're going to see the problem increase" (Sataline, 1991). Moreover, he argued, if it is against the law in South Carolina to use cocaine, then it is against the law for pregnant women to use it, too. If the law applies to pregnant women, then no woman has the right to bear a drug-affected baby (Sataline, 1991)

In the midst of what was shaping up as a major debate on public health policy, the ACLU and the Center for Reproductive Law and Policy publicized details about the women who had been jailed because of the MUSC program (Siegel, 1994). They were black, poor, and as single mothers in their late twenties and thirties, they had used crack or cocaine, and they had several children. On the basis of a positive drug screen, they were arrested on charges of possession and delivery of drugs to a minor.

One example, Theresa Joseph, 35, was the mother of several children, only one of whom lived with her. Although she avoided the hospital throughout her pregnancy for fear of prosecution—she had seen Condon's public service announcement threatening jail for pregnant substance abusers—an infection brought her to MUSC. There the staff told her to get drug treatment, but fearing prosecution, she fled. She returned for further medical care but did not keep the appointment for drug treatment. Back at the hospital for the birth of her baby, she was arrested and taken to jail after the baby tested positive for cocaine.

In addition to fear, the lack of appropriate options in the MUSC program kept women away from treatment. Crystal Ferguson, 31 years old and the mother of three children, was referred late in her pregnancy to MUSC, where she tested positive for cocaine. She was given the option of getting treatment or going to jail, but she felt she could not leave her children, and treatment facilities had no room for children. Ferguson returned to her children, rejecting the offer of treatment, and tried to stop on her own. When she went to the hospital to give birth to her daughter, she tested positive for drugs, and Ferguson was arrested and jailed.

Defense attorneys easily got the charges (drug possession and drug delivery to a minor) against Ferguson and Joseph dismissed (Siegel, 1994). In 1992 an appellate court overturned the child-neglect conviction of a pregnant substance abuser, holding that the law had been misapplied. So when Lynn Paltrow of the Center for Reproductive Law and Policy and the ACLU and Charleston public defender Ted Phillips moved to quash the distribution charges against Joseph and Ferguson, the new ninth circuit solicitor, David Schwacke, who replaced Condon when Condon became state attorney general, did not put up a fight. Schwacke dismissed the charges and rescinded the bench warrants on five other women also charged with possession and delivery of drugs to a minor, hoping to avoid a ruling that the drug delivery charge was misapplied as well.

The Center for Reproductive Law and Policy assembled an impressive array of experts and public health organizations (Siegel, 1994). All had gone on record opposing the MUSC program on public health grounds: prosecution was the least effective way to deal with maternal drug use. Dr. Barry Zuckerman, chairman of the department of pediatrics at the Boston University School of Medicine and Boston City Hospital, and Dr. Jay Katz, professor emeritus of law, medicine, and psychiatry at the Yale University, raised objections to the MUSC program. The American Medical Association, American Academy of Pediatrics, American Public Health Association, American Nurses Association, March of Dimes, and other groups opposed the threat of arrest to force pregnant women into drug treatment programs. Women's groups, including the National Organization for Women, opposed prosecution for public health reasons and because it threatened women's right to make reproductive decisions free of government interference. They were also concerned because prosecution might give anti-abortion advocates grounds for expanding fetal rights.

The Center for Reproductive Law and Policy devised a two-pronged strategy in South Carolina (Siegel, 1994). It first complained to the National Institutes of Health that the evaluation of the MUSC program had not met federal guidelines requiring the consent of human subjects in research. Subjects had not consented to participate in the evaluation research that was later published in a medical journal. MUSC and the study's authors (Dr Edgar Horger, nurse Shirley Brown, and circuit solicitor Charles Condon) stood accused of conducting unethical experiments on African American women. The U.S. Department of Health and Human Services reviewed the charges and threatened to cut off federal funding unless MUSC corrected its procedures. To avoid losing federal funding, MUSC shut down the program in 1994.

Second, the Center for Reproductive Law and Policy filed a $3-million class-action suit against MUSC, the city of Charleston, and local law enforcement officials and agencies (Siegel, 1994). The suit asked for compensatory and punitive damages for 10 women whose civil rights had been violated by

MUSC's arrest-and-jail policy. In January 1997 a federal jury decided, however, that the choice between drug treatment or jail was not racially motivated, nor did the conduct of the hospital in turning over the results of drug tests to prosecutors amount to an illegal search. The U.S. district judge, Westin Houck, had six months to determine whether the search itself was unconstitutional, whether MUSC violated confidentiality of medical information, women's right to procreate, and the Federal Civil Rights Act (Baxley, 1997). Although Lynn Paltrow did not believe that the case was over, the judge failed to act within the time limit, and the issues remain unresolved.

The federal suit in Charleston stirred up local prejudices against the outsiders who defended cocaine mothers (Siegel, 1994). The ACLU, feminists, and "California-type liberals" were rebuked by officials for moralizing and interfering with the way things were done in Charleston. "The left-wing ACLU doesn't represent the American people," said Condon at a press conference during a break in the federal class-action suit. "MUSC deserves an award. If the plaintiff [the women jailed by MUSC] prevails, in effect we'd be legalizing the use of crack cocaine during pregnancy" (Siegel, 1994). As Condon turned back to his private conversation, *Los Angeles Times* correspondent Barry Siegel recorded his comments: "Tell Lynn [Paltrow] thanks for suing me. Running in South Carolina for attorney general, the best thing you can have happen is to be sued by the ACLU" (1994).

⌁❀⌁

With the 1996 federal court decision in South Carolina, the moral panic ground to a halt. One by one, the cases built by prosecutors had unraveled. While the media and the public understood the prosecutions as legitimate attempts to deal with the problem, the judiciary cast a more critical eye. The Rockford grand jury doubted the wisdom of Logli's manslaughter strategy, and in an unusual move for any grand jury, refused to indict Melanie Green. The grand jury in Brockton, less suspicious of O'Malley's drug-delivery strategy, indicted Josephine Pelligrini, and O'Malley managed to get the case to court, but the judge quickly dismissed it and effectively ended such prosecutions in Massachusetts. Tague took advantage of sympathetic lower-court judges to get both his cases bound over for trial, but the Michigan Court of Appeals threw out the charges. The prosecutor in Florida managed to convict Jennifer Johnson, but the Supreme Court of Florida refused to uphold it and ended the cocaine baby cases there.

The five prosecutors had surprisingly little support within their own professional circles. In the National District Attorneys Association (NDAA), one subcommittee, Substance Abused Infants and Children, strongly endorsed their efforts. But most other NDAA sections were less enthusiastic, including the American Prosecutors Research Institute (APRI), the research arm of the association ("Substance Abused Infants," 1990). Charles Condon, Anthony Tague, and Jeffrey Deen figured prominently in an APRI conference, "Substance Abused Infants: A Prosecutor's Dilemma," held in Chicago in July 1990. But the conference failed to endorse the high-profile prosecutions. Jill Hiatt and Janet Dinsmore, spokespeople for the National Center for Prosecution of Child Abuse, distanced APRI and NDAA from the "very few but highly publicized cases, involving novel use of laws to prosecute women who have given birth to drug-affected babies" ("Pregnant Addicts," 1990).

Prosecutors made it easier both morally and politically to cut social service spending, to push fetal rights, and to attack racial preferences. Their crusade appealed to the prejudices of white audiences who watched the panic unfold on the nightly news, but their limited racial experience blinded them to the racial implications of the prosecutions (Greene, 1991). Misconceptions fit into a long line of stereotypes about black sexuality and incompetent mothering (Roberts, 1991). As another dehumanizing wave of restrictions on reproduction, the prosecutions showed that state officials were all too willing to punish black women for having babies. Under slavery, an owner's profit dictated the reproductive choices of black women. Later, involuntary sterilization eliminated the choices arising from fertility. Pronatalist attitudes combined with restrictions on Medicaid abortions made termination unlikely. The crusade against crack mothers, consequently, served as punishment for women who carried their pregnancies to term and delivered babies (Roberts, 1991).

POSTSCRIPT

Should Pregnant Drug Users Be Prosecuted?

Babies born with health problems as a result of their mothers' drug use is a tragedy that needs to be rectified. The issue is not whether or not this problem needs to be addressed but what course of action is best. The need for medical intervention and specialized treatment programs serving pregnant women with drug problems has been recognized. The groundwork has been set for funding and developing such programs. The Office of Substance Abuse Prevention is funding chemical dependency programs specifically for pregnant women in several states.

It has been argued that drug use by pregnant women is a problem that requires medical, not criminal, attention. One can contend that pregnant drug users and their drug-exposed infants are victims of drug abuse. Humphries contends that there is an element of discrimination in the practice of prosecuting women who use drugs during pregnancy because these women are primarily low-income, single, members of minority groups, and recipients of public assistance. Possible factors leading to their drug use—poverty, unemployment, poor education, and lack of vocational training—are not addressed when the solution to drug use during pregnancy is incarceration. Moreover, many pregnant women are denied access to treatment programs.

Prosecution proponents contend that medical intervention is not adequate in preventing pregnant women from using drugs and that criminal prosecution is necessary. Logli argues that "eliminating the pain, suffering and death resulting from drug exposure in newborns must be a prosecutor's priority." He maintains that the criminal justice system should protect newborns and, if legal cause does exist for prosecution, then statutes should provide protection for the fetus. However, will prosecution result in more protection or less protection for the fetus? If a mother stops using drugs for fear of prosecution, then the fetus benefits. If the mother avoids prenatal care because of potential legal punishment, then the fetus suffers.

If women can be prosecuted for using illegal drugs such as cocaine and narcotics during pregnancy because they harm the fetus, then should women who smoke cigarettes and drink alcohol during pregnancy also be prosecuted? The evidence is clear that tobacco and alcohol place the fetus at great risk; however, most discussions of prosecuting pregnant drug users overlook women who use these drugs. Also, the adverse health effects from secondhand smoke are well documented. Should people be prosecuted if they smoke around pregnant women?

An excellent review of the effects of prenatal exposure to alcohol is "Alcohol and Pregnancy, Highlights From Three Decades of Research," by Carrie L. Randall, *Journal of Studies on Alcohol* (vol. 62, 2001). Three articles that examine this issue thoroughly are "The Rights of Pregnant Women: The Supreme Court and Drug Testing," by Lawrence O. Gostin, *The Hastings Center Report* (September/October 2001); "Inside the Womb: Interpreting the Ferguson Case," by Samantha Weyrauch, *Duke Journal of Gender Law and Policy* (Summer 2002); and "Who Is the Guilty Party? Rights, Motherhood, and the Problem of Prenatal Drug Exposure," by Karen Zivi, *Law and Society Review* (vol. 34, no. 1, 2000).

ISSUE 6

Is Drug Addiction a Choice?

YES: Jeffrey A. Schaler, from *Addiction Is a Choice* (Open Court, 2000)

NO: Alan I. Leshner, from "Addiction Is a Brain Disease," *Issues in Science and Technology* (Spring 2001)

ISSUE SUMMARY

YES: Psychotherapist Jeffrey A. Schaler maintains that drug addiction should not be considered a disease, a condition over which one has no control. He states that diseases have distinct characteristics and that drug addiction does not share these characteristics. Classifying behavior as socially unacceptable does not prove that it is a disease, according to Schaler.

NO: Alan I. Leshner, former director of the National Institute on Drug Abuse, contends that drug addiction is not a failure of will nor a sign of weak character. One's initial use of drugs may be voluntary, he says, but over time one cannot stop through force of will alone. Leshner notes that biological and chemical changes within the brain are important components in drug addiction.

Is drug addiction caused by an illness or disease, or is it caused by inappropriate behavioral patterns? This distinction is important because it has both legal and medical implications. Should people be held accountable for behaviors that stem from an illness over which they have no control? For example, if a person cannot help being an alcoholic and hurts or kills someone as a result of being drunk, should that person be treated or incarcerated? Likewise, if an individual's addiction is due to lack of self-control, rather than due to a disease, should taxpayer money go to pay for that person's treatment?

It can be argued that the disease concept of drug addiction legitimizes or excuses behaviors. If addiction is an illness, then blame for poor behavior can be shifted to the disease and away from the individual. Moreover, if drug addiction is incurable, can people ever be held responsible for their behavior?

Jeffrey A. Schaler contends that addicts should be held responsible for their behavior and that loss of control is not inevitable. He asserts that the ability of alcoholics to stop their excessive alcohol consumption is not determined by a physiological reaction to alcohol. Moreover, it has been shown that many cocaine and heroin users do not lose control while using these drugs. In their study of U.S. service personnel in Vietnam, epidemiologist Lee N. Robins and colleagues showed that most of the soldiers who used narcotics regularly during the war did not continue using them once they returned home. Many service personnel in Vietnam reportedly used drugs because they were in a situation they did not want to be in. Additionally, without the support of loved ones and society's constraints, they were freer to gravitate toward behaviors that would not be tolerated by their families and friends.

Attitudes toward treating drug abuse are affected by whether it is perceived as an illness or as an act of free will. According to the disease perspective, an important step for addicts to take in order to benefit from treatment is to admit that they are powerless against their addiction. They need to acknowledge that their drug addiction controls them and that drug addiction is a lifelong problem. The implication of this view is that addicts are never cured. Addicts must therefore abstain from drugs for their entire lives. The disease concept implies that one needs help in overcoming addiction. By calling drug addiction a medical condition, the body is viewed as a machine that needs fixing; character and will become secondary. Also, by calling addiction a disease, the role of society in causing drug addiction is left unexplored. What roles do poverty, crime, unemployment, inadequate health care, and poor education have in drug addiction? Schaler contends that psychological and environmental factors account for drug addiction.

Alan I. Leshner argues that there are certain neurotransmitters in the brain that contribute to the reward response. Humans repeatedly engage in behaviors that produce pleasurable feelings. Psychology tells the body to repeat such behaviors, but biology contributes the concept of chemical communication systems in the brain. These systems are critical to learning and memory. Leshner contends that drugs produce the changes in the brain that provide a pleasurable response.

Is addiction caused by psychological or biological factors? Can drugs produce changes in the brain that result in drug addiction? How much control do drug addicts have over their use of drugs? In the following selections, Schaler argues that drug use is a matter of free will while Leshner contends that drugs produce changes in the brain that result in repeating behaviors that lead to drug addiction.

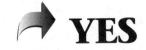 **YES**

Is Addiction Really a Disease?

Being addicted to a melancholy as she is.

—William Shakespeare, *Twelfth Night*

If you watch TV, read the newspaper, or listen to almost any social worker or religious minister, you soon pick up the idea that addiction is a condition in which addicts just physically cannot control themselves, and that this condition is a medical disease.

The federal government views alcohol addiction as a disease characterized by *loss of control,* with a physiological 'etiology' (cause) independent of volition. According to a typical statement of the government's view by Otis R. Bowen, former secretary of health and human services,

> millions of children have a genetic predisposition to alcoholism . . . alcohol use by young people has been found to be a 'gateway' drug preceding other drug use . . . about 1 out of every 15 kids will eventually become an alcoholic. . . . alcoholism is a disease, and this disease is highly treatable. (Bowen 1988, pp. 559, 563)

You may easily conclude that all the experts agree with this kind of thinking. Most people with no special interest in the subject probably never get to hear another point of view.

The true situation is a bit more complicated. Public opinion overwhelmingly accepts the claim that addiction is a disease, but the general public's views are seriously inconsistent. A 1987 study of public views on alcoholism showed that over 85 percent of people believe that alcoholism is a disease, but most of them also believe things that contradict the disease theory. Many people seem to support and reject the disease theory at the same time. For instance, they often say they believe that alcoholism is a disease and also that it is a sign of moral weakness (Caetano 1987, p. 158).

The addiction treatment providers, the many thousands of people who make their living in the addiction treatment industry, mostly accept the disease theory. They are, in fact, for the most part, 'recovered addicts' themselves, redeemed sinners who spend their lives being paid to preach the gospel that social deviants are sick.

Among those psychologists and others who think, write, discuss, and conduct research in this area, however, opinion is much more divided. In this small world, there is an ongoing battle between the 'disease model' and the 'free-will model'.

Biomedical and psychosocial scientists range across both sides of the controversy (Fillmore and Sigvardsson 1988). Some biomedical researchers accept the disease model and assert that genetic and physiological differences account for alcoholism (for example, D.W. Goodwin 1988; F.K. Goodwin 1988; Blum et al. 1990; Tabakoff and Hoffman 1988). Other biomedical researchers have investigated their claims and pronounced them invalid (Lester 1989; Bolos et al. 1990; Billings 1990). Many social scientists reject the idea that alcoholics or other addicts constitute a homogeneous group. They hold that individual differences, personal values, expectations, and environmental factors are key correlates to heavy drinking and drug-taking. Others reject strictly psychological theories (Maltzman 1991; Madsen 1989; Vaillant 1983; Milam and Ketcham 1983; Prince, Glatt, and Pullar-Strecker 1966). Some sociologists regard the disease model of alcoholism as a human construction based on desire for social control (Room 1983; Fillmore 1988). Some embrace the disease model even while agreeing that addiction may not be a real disease—they hold that utility warrants labeling it as such (Kissin 1983; Vaillant 1990). Their opponents believe the disease model does more harm than good (Szasz 1972; Fingarette 1988; Alexander 1990a; 1990b; Crawford et al. 1989; Fillmore and Kelso 1987; Heather, Winton, and Rollnick 1982; Schaler 1996b).

My impression is that the disease model is steadily losing ground. It may not be too much to hope that the notion of addiction as a disease will be completely discredited and abandoned in years to come, perhaps as early as the next 20 years.

If this seems like a fanciful speculation, remember that other recognized 'diseases' have been quite swiftly discredited. The most recent example is homosexuality. Being sexually attracted to members of one's own sex was, overwhelmingly, considered a disease by the psychiatric profession, and therefore by the medical profession as a whole, until the 1960s. Psychiatry and medicine completely reversed themselves on this issue within a few years. Homosexuality was declassified as an illness by the American Psychiatric Association in 1973. It is now officially considered a non-disease, unless the homosexual wishes he were not a homosexual. This doesn't go far enough, but imagine the same principle extended to drug addiction: the addict is not at all sick unless he says he is unhappy being addicted!

Before homosexuality, there were the recognized diseases of masturbation, negritude (having a black skin), Judaism (described as a disease by the German government in the 1930s), and being critical of the Soviet government, which 'treated' political dissidents in mental hospitals (see Rush 1799; Szasz 1970; Robitscher 1980; Lifton 1986; Conrad and Schneider 1992; and Breggin 1993). A similar fate may be in store for the 'disease' of drug addiction.

Many people accept the disease model of addiction on the basis of respect for the messenger. Addiction is a disease because doctors say it's a disease (social psychologists call this peripheral-route processing) rather than critical evaluation of the message itself (central-route processing). Peripheral-route processing has more in common with faith than reason, and research shows that in general its appeal is greatest among the less educated. Reason and faith are not always compatible. Reason requires evidence, faith does not.

Clinical and public policy should not be based on faith, whether the source is drunken anecdote, the proclamations of self-assigned experts, or the measured statements of addiction doctors. Rather, empirical evidence and sound reasoning are required. Both are lacking in the assertion that addiction is a disease.

If it were ever to be shown that there existed a genetic disease causing a powerful craving for a drug, this would not demonstrate that the afflicted person had no choice as to whether to take the drug. Nor would it show that the action of taking the drug was itself a disease.

There are various skin rashes, for example, which often arouse a powerful urge to scratch the inflamed area. It's usually enough to explain the harmful consequences of scratching, and the patient will choose not to scratch. Though scratching may cause diseases (by promoting infection of the area) and is a response to physiological sensations, the activity of scratching is not itself considered a disease.

What Is a Disease?

Is addiction really a disease? Let's clarify a few matters. The classification of behavior as socially unacceptable does not prove its label as a disease. Adherents of the disease model sometimes respond to the claim that addiction is not a disease by emphasizing the terrible problems people create as a result of their addictions, but that is entirely beside the point. The fact that some behavior has horrible consequences does not show that it's a disease.

The 'success' of 'treatment programs' run by people who view addiction as a disease would not demonstrate that addiction was a disease—any more than the success of other religious groups in converting people from vicious practices would prove the theological tenets of these religious groups. However, this possibility need not concern us, since all known treatment programs are, in fact, ineffective.

I will not go into the claims of a genetic basis for 'alcoholism' or other addictions. A genetic predisposition toward some kind of behavior, say, speaking in tongues, would not show that those with the predisposition had a disease. Variations in skin and eye color, for example, are genetically determined, but are not diseases. Fair-skinned people sunburn easily. The fairness of their skin is genetically determined, yet their susceptibility to sunburn is not considered a disease. Neither would a genetic predisposition toward some kind of behavior necessarily show that the predisposed persons could not consciously change their behavior.

With so much commonsense evidence to refute it, why is the view of drug addiction as a disease so prevalent? Incredible as it may seem, because doctors say so. A leading alcoholism researcher once asserted that alcoholism is a disease simply because people go to doctors for it. Undoubtedly, drug 'addicts' seek help from doctors for two reasons. Many addicts have a significant psychological investment in maintaining this view, having been told, and come to believe, that their eventual recovery depends on believing they have a disease. They may even have come to accept that they will die if they question the disease model of addiction. And treatment professionals have a significant economic investment at stake. The more behaviors are diagnosed as diseases, the more they will be paid by health insurance companies for 'treating' these diseases.

When we consider whether drug addiction is a disease we are concerned with what causes the drug to get *into* the body. It's quite irrelevant what the drug does *after* it's in the body. I certainly don't for a moment doubt that the taking of many drugs *causes* disease. Prolonged heavy drinking of alcoholic beverages can cause cirrhosis of the liver. Prolonged smoking of cigarettes somewhat raises the risk of various diseases such as lung cancer. But this uncontroversial fact is quite distinct from any claim that the activity is itself a disease (Szasz 1989b).

Some doctors make a specialty of occupation-linked disorders. For example, there is a pattern of lung and other diseases associated with working down a coal mine. But this does not show that mining coal is itself a disease. Other enterprising physicians specialize in treating diseases arising from sports: there is a pattern of diseases resulting from swimming, another from football, yet another from long-distance running. This does not demonstrate that these sports, or the inclination to pursue these sports, are themselves diseases. So, for instance, the fact that a doctor may be exceptionally knowledgeable about the effects of alcohol on the body, and may therefore be accepted as an expert on 'alcoholism', does nothing to show that alcoholism itself is a legitimate medical concept.

Addiction, a Physical Disease?

If addiction is a disease, then presumably it's either a bodily or a mental disease. What criteria might justify defining addiction as a physical illness? Pathologists use nosology—the classification of diseases—to select, from among the phenomena they study, those that qualify as true diseases. Diseases are listed in standard pathology textbooks because they meet the nosological criteria for disease classification. A simple test of a true physical disease is whether it can be shown to exist in a corpse. There are no bodily signs of addiction itself (as opposed to its effects) that can be identified in a dead body. Addiction is therefore not listed in standard pathology textbooks.

Pathology, as revolutionized by Rudolf Virchow (1821–1902), requires an identifiable alteration in bodily tissue, a change in the cells of the body, for disease classification. No such identifiable pathology has been found in the bodies of heavy drinkers and drug users. This alone justifies the view that addiction is not a physical disease (Szasz 1991; 1994).

A symptom is subjective evidence from the patient: the patient reports certain pains and other sensations. A sign is something that can be identified in the patient's body, irrespective of the patient's reported experiences. In standard medical practice, the diagnosis of disease can be based on signs alone or on a combination of signs and symptoms, but only rarely on symptoms alone. A sign is objective physical evidence such as a lesion or chemical imbalance. Signs may be found through medical tests.

Sometimes a routine physical examination reveals signs of disease when no symptoms are reported. In such cases the disease is said to be 'asymptomatic'—without symptoms. For example, sugar in the urine combined with other signs may lead to a diagnosis of asymptomatic diabetes. Such a diagnosis is made solely on the basis of signs. It is inconceivable that addiction could ever be diagnosed on the basis of bodily signs alone. (The *effects* of heavy alcohol consumption can of course be inferred from bodily signs, but that, remember, is a different matter.) To speak of 'asymptomatic addiction' would be absurd.

True, conditions such as migraine and epilepsy are diagnosed primarily on the basis of symptoms. But, in general, it is not standard medical practice to diagnose disease on the basis of symptoms alone. The putative disease called addiction is diagnosed solely by symptoms in the form of conduct, never by signs, that is, by physical evidence in the patient's body. (A doctor might conclude that someone with cirrhosis of the liver and other bodily signs had partaken of alcoholic beverages heavily over a long period, and might infer that the patient was an 'alcoholic', but actually the doctor would be unable to distinguish this from the hypothetical case of someone who had been kept a prisoner and dosed with alcohol against her will. So, again, strictly speaking, *there cannot possibly be a bodily sign of an addiction.*)

If you visited your physician because of a dull pain in your epigastric region, would you want her to make a diagnosis without confirming it through objective tests? Wouldn't you doubt the validity of a diagnosis of heart disease without at least the results of an EKG? You would want to see reliable evidence of signs. But in the diagnosis of the disease called addiction, there are no signs, only symptoms (Szasz 1987).

We continually hear that 'addiction is a disease just like diabetes'. Yet there is no such thing as asymptomatic addiction, and *logically there could not be.* Moreover, the analogy cannot be turned around. It would be awkward to tell a person with diabetes that his condition was 'just like addiction' and inaccurate too: When a person with diabetes is deprived of insulin he will suffer and in severe cases may even die. When a heavy drinker or other drug user is deprived of alcohol or other drugs his physical health most often improves.

A Mental or Metaphorical Disease?

Mental illnesses are diagnosed on the basis of symptoms, not signs. Perhaps, then, addiction is a mental illness, a psychiatric disease. Where does it fit into the scheme of psychiatric disorders?

Psychiatric disorders can be categorized in three groups: organic disorders, functional disorders, and antisocial behavior (Szasz 1988). Organic disorders include various forms of dementia such as those caused by HIV-1 infection, acute alcohol intoxication, brain tumor or injury, dementia of the Alzheimer's type, general paresis, and multi-infarct dementia. These are physical diseases with identifiable bodily signs. Addiction has no such identifiable signs.

Functional disorders include fears (anxiety disorders), discouragements (mood disorders), and stupidities (cognitive disorders). These are mental in the sense that they involve mental activities. As Szasz has pointed out, they are diseases "only in a metaphorical sense."

Forms of antisocial behavior categorized as psychiatric illness include crime, suicide, personality disorders, and maladaptive and maladjusted behavior. Some people consider these 'disorders' because they vary from the norm and involve danger to self or others. According to Szasz, however, they are "neither 'mental' nor 'diseases' " (Szasz 1988, pp. 249–251). If addiction qualifies as an antisocial behavior, this does not necessarily imply that it is mental or a disease.

Addiction is not listed in the American Psychiatric Association's Diagnostic and Statistical Manual of Mental Disorders IV (DSM-IV). What was once listed as alcoholism is now referred to as alcohol dependence and abuse. These are listed under the category of substance-related disorders. They would not fit the category of organic disorders because they are described in terms of behavior only. They would conceivably fit the functional disorder category but probably would be subordinated to one of the established disorders such as discouragement or anxiety.

Thus, it's difficult to classify addiction as either a physical or a mental disease. Many human problems may be described *metaphorically* as diseases. We hear media pundits speak of a 'sick economy' or 'sick culture'. Declining empires, such as the Ottoman empire at the end of the nineteenth century and the Soviet empire in the 1980s, are said to be 'sick'. There is little harm in resorting to this metaphor, and therefore describing negative addictions as diseases— except that there is the danger that some people will take the metaphor literally.

Today any socially-unacceptable behavior is likely to be diagnosed as an 'addiction'. So we have shopping addiction, videogame addiction, sex addiction, Dungeons and Dragons addiction, running addiction, chocolate addiction, Internet addiction, addiction to abusive relationships, and so forth. This would be fine if it merely represented a return to the traditional, non-medical usage, in which addiction means being given over to some pursuit. However, all of these new 'addictions' are now claimed to be medical illnesses, characterized by self-destructiveness, compulsion, loss of control, and some mysterious, as-yet-unidentified physiological component. This is entirely fanciful.

People become classified as 'addicts' or 'alcoholics' because of their behavior. 'Behavior' in humans refers to intentional conduct. As was pointed out long ago by Wilhelm Dilthey, Max Weber, and Ludwig von Mises, among others, the motions of the human body are either involuntary reflexes or meaningful human action. Human action is governed by the meaning it has for the acting person. The behavior of heavy drinking is not a form of neurological reflex but is the expression of values through action. As Herbert Fingarette puts it:

> A pattern of conduct must be distinguished from a mere sequence of reflex-like reactions. A reflex knee jerk is not conduct. If we regard something as a pattern of conduct . . . we assume that it is mediated by the mind, that it reflects consideration of reasons and preferences, the election of a preferred means to the end, and the election of the end itself from among alternatives.

> The complex, purposeful, and often ingenious projects with which many an addict may be occupied in his daily hustlings to maintain his drug supply are examples of conduct, not automatic reflex reactions to a singly biological cause. (1975, p. 435)

Thomas Szasz agrees that

> by behavior we mean the person's 'mode of conducting himself' or his 'deportment' . . . the name we attach to a living being's conduct in the daily pursuit of life. . . . bodily movements that are the products of neurophysiological discharges or reflexes are not behavior. . . . behavior implies action, and action implies conduct pursued by an agent seeking to attain a goal. (1987, p. 343)

The term 'alcoholism' has become so loaded with prescriptive intent that it no longer describes any drinking behavior accurately and should be abandoned. 'Heavy drinking' is a more descriptive term (Fingarette 1988). It is imprecise, but so is 'alcoholism'.

If we continue to use the term 'alcoholism', however, we should bear in mind that there is no precisely defined condition, activity, or entity called alcoholism in the way there is a precise condition known as lymphosarcoma of the mesenteric glands, for example. The actual usage of the term 'alcoholism', like 'addiction', has become primarily normative and prescriptive: a derogatory, stigmatizing word applied to people who drink 'too much'. The definition of 'too much' depends on the values of the speaker, which may be different from those of the person doing the drinking.

Calling addiction a 'disease' tells us more about the labeler than the labelee. Diseases are medical conditions. They can be discovered on the basis of bodily signs. They are something people have. They are involuntary. For example, the disease of syphilis was discovered. It is identified by specific signs. It is not a form of activity and is not based in human values. While certain behaviors increase the likelihood of acquiring syphilis, and while the acquisition of syphilis has consequences for subsequent social interaction, the behavior and the disease are separate phenomena. Syphilis meets the nosological criteria for disease classification in a pathology textbook. Unlike addiction, syphilis is a disease that can be diagnosed in a corpse.

Once we recognize that addiction cannot be classified as a literal disease, its nature as an ethical choice becomes clearer. A person starts, moderates, or abstains from drinking because that person wants to. People do the same thing with heroin, cocaine, and tobacco. Such choices reflect the person's values. The person, a moral agent, chooses to use drugs or refrains from using drugs because he or she finds meaning in doing so.

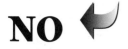
Alan I. Leshner

Addiction Is a Brain Disease

The United States is stuck in its drug abuse metaphors and in polarized arguments about them. Everyone has an opinion. One side insists that we must control supply, the other that we must reduce demand. People see addiction as either a disease or as a failure of will. None of this bumpersticker analysis moves us forward. The truth is that we will make progress in dealing with drug issues only when our national discourse and our strategies are as complex and comprehensive as the problem itself.

A core concept that has been evolving with scientific advances over the past decade is that drug addiction is a brain disease that develops over time as a result of the initially voluntary behavior of using drugs. The consequence is virtually uncontrollable compulsive drug craving, seeking, and use that interferes with, if not destroys, an individual's functioning in the family and in society. This medical condition demands formal treatment.

We now know in great detail the brain mechanisms through which drugs acutely modify mood, memory, perception, and emotional states. Using drugs repeatedly over time changes brain structure and function in fundamental and long-lasting ways that can persist long after the individual stops using them. Addiction comes about through an array of neuroadaptive changes and the laying down and strengthening of new memory connections in various circuits in the brain. We do not yet know all the relevant mechanisms, but the evidence suggests that those long-lasting brain changes are responsible for the distortions of cognitive and emotional functioning that characterize addicts, particularly including the compulsion to use drugs that is the essence of addiction. It is as if drugs have highjacked the brain's natural motivational control circuits, resulting in drug use becoming the sole, or at least the top, motivational priority for the individual. Thus, the majority of the biomedical community now considers addiction, in its essence, to be a brain disease: a condition caused by persistent changes in brain structure and function.

This brain-based view of addiction has generated substantial controversy, particularly among people who seem able to think only in polarized ways. Many people erroneously still believe that biological and behavioral explanations are alternative or competing ways to understand phenomena, when in fact they are complementary and integratable. Modern science has taught that it is much too simplistic to set biology in opposition to behavior or to pit willpower against brain chemistry. Addiction involves inseparable biological and behavioral components. It is the quintessential biobehavioral disorder.

Many people also erroneously still believe that drug addiction is simply a failure of will or of strength of character. Research contradicts that position. However, the recognition that addiction is a brain disease does not mean that the addict is simply a hapless victim. Addiction begins with the voluntary behavior of using drugs, and addicts must participate in and take some significant responsibility for their recovery. Thus, having this brain disease does not absolve the addict of responsibility for his or her behavior, but it does explain why an addict cannot simply stop using drugs by sheer force of will alone. It also dictates a much more sophisticated approach to dealing with the array of problems surrounding drug abuse and addiction in our society.

The Essence of Addiction

The entire concept of addiction has suffered greatly from imprecision and misconception. In fact, if it were possible, it would be best to start all over with some new, more neutral term. The confusion comes about in part because of a now archaic distinction between whether specific drugs are "physically" or "psychologically" addicting. The distinction historically revolved around whether or not dramatic physical withdrawal symptoms occur when an individual stops taking a drug; what we in the field now call "physical dependence."

However, 20 years of scientific research has taught that focusing on this physical versus psychological distinction is off the mark and a distraction from the real issues. From both clinical and policy perspectives, it actually does not matter very much what physical withdrawal symptoms occur. Physical dependence is not that important, because even the dramatic withdrawal symptoms of heroin and alcohol addiction can now be easily managed with appropriate medications. Even more important, many of the most dangerous and addicting drugs, including methamphetamine and crack cocaine, do not produce very severe physical dependence symptoms upon withdrawal.

What really matters most is whether or not a drug causes what we now know to be the essence of addiction: uncontrollable, compulsive drug craving, seeking, and use, even in the face of negative health and social consequences. This is the crux of how the Institute of Medicine, the American Psychiatric Association, and the American Medical Association define addiction and how we all should use the term. It is really only this compulsive quality of addiction that matters in the long run to the addict and to his or her family and that should matter to society as a whole. Compulsive craving that overwhelms all other motivations is the root cause of the massive health and social problems associated with drug addiction. In updating our national discourse on drug abuse, we should keep in mind this simple definition: Addiction is a brain disease expressed in the form of compulsive behavior. Both developing and recovering from it depend on biology, behavior, and social context.

It is also important to correct the common misimpression that drug use, abuse, and addiction are points on a single continuum along which one slides back and forth over time, moving from user to addict, then back to occasional user, then back to addict. Clinical observation and more formal research studies support the view that, once addicted, the individual has moved into a different state of being. It is as if a threshold has been crossed. Very few people appear able to successfully return to occasional use after having been truly addicted. Unfortunately, we do not yet have a clear biological or behavioral marker of that transition from voluntary drug use to addiction. However, a body of scientific evidence is rapidly developing that points to an array of cellular and molecular changes in specific brain circuits. Moreover, many of these brain changes are common to all chemical addictions, and some also are typical of other compulsive behaviors such as pathological overeating.

Addiction should be understood as a chronic recurring illness. Although some addicts do gain full control over their drug use after a single treatment episode, many have relapses. Repeated treatments become necessary to increase the intervals between and diminish the intensity of relapses, until the individual achieves abstinence.

The complexity of this brain disease is not atypical, because virtually no brain diseases are simply biological in nature and expression. All, including stroke, Alzheimer's disease, schizophrenia, and clinical depression, include some behavioral and social aspects. What may make addiction seem unique among brain diseases, however, is that it does begin with a clearly voluntary behavior—the initial decision to use drugs. Moreover, not everyone who ever uses drugs goes on to become addicted. Individuals differ substantially in how easily and quickly they become addicted and in their preferences for particular substances. Consistent with the biobehavioral nature of addiction, these individual differences result from a combination of environmental and biological, particularly genetic, factors. In fact, estimates are that between 50 and 70 percent of the variability in susceptibility to becoming addicted can be accounted for by genetic factors.

Over time the addict loses substantial control over his or her initially voluntary behavior, and it becomes compulsive. For many people these behaviors are truly uncontrollable, just like the behavioral expression of any other brain disease. Schizophrenics cannot control their hallucinations and delusions. Parkinson's patients cannot control their trembling. Clinically depressed patients cannot voluntarily control their moods. Thus, once one is addicted, the characteristics of the illness—and the treatment approaches—are not that different from most other brain diseases. No matter how one develops an illness, once one has it, one is in the diseased state and needs treatment.

Moreover, voluntary behavior patterns are, of course, involved in the etiology and progression of many other illnesses, albeit not all brain diseases. Examples abound, including hypertension, arteriosclerosis and other cardiovascular diseases, diabetes, and forms of cancer in which the onset is heavily influenced by the individual's eating, exercise, smoking, and other behaviors.

Addictive behaviors do have special characteristics related to the social contexts in which they originate. All of the environmental cues surrounding initial drug use and development of the addiction actually become "conditioned" to that drug use and are thus critical to the development and expression of addiction. Environmental cues are paired in time with an individual's initial drug use experiences and, through classical conditioning, take on conditioned stimulus properties. When those cues are present at a later time, they elicit anticipation of a drug experience and thus generate tremendous drug craving. Cue-induced craving is one of the most frequent causes of drug use relapses, even after long periods of abstinence, independently of whether drugs are available.

The salience of environmental or contextual cues helps explain why reentry to one's community can be so difficult for addicts leaving the controlled environments of treatment or correctional settings and why aftercare is so essential to successful recovery. The person who became addicted in the home environment is constantly exposed to the cues conditioned to his or her initial drug use, such as the neighborhood where he or she hung out, drug-using buddies, or the lamppost where he or she bought drugs. Simple exposure to those cues automatically triggers craving and can lead rapidly to relapses. This is one reason why someone who apparently overcame drug cravings while in prison or residential treatment could quickly revert to drug use upon returning home. In fact, one of the major goals of drug addiction treatment is to teach addicts how to deal with the cravings caused by inevitable exposure to these conditioned cues.

Implications

Understanding addiction as a brain disease has broad and significant implications for the public perception of addicts and their families, for addiction treatment practice, and for some aspects of public policy. On the other hand, this biomedical view of addiction does not speak directly to and is unlikely to bear significantly on many other issues, including specific strategies for controlling the supply of drugs and whether initial drug use should be legal or not. Moreover, the brain disease model of addiction does not address the question of whether specific drugs of abuse can also be potential medicines. Examples abound of drugs that can be both highly addicting and extremely effective medicines. The best-known example is the appropriate use of morphine as a treatment for pain. Nevertheless, a number of practical lessons can be drawn from the scientific understanding of addiction.

It is no wonder addicts cannot simply quit on their own.   They have an illness that requires biomedical treatment. People often assume that because addiction begins with a voluntary behavior and is expressed in the form of excess behavior, people should just be able to quit by force of will alone. However, it is essential to understand when dealing with addicts that we are dealing with individuals whose brains have been altered by drug use. They need drug addiction treatment. We know that, contrary to common belief, very few addicts actually do just stop on their own. Observing that there are very few heroin addicts in their 50 or 60s, people frequently ask what happened to those who were heroin addicts 30 years ago, assuming that they must have quit on their own. However, longitudinal studies find that only a very small fraction actually quit on their own. The rest have either been successfully treated, are currently in maintenance treatment, or (for about half) are dead. Consider the example of smoking cigarettes: Various studies have found that between 3 and 7 percent of people who try to quit on their own each year actually succeed. Science has at last convinced the public that depression is not just a lot of sadness; that depressed individuals are in a different brain state and thus require treatment to get their symptoms under control. The same is true for schizophrenic patients. It is time to recognize that this is also the case for addicts.

The role of personal responsibility is undiminished but clarified. Does having a brain disease mean that people who are addicted no longer have any responsibility for their behavior or that they are simply victims of their own genetics and brain chemistry? Of course not. Addiction begins with the voluntary behavior of drug use, and although genetic characteristics may predispose individuals to be more or less susceptible to becoming addicted, genes do not doom one to become an addict. This is one major reason why efforts to prevent drug use are so vital to any comprehensive strategy to deal with the nation's drug problems. Initial drug use is a voluntary, and therefore preventable, behavior.

Moreover, as with any illness, behavior becomes a critical part of recovery. At a minimum, one must comply with the treatment regimen, which is harder than it sounds. Treatment compliance is the biggest cause of relapses for all chronic illnesses, including asthma, diabetes, hypertension, and addiction. Moreover, treatment compliance rates are no worse for addiction than for these other illnesses, ranging from 30 to 50 percent. Thus, for drug addiction as well as for other chronic diseases, the individual's motivation and behavior are clearly important parts of success in treatment and recovery.

Implications for treatment approaches and treatment expectations. Maintaining this comprehensive biobehavioral understanding of addiction also speaks to what needs to be provided in drug treatment programs. Again, we must be careful not to pit biology against behavior. The National Institute on Drug Abuse's recently published *Principles of Effective Drug Addiction Treatment* provides a detailed discussion of how we must treat all aspects of the individual, not just the biological component or the behavioral component. As with other brain diseases such as schizophrenia and depression, the data show that the best drug addiction treatment approaches attend to the entire individual, combining the use of medications, behavioral therapies, and attention to necessary social services and rehabilitation. These might include such services as family therapy to enable the patient to return to successful family life, mental health services, education and vocational training, and housing services.

That does not mean, of course, that all individuals need all components of treatment and all rehabilitation services. Another principle of effective addiction treatment is that the array of services included in an individual's treatment plan must be matched to his or her particular set of needs. Moreover, since those needs will surely change over the course of recovery, the array of services provided will need to be continually reassessed and adjusted.

What to do with addicted criminal offenders. One obvious conclusion is that we need to stop simplistically viewing criminal justice and health approaches as incompatible opposites. The practical reality is that crime and drug addiction often occur in tandem: Between 50 and 70 percent of arrestees are addicted to illegal drugs. Few citizens would be willing to relinquish criminal justice system control over individuals, whether they are addicted or not, who have committed crimes against others. Moreover, extensive real-life experience shows that if we simply incarcerate addicted offenders without treating them, their return to both drug use and criminality is virtually guaranteed.

A growing body of scientific evidence points to a much more rational and effective blended public health/public safety approach to dealing with the addicted offender. Simply summarized, the data show that if addicted offenders are provided with well-structured drug treatment while under criminal justice control, their recidivism rates can be reduced by 50 to 60 percent for subsequent drug use and by more than 40 percent for further criminal behavior. Moreover, entry into drug treatment need not be completely voluntary in order for it to work. In fact, studies suggest that increased pressure to stay in treatment—whether from the legal system or from family members or employers—actually increases the amount of time patients remain in treatment and improves their treatment outcomes.

Findings such as these are the underpinning of a very important trend in drug control strategies now being implemented in the United States and many foreign countries. For example, some 40 percent of prisons and jails in this country now claim to provide some form of drug treatment to their addicted inmates, although we do not know the quality of the treatment provided. Diversion to drug treatment programs as an alternative to incarceration is gaining popularity across the United States. The widely applauded growth in drug treatment courts over the past five years—to more than 400—is another successful example of the blending of public health and public safety approaches. These drug courts use a combination of criminal justice sanctions and drug use monitoring and treatment tools to manage addicted offenders.

Updating the Discussion

Understanding drug abuse and addiction in all their complexity demands that we rise above simplistic polarized thinking about drug issues. Addiction is both a public health and a public safety issue, not one or the other. We must deal with both the supply and the demand issues with equal vigor. Drug abuse and addiction are about both biology and behavior. One can have a disease and not be a hapless victim of it.

We also need to abandon our attraction to simplistic metaphors that only distract us from developing appropriate strategies. I, for one, will be in some ways sorry to see the War on Drugs metaphor go away, but go away it must. At some level, the notion of waging war is as appropriate for the illness of addiction as it is for our War on Cancer, which simply means bringing all forces to bear on the problem in a focused and energized way. But, sadly, this concept has been badly distorted and misused over time, and the War on Drugs never became what it should have been: the War on Drug Abuse and Addiction. Moreover, worrying about whether we are winning or losing this war has deteriorated to using simplistic and inappropriate measures such as counting drug addicts. In the end, it has only fueled discord. The War on Drugs metaphor has done nothing to advance the real conceptual challenges that need to be worked through.

I hope, though, that we will all resist the temptation to replace it with another catchy phrase that inevitably will devolve into a search for quick or easy-seeming solutions to our drug problems. We do not rely on simple metaphors or strategies to deal with our other major national problems such as education, health care, or national security. We are, after all, trying to solve truly monumental, multidimensional problems on a national or even international scale. To devalue them to the level of slogans does our public an injustice and dooms us to failure.

Understanding the health aspects of addiction is in no way incompatible with the need to control the supply of drugs. In fact, a public health approach to stemming an epidemic or spread of a disease always focuses comprehensively on the agent, the vector, and the host. In the case of drugs of abuse, the agent is the drug, the host is the abuser or addict, and the vector for transmitting the illness is clearly the drug suppliers and dealers that keep the agent flowing so readily. Prevention and treatment are the strategies to help protect the host. But just as we must deal with the flies and mosquitoes that spread infectious diseases, we must directly address all the vectors in the drug-supply system.

In order to be truly effective, the blended public health/public safety approaches advocated here must be implemented at all levels of society—local, state, and national. All drug problems are ultimately local in character and impact, since they differ so much across geographic settings and cultural contexts, and the most effective solutions are implemented at the local level. Each community must work through its own locally appropriate antidrug implementation strategies, and those strategies must be just as comprehensive and science-based as those instituted at the state or national level.

The message from the now very broad and deep array of scientific evidence is absolutely clear. If we as a society ever hope to make any real progress in dealing with our drug problems, we are going to have to rise above moral outrage that addicts have "done it to themselves" and develop strategies that are as sophisticated and as complex as the problem itself. Whether addicts are "victims" or not, once addicted they must be seen as "brain disease patients."

Moreover, although our national traditions do argue for compassion for those who are sick, no matter how they contracted their illnesses, I recognize that many addicts have disrupted not only their own lives but those of their families and their broader communities, and thus do not easily generate compassion. However, no matter how one may feel about addicts and their behavioral histories, an extensive body of scientific evidence shows that approaching addiction as a treatable illness is extremely cost-effective, both financially and in terms of broader societal impacts such as family violence, crime, and other forms of social upheaval. Thus, it is clearly in everyone's interest to get past the hurt and indignation and slow the drain of drugs on society by enhancing drug use prevention efforts and providing treatment to all who need it.

POSTSCRIPT

Is Drug Addiction a Choice?

There is little debate that drug addiction is a major problem. Drug addiction wreaks havoc for society and ruins the lives of numerous individuals. The causes of drug addiction are divergent. Because drug abuse can be viewed as a matter of free will or as a brain disorder, there are also different views on how society should deal with drug abusers. Should drug addicts be incarcerated or treated?

One could argue that free will and the concept of a brain disorder both apply to drug addiction. What may start out as a matter of free will may turn into an illness. What may start out as an occasional behavior may become abusive. For example, a person may use alcohol for social purposes, but his or her use may develop into a chronic pattern—one that the person cannot easily overcome. Initially, one can stop using alcohol without too much discomfort. As time passes, however, and drinking becomes heavier, stopping for some becomes difficult. By its very definition, social drinkers can stop drinking at will. Alcoholics drink out of necessity.

Many people use addictive drugs and do not become dependent on them. Perhaps there are factors beyond free will and changes in the brain that account for those who become dependent. Is it possible that social factors come into play? Can friends and colleagues and their attitudes about drugs influence whether or not a drug user becomes a drug abuser? In the final analysis, drug addiction may result from the interaction of numerous factors and not simply be a dichotomy between psychology and biology.

Leshner states that there are 72 risk factors for drug abuse and addiction, although one may have many of these risk factors yet not become drug dependent. Not all risk factors are equally important, says Leshner. Stanton Peele, an outspoken critic of the disease concept, discusses this issue in "Hungry for the Next Fix," *Reason* (May 2002). Another article that explores whether or not addiction is a matter of biology is "Addiction and Responsibility," by Richard J. Bonnie, *Social Research* (Fall 2001). Sally Satel, in "The Fallacies of No-Fault Addiction," *The Public Interest* (Winter 1999), describes the views of numerous drug addiction experts. An article that contends that drug addiction is primarily genetic is Ronald Kotaluk's "Nearly Everyone Inherits Genetic Vulnerability to Drug Abuse," *Chicago Tribune* (March 14, 1999).

ISSUE 7

Are Athletes Who Use Anabolic Steroids Engaging in High-Risk Behavior?

YES: William N. Taylor, from *Anabolic Steroids and the Athlete,* 2d ed. (McFarland, 2002)

NO: Charles E. Yesalis, Michael S. Bahrke, and James E. Wright, from "Societal Alternatives," in Charles E. Yesalis, ed., *Anabolic Steroids in Sport and Exercise,* 2d ed. (Human Kinetics, 2000)

ISSUE SUMMARY

YES: Physician William N. Taylor opposes athletes using anabolic steroids due to the tremendous risks associated with the drugs. He argues that rather than helping themselves, many athletes are shortening their athletic careers because of the adverse effects of anabolic steroids and that many of the harmful effects of steroids may not be known for years.

NO: Charles E. Yesalis, a professor of health policy and administration, exercise, and sport science; acquisitions editor Michael S. Bahrke; and exercise physiologist James E. Wright acknowledge that there are problems with the use of steroids, but they assert that those problems are exaggerated. They also maintain that many of the problems related to steroids come from the lack of regulation of these drugs; the quality of illegally purchased anabolic steroids is questionable.

Anabolic steroids are synthetic derivatives of the male hormone testosterone. Although they have legitimate medical uses, steroids are increasingly being used by individuals to build up muscle quickly and to increase personal strength. Concerns over the potential negative effects of steroid use seem to be justified: an estimated 1 million Americans, half of whom are adolescents, have used illegally obtained steroids. Anabolic steroid users span all ethnic groups, nationalities, and socioeconomic groups. The emphasis on winning has led many athletes to take risks with steroids that are potentially destructive. Despite the widespread belief that anabolic steroids are used primarily by athletes, up to one-third of users are nonathletes who use these drugs to improve their physiques and self-images.

Society places much emphasis on winning, and to come out on top, many individuals are willing to make sacrifices—sacrifices that might compromise their health. Sports headlines in many newspapers mention how various athletes have used steroids. Because of widespread steroid use, drug testing is a major issue every time the Olympic competition is held. Besides the adverse physical consequences of steroids, there is the ethical question regarding fair play. Do steroids give competitors an unfair advantage? Should they be banned even if the side effects are *not* harmful? Do nonusers feel pressured to use these drugs to keep up with the competition?

The short-term consequences of anabolic steroids are well documented. Possible short-term effects among men include testicular atrophy, sperm count reduction, impotency, baldness, difficulty urinating, and breast enlargement. Among women, some potential effects are deepening of the voice, breast reduction, menstrual irregularities, the growth of body hair, and clitoral enlargement. Both sexes may develop acne, swelling in the feet, reduced levels of high-density lipoproteins (the type of cholesterol that is good for the body), hypertension, and liver damage. Taking steroids as an adolescent will stunt one's growth. Also related to steroid use are psychological changes, including mood swings, paranoia, and violent behavior.

Steroids' short-term effects have been researched thoroughly; however, their long-term effects have not been substantiated. The problem with identifying the long-term effects of anabolic steroids is the lack of systematic, long-term studies. Much of the information regarding steroids' long-term effects comes from personal reports, not well-conducted, controlled studies. However, personal stories and anecdotal evidence are often accepted as fact.

The American Medical Association opposes stricter regulation of anabolic steroids on two grounds. First, anabolic steroids have been used medically to improve growth and development and to treat certain types of anemia, breast cancer, endometriosis, and osteoporosis. If stricter regulations are imposed, people who might benefit medically from these drugs will have more difficulty acquiring them. Second, it is highly unlikely that illicit use of these drugs will cease if they are banned. By maintaining legal access to these drugs, more studies regarding their long-term consequences can be conducted.

In the following selections, William N. Taylor contends that people who use anabolic steroids are risking their lives as well as their athletic careers. He maintains that stricter control of these substances is essential. Charles E. Yesalis, Michael S. Bahrke, and James E. Wright argue that the effects of steroids are overstated. They do not advocate the use of steroids, but they argue that better regulation of these drugs can occur if they are legal. Obtaining anabolic steroids through a legitimate pharmaceutical company, they conclude, is far better than buying steroids from a questionable source.

William N. Taylor

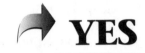

Adverse Physical Effects Associated With Anabolic Steroid Abuse

Introduction: Anabolic Steroid Abuse: A Dangerous "Breakfast of Champions"

Clinical doses of anabolic steroids for medically supervised patients are as safe and effective as any other prescription drug. This is strongly emphasized, *anabolic steroids when taken in clinically approved doses under medical supervision are both effective and safe!* However, the prolonged abuse of anabolic steroids in doses well above the clinically acceptable is a dangerous "breakfast of champions."

Since the peak of the anabolic steroid epidemic in the early 1990s, evidence of the adverse physical effects of anabolic steroid abuse by athletes and bodybuilders has been mounting. The available information has come from cross-sectional, short-term longitudinal, and case studies. To fully investigate the adverse physical effects the needs are: a) to develop a comprehensive battery of sensitive and specific markers of the adverse effects, particularly ones able to detect the onset of adverse reactions; and, b) to conduct controlled and long-term longitudinal studies designed to understand the mechanisms involved in the doses and duration regimes athletes employ that cause adverse physical effects.

Anabolic steroids function as hormones, and when abused have potentially detrimental effects on many of the body's systems, including the hepatic (liver), endocrine, cardiovascular, reproductive, neuroendocrine, and immune systems. There is a wide range of concomitant temporary and permanent adverse effects that can occur with high-dose anabolic steroid use. Several adverse reactions may develop rapidly, within several weeks or less, while others require several years of anabolic steroid intake. Recent case studies of athletic anabolic steroid users indicate a plethora of adverse physical effects.

Anabolic Steroid-Induced Risk-Taking Behaviors

There are over 50 prescription drugs that pose potential adverse drug interactions when taken simultaneously (and unknowingly to the physician) with anabolic steroids. This can place both medical care providers and anabolic steroid users in danger. A recent study reported that among patients who receive frequent medical care and are prescribed an assortment of prescription drugs, less than one-third of anabolic steroid users inform their physicians about their anabolic steroid use. The anabolic steroid users who are prescribed prescription drugs and do not inform their physicians may be making a deadly mistake.

It is impossible to discuss the potential risks associated with anabolic use without discussing anabolic steroid–induced risk-taking behaviors. Anabolic steroid abuse promotes the use of a variety of prescription drugs without medical supervision in an attempt to treat the pesky anabolic steroid–induced side effects. Anabolic steroid users also use non-prescription drugs and substances, both legal and illegal ones, This polypharmacy behavior is practiced by over 80 percent of anabolic steroid users. Anabolic steroid users also consume dramatically more alcohol and demonstrate higher rates of binge drinking than do non-users. In addition, anabolic steroid users are more likely to use tobacco products, marijuana, cocaine, amphetamines, sedatives, hallucinogens, heroin and other opiates, inhalants, and designer drugs. Recently it has been reported that anabolic steroid use can be a gateway to opioid dependence, including heroin.

For anabolic steroid users, experimentation with other drugs can be a lethal mixture. Of great concern is the use of gamma-hydroxybutyrate (GHB) as a "bodybuilding supplement" and rave party drug. A number of deaths and near-deaths have occurred when anabolic steroid users took GHB. Homicides, suicides, and lethal poisonings have been implicated, due to disinhibited behavior, in the deaths of dozens of anabolic steroid users.

The out-of-control aggressive behavior seen in some anabolic steroid users can result in negligent homicide, especially when a user exhibits this behavior in an automobile. Police officers on anabolic steroids act in aberrant, erratic, and bizarre manners when engaged in automobile chases and brutality excursions, some of which end with lethal consequences. Imagine the disastrous results occurring from the combination of anabolic steroid–using police officers attempting to apprehend anabolic steroid–using assailants.

Another potentially lethal form of anabolic steroid–induced risk-taking behavior is the spread of life-threatening and often lethal infections. Needle and multi-dose vial sharing have been reported among anabolic steroid users resulting in the transmission of viral hepatitis, AIDS, bacterial, and fungal infections.

Perhaps the most common result of the risk-taking behaviors of anabolic steroid users is incarceration. America's prison system is overloaded with anabolic steroid users who have acted in risky and violent manners. Child sexual abuse and murder has a high correlation with anabolic-androgenic steroid use.

A recent study evaluating high-risk behaviors of high school students found that anabolic steroid use was associated with all the high-risk categories studied. These high-risk behaviors included risky sexual behavior, suicidal behaviors, not wearing a passenger seat belt, riding a motorcycle without a helmet, driving and drinking, fighting, and carrying a weapon.

Underreporting of Anabolic Steroid–Induced Adverse Effects

Anabolic steroid users eventually seek medical attention. However, the true incidence of adverse physical effects due to anabolic steroid self-use is unknown. This has resulted in an underreporting by physicians and researchers. The reasons for this phenomenon include:

a) the fact that nearly two-thirds of anabolic steroid users do not inform their primary physicians of their use;

b) the fact that over 80 percent of anabolic steroid users take other drugs along with their anabolic steroid use;

c) the fact that many anabolic steroid users deny their use;

d) the fact that local, regional and state laboratories, including those used by coroners and medical examiners, do not have the means to test for anabolic steroids;

e) the fact that many physicians do not ask their patients about anabolic steroid use;

f) the fact that some physicians are unaware of some or all of the potential health risks of anabolic steroids and do not know how to recognize use in their patients. This is illustrated by reports indicating "no side effects" with prolonged anabolic steroid use, or "the incidence of serious health problems associated with the use of androgens by athletes has been overstated"; and,

g) the fact that there is still a substantial "credibility gap" between anabolic steroid users and physicians. Some physicians still believe that anabolic steroids are just placebos or "fool's gold" for athletes.

Despite these shortcomings, considerable progress has been made in identifying the adverse physical effects associated with anabolic steroid use. In this [selection], these adverse physical effects will be arbitrarily divided into categories even though some of the adverse effects are more of a continuum of factors that may take years to fully develop. These categories include: lethal, serious and life-threatening, serious but not life-threatening, and less serious adverse physical effects.

Lethal Adverse Physical Effects

A number of adverse anabolic steroid–induced effects are lethal. Most of these lethal effects have involved the cardiovascular system and have been reported in case studies. The cases that have occurred in young (ages 20–39) anabolic steroid users include:

a) sudden death from myocardial infarction (heart attack),

b) sudden death from pulmonary embolism (blood clot in the lungs),

c) sudden death from cerebral edema and cerebellar hemorrhage (stroke),

d) sudden death from intra-abdominal hemorrhage, and,

e) sudden death from suicides, homicides, and accidental drug overdoses.

These published reports probably represent just the tip of a huge iceberg. When anabolic steroid users die of cardiovascular insult, suicide, homicide, or accidental drug overdose, it is usually very difficult to obtain an accurate history. Since anabolic steroid users tend to hang out together, the surviving users deny anabolic steroid use as a possible factor, especially if the survivors are dealing anabolic steroids, since an admission could implicate them in murder, practicing medicine without a license, or dealing in controlled substances.

There is no doubt that some anabolic steroid users have died and will die of heart attacks caused by the drugs. Some will die early from a sudden death from myocardial infarction while others will die later due to the acceleration of atherogenic effects.

There are at least five hypothetical mechanisms of anabolic steroid–induced adverse cardiovascular effects. These include:

a) an atherogenic (plaque-forming) model involving the effects of anabolic steroids on lipoprotein concentrations in the blood;

b) a thrombus (clot) model involving the effects of anabolic steroids on clotting factors and platelets;

c) a vasospasm (spasm of the arteries) model involving the effects of anabolic steroids on the vascular nitric oxide system;

d) a direct myocardial injury model involving the effects of anabolic steroids on myocardial cells; and,

e) a combination of all of the above models.

Besides the acute nature of the adverse lethal conditions, anabolic steroid users also show an increase in premature mortality rates. A recent study compared mortality rates of non-users to elite anabolic steroid–using power-lifters from Finland. A 12-year follow-up study was conducted on 62 of the power-lifters. The study results showed that the premature death rate of the anabolic steroid–using powerlifters was 12.9 percent compared to 3.1 percent of non-users. Eight of the 62 anabolic steroid users died before the age of 40 years. The causes of the premature death among the anabolic steroid users were: suicide (3), acute myocardial infarction (3), hepatic coma (1), and non-Hodgkin's lymphoma (1).

Evidence is mounting that indicates a strong correlation between anabolic steroid abuse and premature death. Some of these serious and life-threatening adverse physical effects leading to premature death are discussed in the next section.

Serious and Life-Threatening Adverse Physical Effects

Liver Conditions and Other Cancers

It has been known for decades that patients who have been treated with high-dose prolonged anabolic steroid therapy have been at a greater risk for liver cancer and other serious liver conditions. These include peliosis hepatitis,

hepatomas, hepatocellular carcinomas, hepatitis, severe cholestasis, hepatic angiosarcoma, and fatal hepatic coma.

Long-term anabolic steroid use is the fourth leading cause of a highly
lethal form of liver cancer, hepatic angiosarcoma. Peliosis hepatitis is a condition that describes the presence of blood-filled sacs or spaces within the liver.
Documented case reports of severe liver abnormalities and other types of cancers suggest that these conditions occur in anabolic steroid users. These conditions, while currently considered rare, include:

a) hepatocellular carcinoma (liver cancer),

b) severe cholestasis (bile build up in the liver),

c) renal cell carcinoma (kidney cancer),

d) intratesticular leiomyosarcoma (rare form of testicular cancer), and,

e) adenocarcinoma of the prostate (prostate cancer).

Some argue that the underlying diseases and not anabolic steroids are responsible for these conditions.

Serious Cardiovascular Conditions

As previously presented, anabolic steroid use can cause lethal cardiovascular
events. It can also cause other cardiovascular conditions that can be life threatening. Documented case reports of these cardiovascular events in young anabolic steroid users include:

a) severe coronary artery disease,

b) severe cardiomyopathy (weakening of the heart muscle),

c) congestive heart failure and ventricular fibrillation (irregular heart
   beating),

d) cardiac tamponade (blood that accumulates in the space between the
   heart muscle and the outer heart lining preventing the heart from
   properly beating),

e) ascending aortic dissection (tearing of the muscle lining of the aorta).

These life-threatening cardiovascular events occur in some young anabolic steroid users, and are currently considered rare events.

Serious, Non–Life Threatening Adverse Physical Effects

A number of anabolic steroid–induced conditions are serious and may even require surgical intervention and rehabilitation. Others, such as serious viral infections, may require prolonged medical care and may lead to premature death.

Over the past decade a number of serious, non−life threatening conditions have been reported in case studies of anabolic steroid users. These serious, non−life threatening conditions include:

a) avascular necrosis of the femoral heads. Avascular necrosis means that the blood supply to a region (in these cases the head of the femur) has been disrupted resulting in tissue (femoral head) death. Treatment is usually a surgical hip replacement. Avascular necrosis of the femoral head has been associated with high-dose corticosteroid therapy and trauma. Bo Jackson, a college Heisman Trophy winner, NFL and MLB player, had this condition. After receiving an artificial hip, he continued to play professional baseball for a short while, but his athletic career was both limited and shortened by avascular necrosis.

b) spontaneous rupture of the anterior cruciate ligament of the knee. This is a condition almost always associated with significant trauma. The anterior cruciate ligament provides major support for the knee joint. Even with surgical intervention, a ruptured anterior cruciate ligament can be a career-ending injury for an athlete.

c) atrial fibrillation (a non-lethal heart beat abnormality).

d) systemic lupus erythematosus (SLE). This disease can affect nearly every system in the body. It is thought to be initiated by a disruption of or abnormality in the immune system. Patients with SLE usually have severely abbreviated life spans.

e) multi-compartment syndrome following surgery. In several areas of the body, muscles are contained by fibrous tissue, thus compartmentalized. When large muscles swell, usually due to trauma, there is very little room available for the swelling processes to occur. Blood and nerve supply to the compartment may be compromised due to the mounting pressure within the compartment. This is a condition that may require emergency surgical intervention.

f) spinal epidural lipomatosis with radiculopathy. This is a rare condition in which excess fat tissue is deposited circumferentially about the epidural space in the spinal cord. It is most commonly seen in patients on chronic corticosteroid therapy for a variety of medical conditions. This condition can cause muscle weakness and chronic pain.

g) neuropathies of the upper extremities. This condition (in these cases) is probably caused by excessive muscle enlargement squeezing the nerves to the muscles in the upper extremities. This condition can cause muscle weakness and chronic pain.

These case studies represent areas where physicians have linked anabolic steroid use with adverse physical conditions. It is likely that these studies represent only a small portion of the adverse physical effects caused by anabolic steroid use. The true incidence of these conditions is unknown.

Less Serious Physical Health Risks

Anabolic steroid use can cause alterations in almost every system within the body because cellular receptors for these drugs are in almost every tissue in the body. Therefore, it should not be surprising that many of these alterations appear as qualitative or quantitative adverse effects. Some of these adverse effects are seen only in male users or are more prevalent in males than females.

In general, the less severe anabolic steroid–induced adverse effects are dose and duration related. However, there is a wide variance to this generality. Less severe adverse effects may occur in one user and not another. These side effects may occur in moderate doses in some users but require larger doses in others. In short, anabolic steroid abuse is a form of self-experimentation with controlled substances.

There are hundreds of scientific articles that report adverse effects of a less serious nature in anabolic steroid users. Many of these are listed in Tables 1 and 2.

Summary: Anabolic Steroid Abuse Is "'Roid" Roulette

In this [selection] the adverse physical effects that anabolic steroid users can and have experienced have been presented. No other form of drug abuse has such a wide variety of associated adverse physical effects. Some of these effects

Table 1

Minor Abnormalities Due to Anabolic Steroid Use in Men

Hypertension	Disturbances in sleep cycles
Acne	Increased appetite
Fluid retention	Gynecomastia
Abnormal liver function tests	Deepening of the voice
Reduction in testicular size & function	Increased sebaceous gland size and secretion
Psychological disturbances	Viral illness after steroid cessation
Penile enlargement	Increased energy level
Increased libido	Cessation of mental depression
Changes in hair growth & distribution	Rebound resetting of hormonal balance
Epistaxis (nose bleeds)	Increased aggressiveness
Alterations in coping mechanisms	Withdrawal reduction in libido
Withdrawal depression	Atherogenic lipoprotein profiles
Altered thyroid function tests	Altered immune system tests
Altered healing capacity for injuries	Increased bone mineral density
Reduced inhibitions for risky behaviors	Abnormal blood clotting tests
Increased risk for drug abuse	Increased hemoglobin concentration
Benign prostate enlargement	Heart enlargement

Table 2

Minor Abnormalities Due to Anabolic Steroid Self-Use in Women

Hypertension	Disturbance in sleep cycles
Acne	Increased appetite
Fluid retention	Reduction in body fat
Abnormal liver function tests	Menstrual disturbances
Psychological disturbances	Increased energy level
Reduction in breast tissue	Deepening tone of the voice
Clitoral enlargement and sensitivity	Cessation of mental depression
Epistaxis (nose bleeds)	Increased aggression
Changes in hair growth and distribution	Increased sebaceous gland size and secretion
Viral illness after steroid cessation	Withdrawal depression
Ruddiness of the face	Rebound estrogenization
Increased muscle vascularity	Withdrawal reduction in libido
Abnormal liver function tests	Atherogenic lipoprotein profiles
Altered thyroid function tests	Altered immune system tests
Reduced inhibitions for risky behaviors	Abnormal blood clotting tests
Altered endocrine function tests	Increased risk for drug abuse
Altered healing capacity from injuries	Increased hemoglobin concentration
Increased libido and orgasmic responses	Increased bone mineral density
Heart enlargement	

---

can be lethal and some of them, while chronic, are life shortening nonetheless. Other side effects are more benign, subtle, or minor irritations. No one can predict which adverse physical effects will happen to any given user.

Anabolic steroid use is endocrine experimentation. No qualified endocrinologist would ever perform such experimentation with patients. Every anabolic steroid user is participating in an experiment that could lead to lethal and or legal consequences. The fallout of these experiments is accumulating. Some of the health consequences of these self-experiments will not be known for a decade or more.

The use of anabolic steroids is unsafe. It sets bad examples for society. For a select few lucky users, anabolic steroids *are* the breakfast of champions. For the rest, their abuse is a health hazard, a "'roid roulette." Have body image and athletic fame, fortune, and glory reached the point in society that we must continue to bet our health and futures on the "'roid" roulette wheel? Sadly, for many, it is probably so.

Charles E. Yesalis, Michael S. Bahrke, and James E. Wright

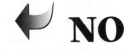 **NO**

Societal Alternatives

When the first edition of this book [*Anabolic Steroids in Sport and Exercise*] was published in 1993, this chapter opened with a quote from Robert Voy, MD (1991), former Chief Medical Officer of the U.S. Olympic Committee:

> If we will have reached a point of no return with this win at all costs attitude, the gold medals won't shine as brightly, the flags won't wave as boldly, the torch will flicker dimly, and we will have lost one of the greatest treasures ever known.

With this second edition, it appears that Dr. Voy's predictions have already come to pass. In 1998 alone, the public was bombarded with continual reports of drug scandals (Dickey, Helmstaedt, Nordland, & Hayden, 1999; "Drug Trial, Take II," 1998; "Snowboarder Loses Medal," 1998; "Drugs and Cycling," 1998; "Track Star Blazed Trail," 1998), including the following:

1. Chinese swimmers being ejected from the World Championships in Australia after having tested positive for banned substances.
2. Former East German coaches and physicians tried for their roles in the systematic doping of East German athletes over three decades.
3. Canadian snowboarder Ross Rebagliati testing positive for marijuana after having won a gold medal at the Winter Olympics in Nagano, Japan.
4. Olympic gold medalist Michelle Smith de Bruin accused of "manipulating" her urine sample in an out-of-competition drug test.
5. Cyclists, coaches, physicians, and trainers participating in the Tour de France implicated in a widespread, systematic doping scheme.
6. Olympic champion Randy Barnes testing positive for androstenedione.
7. Home run king Mark McGwire admitting the use of androstenedione.
8. Olympic champion Florence Griffith Joyner dying at age 38. Rumors of prior performance-enhancing drug use that surrounded her victories at the Seoul Olympic Games are resurrected.

9. Uta Pippig, three-time winner of the Boston Marathon, testing positive for a high level of testosterone.
10. Australian Open champion Petr Korda testing positive for an anabolic steroid.

When discussing the problem of performance-enhancing drug use, it is important to remember that sport is a microcosm of our society and the problems in sport are not limited to drug use. During the 1980s, 57 of 106 universities in Division I-A were punished by the NCAA via sanctions, censure, or probation for rule violations (Leaderman, 1990). These offenses did not involve illicit drug use by athletes but rather the unethical behavior of coaches, athletic administrators, staff, and faculty, the very men and women who should be setting the example. More recently, collegiate athletes have been convicted of criminal offences related to sports gambling (Lassar, 1998; Saum, 1998). In addition, an NCAA survey of 2,000 Division I male football and basketball players found 72% had gambled in some form, and 25% reported gambling on collegiate sports; 4% bet on games in which they played (Saum, 1998; "Study: Gambling in NCAA Rampant," 1999). Among members of the International Olympic Committee (IOC), bribery, graft, and other corruption appear entrenched in the culture of the organization (Simson & Jennings, 1992; Swift, 1999). A common factor among all these scandals is money. In the 1990s there is no doubt sport has become a multinational industry of huge proportions. The IOC, NCAA, NFL, NBA, and MLB, among others, are all billion-dollar businesses ("A Survey of Sport," 1998; Hiestand, 1999).

A free society relies on the news media to inform the populace of the incidence and magnitude of social problems such as doping in sport. Even though the epidemic of drug use in sport has been common knowledge among insiders, the news media, especially in the United States, have not engaged in a widespread concerted effort to chronicle this issue. Unfortunately the media, in particular television news, are often influenced by conflicts of interest within their parent companies between those reporting the news and those responsible for the broadcast of major sporting events. Few would argue that an in-depth exposé of drug use, for example, in the NFL or the Olympics, would enhance the marketing of these highly lucrative sporting events.

Before any effort can be made to address the issue of doping in sport, it is critical that all of the stakeholders acknowledge that a problem exists. In this regard, we need to fully appreciate the high entertainment value placed on sport by society. Some go so far as to argue that sport is the opiate of the masses—a contention made earlier by Karl Marx regarding religion. If sport has become the opiate of the masses, then we must be prepared for the public to be indifferent to drug use in sport, at least at the elite level. Moreover, it could be argued that if substantial progress is made in the fight against epidemic doping, fans may express anger, rather than appreciation, toward those fighting drug use. Many people view competitive sports to escape from the problems of daily life and do not wish to be confronted with the moral and ethical aspects of doping. Besides, if antidoping efforts are successful, the once bigger-than-life idols could begin to appear all too human in stature and the eclipsing of records at national, Olympic, and world levels could become so rare that the fervor of fans would wane and the business of sports would suffer. Even high school sport appears to be expanding as a source of entertainment for adults, as shown by the increasing level of television coverage of high school football and basketball games. Consequently, it can be argued that the growth of the high school sport entertainment business is contributing to the increase in anabolic steroid use among adolescents during the 1990s.

Sport has also been used by governments as a tool to control the masses or as justification for their social, political, and economic systems. "Bread and circuses" (panem et circenses) were used in this fashion by the emperors of Rome (Benario, 1983). Nazi Germany, the Soviet Union, East Germany, and Communist China all used sport for political advantage (Hoberman, 1984). Consequently, such governments, arguably, would be less than enthusiastic participants in the fight against doping or, for that matter, even in publicly acknowledging the existence of widespread doping. On the contrary, there is a reasonable amount of evidence that the governments of the Soviet Union, East Germany, and Communist China all played significant roles in the systematic doping of their athletes.

With many societal problems, identifying potential solutions is easy, but agreeing on a proper course of action and successfully completing it are difficult. The following are our alternatives for dealing with the use of anabolic steroids and other performance-enhancing drugs: legalization, interdiction, education, and alteration of societal values and attitudes related to physical appearance and winning in sport.

Legalization: An End to Hypocrisy?

The legalization of illicit drugs has for some time been the subject of heated debate: comments range from "morally reprehensible" to "accepting reality." Legalization would reduce the law enforcement costs associated with illicit anabolic steroid use as well as the substantial cost of drug testing. Even some opponents of legalization must concede that such an action would lessen the level of hypocrisy in sport. It can be argued that society and sports federations have turned a blind eye or have subtly encouraged drug use in sport as long as the athletes have not been caught or spoken publicly about their use of anabolic steroids (Bamberger & Yaeger, 1997; Dubin, 1990; Lemonick, 1998; "Drugs and Cycling," 1998; "Longtime Drug Use," 1999; Voy, 1990; Yesalis & Friedl, 1988).

Legalization of anabolic steroid use in sport would involve two levels of authority. At one level, federal and state laws related to the possession, distribution, and prescription of anabolic steroids would have to be changed. If in the future anabolic steroids become an accepted means of contraception or as treatment for "andropause," it is difficult to understand how anabolic steroids could remain a Schedule III controlled substance. At the second level, bans on anabolic steroids now in place in virtually every sport would have to be rescinded. Legalization would bring cries that the traditional ideals of sport and competition were being further eroded. On the other hand, given the continued litany of drug and other sport scandals (see above) that have taken pace in full public view, it is hard to imagine in this jaundiced age that many people believe that the so-called traditional ideals in elite sports even exist.

It has long been asserted that the legalization of anabolic steroids would force athletes to further expose themselves to possible physical harm or else to compete at a disadvantage. Others have even questioned the basic premise that banning drugs in sport benefits the health of athletes and have argued that "the ban has in fact increased health risks by denying users access to medical advice and caused users to turn to high risk black market sources" (Black, 1996).

Further, legalization would allow athletes to use pharmaceutical grade steroids while being monitored by a physician. It can also be argued that the "danger" of steroid use is not, in itself, a realistic deterrent given the existing levels of tobacco, alcohol, and other illicit drug use.

In 1999 it seems that legalization of anabolic steroid use in sport is not acceptable. However, if the impotence of drug testing, now in full public view, persists for much longer, it is easy to imagine the IOC or other sport federations throwing up their hands in frustration and allowing the athlete with the best chemist to prevail.

Interdiction: A Question of Cost-Effectiveness

The U.S. federal government and all state governments currently have laws regarding the distribution, possession, or prescription of anabolic steroids (USDHHS, 1991). The Federal Food, Drug, and Cosmetic Act (FFDCA) was amended as part of the Anti-Drug Abuse Act of 1988 such that distribution of steroids or possession of steroids with intent to distribute without a valid prescription became a felony. This legislation not only increased the penalties for the illicit distribution of steroids but also facilitated prosecution under the FFDCA. In 1990 the Anabolic Steroids Control Act was signed into law by President [George H. W.] Bush and added anabolic steroids to Schedule III of the Controlled Substances Act. This law institutes a regulatory and criminal enforcement system whereby the Drug Enforcement Administration (DEA) controls the manufacture, importation, exportation, distribution, and dispensing of anabolic steroids. However, the act did not provide extra resources to the DEA to shoulder the added responsibility.

Furthermore, as the use of anabolic steroids is increasingly criminalized, drug use will likely be driven further underground, and the source of the drugs will increasingly be clandestine laboratories, the products of which are of questionable quality. It also appears that in some areas criminalization has already altered the distribution network for anabolic steroids; athletes used to sell to other athletes, but sellers of street drugs are now becoming a major source (U.S. Department of Justice, 1994).

Even though the legal apparatus to control steroid trafficking exists, enforcement agents already are struggling to handle the problems of importation, distribution, sales, and use of other illicit drugs such as cocaine and heroin (U.S. Department of Justice, 1994). Based on what we know about the physical, psychological, or social effects of steroids, it is neither realistic nor prudent that enforcement efforts for steroids take precedent over those for more harmful drugs. On the other hand, this line of reasoning should not be used as a rationale for a lack of effective action against steroids. Nevertheless, the outlook that limited resources can be stretched to cover yet another class of drugs is not optimistic (U.S. Department of Justice, 1994), especially given the increase in recreational drug use among adolescents (Office of Applied Studies, 1999). The availability of anabolic steroids in this country suggests there is some reason to believe the United States may simply not have sufficient law enforcement personnel to deal with apprehending and punishing sellers of anabolic steroids and other performance-enhancing drugs.

Nonetheless, between February 1991 and February 1995, 355 anabolic steroid investigations were initiated by the DEA (Yesalis & Cowart, 1998). There have been more than 400 arrests, and more than 200 defendants have been convicted. However, because of the way criminal penalties were developed for steroid infractions, an individual brought to court on charges of distribution or selling must be a national-level dealer to receive more than a "slap on the wrist" and perhaps a short visit to a "country club" prison. For this reason, law enforcement agents often do not bother pursuing small cases because the costs of prosecution vastly outweigh any penalties that will be assessed.

Drug testing by sport federations is yet another form of interdiction. Such testing has been partially successful when directed at performance-enhancing drugs that, to be effective, must be in the body at the time of competition, such as stimulants and narcotics. . . . [D]rug testing has been even less effective against anabolic steroids that are used during training or used to enhance an athlete's capacity to train. Testing can be circumvented by the steroid user in several ways. Generally, to avoid a positive test, athletes can determine when to discontinue use prior to a scheduled test, or, in the case of an unannounced test, they titrate their dose using transdermal patches or skin creams containing testosterone so as to remain below the maximum allowable level. Further confounding the testing are other drugs used by athletes, such as human growth hormone and erythropoietin, for which no effective tests currently exist. Moreover, testing for anabolic steroids is expensive (approx. $120 per test), and although organizations like the IOC, NFL, or NCAA may be able to institute such procedures, the cost is prohibitive for the vast majority of secondary schools. Consequently, only a handful of secondary school systems test for anabolic steroids.

In summary, although interdiction through law enforcement and drug testing has intuitive appeal, its impact on the nonmedical use of anabolic steroids and other performance-enhancing drugs is open to debate. Since the flurry of legislative activity at the state and national levels regarding the control of the manufacture, distribution, prescription, and possession of steroids in the late 1980s and the early 1990s, use among adolescents has increased significantly. As for the future of testing, it is difficult to be optimistic: over the past 30 years, drug users have consistently outplayed the drug testers. In addition, one can only speculate as to the future challenges to testing created by impending advances in genetic engineering. Will we be able to genetically enhance muscle mass, aerobic capacity, vision, and neurological response (Barton-Davis, Shoturma, Musaro, Rosenthal, & Sweeney, 1998)?

Education: Is Anybody Listening?

Since the 1980s, the U.S. Public Health Service, the U.S. Department of Education, as well as many state education departments, state and local medical societies, private foundations, and sport federations have been involved in prevention efforts related to steroid abuse. For the most part, these have centered on the development and distribution of educational materials and programs such as posters, videos, pamphlets, and workshops. For example, the Iowa High School Athletic Association has developed an educational booklet that provides information on the effects of steroid use, but also includes strength-enhancing alternatives to steroids and prevention ideas (Beste, 1991). The U.S. Department of Education and other sources have developed a variety of informational posters targeted at high school students to provide facts about steroids, their adverse effects, alternatives to their use, and their illegal status (American Academy of Orthopaedic Surgeons; U.S. Department of Health & Human Services [USDHHS], 1988). Video distributors now have a wide range of videotape programs available on steroid use prevention as well as bodybuilding techniques (William C. Brown Communications Inc., 1993). Educational consulting firms provide antisteroid training, program, and curriculum development to junior and senior high schools across the United States (Griffin & Svendsen, 1990; Harding Ringhofer, 1993). Major television networks have presented special programming targeted at adolescent audiences to relay the possible consequences of steroid use (*ABC Afterschool Special:* "Testing Dirty" and *CBS Schoolbreak Special:* "The Fourth Man"; Disney Educational Productions: "Benny and the Roids").

Health educators have made some inroads in changing several high-risk behaviors, such as high-fat diets, sedentary lifestyles, and smoking. Educators are well armed with vast quantities of scientific data regarding the deleterious nature of these activities. Furthermore, these are behaviors on which society has increasingly frowned. In sports, on the other hand, athletes who use anabolic steroids have enjoyed significant improvements in physical performance and appearance. Society is much less likely to shun these people. The adulation of fans, the media, and peers is a strong secondary reinforcement, as are financial, material, and sexual rewards.

Another fly in the education ointment is the possibility that anabolic steroids taken intermittently in low to moderate doses may have only a negligible impact on health, at least in the short term. In 1989, several experts at the National Steroid Consensus Meeting concluded that according to the existing evidence, these drugs represent more of an ethical dilemma than a public health problem (Yesalis, Wright, & Lombardo, 1989). Although there is still little available evidence regarding the long-term health effects of anabolic steroids, many current or potential anabolic steroid users unfortunately mistake absence of evidence for evidence of absence. Even more frustrating is the fact that in two national studies, a substantial minority of the anabolic steroid users surveyed expressed no intention to stop using anabolic steroids if deleterious health effects were unequivocally established (Yesalis, Herrick, Buckley, Friedl, Brannon, & Wright, 1988; Yesalis, Streit, Vicary, Friedl, Brannon, & Buckley, 1989). Clearly, the paucity of scientific information has impeded the formulation of effective health education strategies. Far more than that, the unsubstantiated claims of dire health effects made by some in sports medicine and sensationalized by the news media have further eroded communication between athletes and doctors. However, even if long-term deleterious effects were well documented for anabolic steroids, our experience with teenagers and smoking suggests that substantial abuse would probably persist (Centers for Disease Control and Prevention, 1994; U.S. Department of Health and Human Services, 1989).

All of these problems and limitations in developing and disseminating effective prevention and intervention strategies could largely explain the significant increase in anabolic steroid use among adolescents since 1990.

Changing a behavior that has resulted in major benefits to the user, such as improved appearance and athletic performance, presents a monumental challenge. Traditional cognitive and affective education approaches to tobacco, alcohol, and drug abuse prevention have not been effective (Schaps, Bartolo, Moskowitz, Palley, & Churgin, 1981). In fact, there is evidence that providing a prevention program that uses "scare tactics" to dissuade adolescents from becoming involved with anabolic steroids may actually lead to increased usage, possibly because additional information stimulated curiosity (Goldberg, Bents, Bosworth, Trevisan, & Elliot, 1991). This observation helped lead to a prevention program (ATLAS) focused, in part, on positive educational initiatives related to nutrition and strength training. The program also focused on increasing adolescents' awareness of the types of social pressures they are likely to encounter to use anabolic steroids, and attempts to "inoculate" them against these pressures. Adolescents are taught specific skills for effectively resisting both peer and media pressures to use anabolic steroids. Periodic monitoring and reporting of actual anabolic steroid use among adolescents was conducted in an effort to dispel misinformation concerning the widespread use of anabolic steroids among peers. Using peers as program leaders is an additional component. This program has been successful in significantly affecting attitudes and behaviors related to steroid use and remained effective over several years (Goldberg et al., 1996).

Unfortunately, the generalizability of the ATLAS program is open to question. The program focused on male high school football players and was not designed specifically to address anabolic steroid use among teenage girls, whose rate of steroid use . . . has doubled since 1990. In addition, the long-term effectiveness of this school-based program is still unknown and the program has yet to be replicated in other states. Moreover, there are two important and, as yet, unanswered questions regarding the ATLAS program. First, are school boards, in an age of constrained resources, willing to commit time and money to this relatively demanding program? Efficacy aside, it would be far easier and cheaper to continue to give only "lip service" to this problem and limit efforts to an occasional talk by the coach and the use of readily available educational videos and posters.

The second question is even more threatening to school officials. In an era when some believe that the "win at all costs" philosophy is gaining the upper hand, will some schools hesitate to unilaterally "disarm"? That is, will some schools hesitate to institute a program that could significantly reduce steroid use at the cost of conferring an advantage to an opponent who chooses to maintain a "see no evil" stance on the use of performance-enhancing drugs? This question is given some legitimacy by pervasive anecdotal accounts of high school coaches encouraging the use of, and in some instances selling, so-called supplements such as creatine, DHEA, and androstenedione to their athletes.

In summary, although educating athletes about the health risks and ethical issues associated with anabolic steroid use can help reduce use, this strategy is not a panacea.

Conclusion: Our Values Must Change

Compared with legalization, interdiction, and education, the influence of our social environment on anabolic steroid use receives far less attention. Yet in many ways the social environment exerts a more fundamental influence on drug use in sport than do the more superficial strategies to reduce use described earlier.

A number of performance-enhancing drugs, including anabolic steroids, are not euphorigenic, or mood altering, immediately following administration. Instead, the appetite for these drugs was created predominantly by our societal fixation on winning and physical appearance. An infant does not innately believe that a muscular physique is desirable—our society teaches this. Likewise, children play games for fun, but society preaches the importance of winning—seemingly, at an increasingly younger age.

Ours is a culture that thrives on competition, both in business and in sport. However, we long ago realized that competition of all types must exist within some boundaries. A primary goal of competition is to win or be the very best in any endeavor. Philosophically, many in our society appear to have taken a "bottom-line" attitude and consider winning the *only* truly worthwhile goal of competition. If we accept this philosophy, then it becomes easy to justify, or be led to the belief, that one should win at any cost. At that point doping becomes a very rational behavior, with the end (winning) justifying the means (use of anabolic steroids and other drugs).

This "win at any cost/winner take all" philosophy is not new. The winners in the ancient Greek Olympics were handsomely rewarded, and episodes of athletes cheating to obtain these financial rewards are well documented (Thompson, 1986a, 1986b; Young, 1985). Smith (1988) argued persuasively that the level of cheating in college athletics at the turn of the century exceeded what we see today. Even the legendary Knute Rockne was quoted as saying, "Show me a good and gracious loser and I'll show you a failure." Vince Lombardi went a step further with his philosophy that winning isn't everything—it's the only thing. Indeed episodes of cheating, including drug use, have been commonplace at the collegiate, professional, and Olympic levels over the past four decades (Dealy, 1990; Dickey et al., 1999; Dubin, 1990; Francis, 1990; Sperber, 1990; Swift, 1999; Telander, 1989; Voy, 1990). Moreover, because of reports in the news media as well as written and oral testimonials by athletes, adolescents are aware that anabolic steroids and other performance-enhancing drugs have played a part in the success of many so-called role-model athletes (Alzado, 1991; Bamberger & Yaeger, 1997; Dickey et al., 1999).

Our fixation on appearance, especially the muscularity of males, is also long lived. An entire generation of young men aspired to the physique of Charles Atlas, followed by yet another generation who marveled at the muscles of Mr. Universe, Steve Reeves, who played Hercules in several movies in the 1950s. Today's children look with envy at the physiques of Sylvester Stallone, Jean-Claude Van Damme, Wesley Snipes, Linda Hamilton, and other actors *and actresses* whose movie roles call for a muscular athletic build. In addition, a number of professional wrestlers such as Hulk Hogan and "Stone Cold" Steve Austin as well as some elite athletes like Mark McGwire are admired in part for their bigger-than-life muscularity. Anabolic steroid use among professional wrestlers, including Hulk Hogan, was given national attention during a steroid trafficking trial in 1991 (Demak, 1991). President Bush's appointment of Arnold Schwarzenegger, an individual who attained his prominence as a bodybuilder and movie star at least in part as a result of steroid use, as chair of the President's Council on Physical Fitness and Sports was yet another inappropriate message sent to our children. Such messages of material reward and fame as a result of drug-assisted muscularity and winning grossly overshadow posters on gym walls and videos that implore "Just Say No to Steroids."

Some might argue that our attitudes and values related to sports and appearance are too deeply entrenched to change. That may be so, in particular when it comes to elite sport—there is simply too much money involved. However, if we cannot control our competitive and narcissistic natures, we then must resign ourselves to anabolic steroid use, even among our children.

Society's current strategy for dealing with the use of anabolic steroids in sport is multifaceted and primarily involves interdiction and education. However, 10 years after our society was made aware that our children were using steroids, our efforts to deal with this problem have not been very successful. Since 1989 a number of national conferences on anabolic steroid use have been held, sponsored by either the U.S. federal government or sport and educational organizations. The purpose of these meetings was to gather and or disseminate information or to achieve a consensus for action. At this point all these activities appear to have been a sincere effort to deal with the problem, but this strategy of attacking the symptoms while ignoring the social influence of drug use in sport is obviously ineffective. If we maintain our current course in the face of increased high levels of anabolic steroid use (or use of other performance-enhancing drugs), then we as sports medicine professionals, parents, teachers, and coaches are guilty of duplicity—acting for the sake of acting. We plan and attend workshops, distribute educational materials, lobby for the passage of laws, and seek the assistance of law enforcement. All these activities merely soothe our consciences in the face of our inability, or unwillingness, to deal with our addiction to sport and our fixations on winning and appearance.

References

Alzado, L. (1991, July 8). I'm sick and I'm scared. *Sports Illustrated,* 20–27.

American Academy of Orthopaedic Surgeons and the U.S. Department of Health and Human Services. *STEROIDS DON'T WORK OUT!* (a poster). Washington, DC: Center for Substance Abuse Prevention, Substance Abuse and Mental Health Services Administration.

Bamberger, M., & Yaeger, D. (1997, April 14). Over the edge. *Sports Illustrated,* 60–70.

Barton-Davis, E.R., Shoturma, D.I., Musaro, A., Rosenthal, N., & Sweeney. H.L. (1998). Viral mediated expression of insulin-like growth factor I blocks the aging-related loss of skeletal muscle function. *Proceedings of the National Academy of Sciences, 95,* 15603–15607.

Benario, H. (1983). Sport at Rome. *The Ancient World, 7,* 39.

Beste A. (1991). *Steroids: You make the choice.* N.p.: Iowa High School Athletic Association Printing Department.

Black, T. (1996). Does the ban on drugs in sport improve societal welfare? *International Review for Sociology of Sport, 31,* 367–380.

Centers for Disease Control and Prevention (1994). *Preventing tobacco use among young people: A report of the Surgeon General.* Atlanta: Author.

Dealy, F (1990). *Win at any cost: The sell out of college athletics.* New York: Birch Lane Press Books.

Demak, R. (1991, July). The sham is a sham. *Sports Illustrated,* 8.

Dickey. C., Helmstaedt, K., Nordland, R., & Hayden, T. (1999, February 15). The real scandal. *Newsweek,* pp. 48–54.

Drug trial, take II. (1998, August 19). *USA Today,* p. 3C.

Drugs and cycling. (1998, September 29). *USA Today,* p. 1C.

Dubin, C. (1990). *Commission of inquiry into the use of drugs and banned practices intended to increase athletic performance* (Catalogue No. CP32-56/1990E, ISBN 0-660-13610-4). Ottawa, ON: Canadian Government Publishing Centre.

Francis, C. (1990). *Speed trap.* New York: St. Martin's Press.

Goldberg, L., Bents, R., Bosworth, E., Trevisan, L., & Elliot, D. (1991). Anabolic steroid education and adolescents: Do scare tactics work? *Pediatrics, 87,* 283–286.

Goldberg, L., Elliot D.L., Clarke G., MacKinnon, D., Zoref, L., Moe, E., Green, C., & Wolf, S. (1996). The Adolescents Training and Learning to Avoid Steroids (ATLAS) prevention program: Background and results of a model intervention. *Archives of Pediatrics and Adolescent Medicine, 150,* 713–721.

Griffin T., & Svendsen R. (1990). *Steroids and our students: A program development guide.* St. Paul: Health Promotion Resources and WBA Ruster Foundation.

Harding Ringhofer & Associates and Media One. (1993). *Students and steroids: The facts . . . straight up* (a steroid use prevention program for adolescents). Minnetonka, MN: Author.

Hiestand, M. (1999, January 12). The B word—billion—no longer out of bounds. *USA Today,* pp. 1–2a.

Hoberman, J. (1984). *Sport and political ideology.* Austin, TX: University of Texas Press.

Lassar, S. (1998, December 3). Four former Northwestern football players indicted on perjury charges related to sports gambling investigation (press release). U.S. Justice Department, U.S. Attorney, Northern District of Illinois.

Leaderman, D. (1990, January 3). 57 of 106 universities in NCAA's top unit punished in 1980s. *Chronicle of Higher Education,* p. A31.

Lemonick, M. (1998, August 10). Le Tour des Drugs. *Time,* p. 76.

Longtime drug use. (1999, January 28). *USA Today,* p. 3C.

Office of Applied Studies (1999). *National Household Survey on Drug Abuse: Main findings, 1997* (SMA # 99-3295). Rockville, MD: U.S. Department of Health and Human Services, Substance Abuse and Mental Health Services Administration.

Saum, B. (1998, November 10). Written testimony of Bill Saum, Director of Agent and Gambling Activities, National Collegiate Athletic Association, before the National Gambling Impact Study Commission, Las Vegas, Nevada.

Schaps, E.. Bartolo, R., Moskowitz, J., Palley, C., & Churgin, S. (1981). Review of 127 drug abuse prevention program evaluations. *Journal of Drug Issues, 2,* 17–43.

Simson, V., & Jennings, A. (1992). *The lords of the rings: Power, money, and drugs in the modern Olympics.* London: Simon & Schuster.

Smith, R. (1988). *Sports and freedom: The rise of big-time college athletics.* New York: Oxford University Press.

Snowboarder loses medal after drug test. (1998, February 11). *USA Today,* p. 9E.

Sperber. M. (1990). *College sports inc.* New York: Holt.

Study: Gambling in NCAA rampant. (1999, January 12). *USA Today,* p. 3C.

A survey of sport: Not just a game. (1998). *Economist, 347,* 2–23.

Swift. E. (1999, February 1). Breaking point. *Sports Illustrated,* 34–35.

Telander, R. (1989). *The hundred yard lie.* New York: Simon & Schuster.

Thompson, J. (1986a). Historical errors about the ancient Olympic games. *Gamut, 17*(winter), 20–23.

Thompson, J. (1986b). The intrusion of corruption into athletics: An age-old problem. *Journal of General Education, 23,* 144–153.

Track star blazed trail. (1998, September 22). *USA Today,* pp. 1–2C.

U.S. Department of Health and Human Services, Department of Education. (1988). *Steroids: Playing with trouble* (a poster). Washington, DC: U.S. Government Printing Office, 1988-0-208-087.

U.S. Department of Health and Human Services. (1989, March). *Health United States: 1988* (DHHS Publication [PHS] 89-1232, U.S.). Hyattsville, MD: USDHHS, National Center for Health Statistics.

U.S. Department of Health and Human Services, Public Health Service. (1991, January). *Interagency Task Force on Anabolic Steroids.* Washington, DC: Author.

U.S. Department of Justice (1994). *Report of the International Conference on the Abuse and Trafficking of Anabolic Steroids.* Washington, DC: Drug Enforcement Administration.

Voy, R. (1990). *Drugs, sport, and politics.* Champaign, IL: Leisure Press.

Wm. C. Brown Communications. (1993). *1992–1993 Weight training fitness and conditioning catalog.* Dubuque, IA: Brown and Benchmark.

Yesalis, C., & Cowart, V. (1998). *The steroids game.* Champaign, IL: Human Kinetics.

Yesalis, C., & Friedl, K. (1988). Anabolic steroid use in amateur sports: An epidemiologic perspective. In R. Kretchmar (Ed.), *Proceedings of the US Olympic Academy XII* (pp. 83–89). Colorado Springs: U.S. Olympic Committee.

Yesalis, C.E., Herrick, R.T., Buckley, W.E., Friedl, K.E., Brannon, D., & Wright, J.E. (1988). Self-reported use of anabolic-androgenic steroids by elite power lifters. *The Physician and Sportsmedicine, 16,* 91–100.

Yesalis, C., Wright, J., & Lombardo, J. (1989, July 30–31). *Anabolic androgenic steroids: A synthesis of existing data and recommendations for future research.* Keynote research address, National Steroid Consensus Meeting, Los Angeles.

Yesalis, C., Streit, A., Vicary, J., Friedl, K., Brannon, D., & Buckley, W. (1989). Anabolic steroid use: Indications of habituation among adolescents. *Journal of Drug Education, 19,* 103–116.

Young, D. (1985). *The Olympic myth of Greek amateur athletics.* Chicago: Ares.

POSTSCRIPT

Are Athletes Who Use Anabolic Steroids Engaging in High-Risk Behavior?

There are several reasons why long-term research into the effects of steroids is lacking. First, it is unethical to give drugs that may prove harmful, even lethal, to people. Also, the amount of steroids given to subjects in a laboratory setting may not replicate what illegal steroid users actually take. Users who take steroids illegally may take substantially more than that which subjects are given in a clinical trial.

Second, to determine the true effects of drugs, double-blind studies need to be conducted. This means that neither the researcher nor the people receiving the drugs know whether the subjects are receiving the steroids or the placebos (inert substances). This is not practical with steroids because subjects can always tell if they received the steroids or the placebos. The effects of steroids could be determined by following up with people who are known steroid users. However, this method lacks proper controls. If physical or psychological problems appear in a subject, for example, it cannot be determined whether the problems are due to the steroids or to other drugs the person might have been taking. Also, the type of person who uses steroids might be the type of person who has emotional problems in the first place.

Even though the Drug Enforcement Administration estimates the black market trade in anabolic steroids to be several hundred million dollars a year, one could argue that steroids are symptomatic of a much larger social problem. Society places much emphasis on appearance and performance. From the time we are children, we are bombarded with constant reminders that we must do better than the next person. We are also constantly reminded of the importance of appearance—to either starve ourselves or pump ourselves up (or both) in order to satisfy the cultural ideal of beauty. If we cannot achieve these cultural standards through exercising, dieting, or drug use, then we can turn to surgery. Many males growing up are given the message that they should be "big and strong." One shortcut to achieving that look is through the use of steroids. Steroid use fits into the larger social problem of people not accepting their physical selves and their limitations.

Campbell Aitken deals with the use of steroids in sports in "Lifting Your Game: Campbell Aitken Probes the Use of Steroids in Sports," *Meanjin* (June 2002), as do Kieran Hogan and Kevin Norton in "The 'Price' of Olympic Gold," *Journal of Science and Medicine in Sport* (vol. 3, no. 2, 2000). An article that focuses on steroid use during the 2000 Summer Olympics is "Drug Testing at the Sydney Olympics," by Brian Corrigan and Ray Kazlauskas, *Medical Journal of Australia* (vol. 173, 2000), pp. 312–313.

On the Internet . . .

American Medical Association (AMA)

Information regarding the development and promotion of standards in medical practice, research, and education are included on this Web site.

http://www.ama-assn.org

The Columbia University College of Physicians and Surgeons Complete Home Medical Guide

This site provides information about health and medicine, including information on psychotherapeutic drugs.

http://cpmcnet.columbia.edu/texts/guide/

American Psychological Association (APA)

Research concerning different psychological disorders and the various types of treatments, including drug treatments, can be accessed through this site.

http://www.apa.org

CDC's Tobacco Information and Prevention Source

This location contains current information on smoking prevention programs. Much data on teen smoking can be found at this site.

http://www.cdc.gov/tobacco/

PART 2

Drugs and Social Policy

*E*xcept *for the debate over legalizing marijuana for medical use, each debate in this section focuses on drugs that are already legal. Despite concerns over the effects of illegal drugs, the most frequently used drugs in society are legal drugs. Because of their prevalence and legal status, the social, psychological, and physical impact of drugs like tobacco, caffeine, alcohol, and prescription drugs are often minimized or negated. However, tobacco and alcohol cause far more death and disability than all illegal drugs combined.*

The recent trend toward medical self-help raises questions of how much control one should have over one's health. In the last several years the increase in consumers' requesting prescription drugs for themselves and Ritalin for their children has created much concern. The current tendency to identify nicotine as an addictive drug and to promote the moderate use of alcohol to reduce heart disease has also generated much controversy. Lastly, should marijuana be prescribed for people with certain illnesses for which some have suggested the drug could be beneficial?

- Are the Adverse Effects of Smoking Exaggerated?

- Should Marijuana Be Legal for Medicinal Purposes?

- Do the Advantages of Psychiatric Medicines Outweigh Their Disadvantages?

- Do the Consequences of Caffeine Outweigh the Benefits?

- Are Too Many Children Receiving Ritalin?

- Do Consumers Benefit When Prescription Drugs Are Advertised?

ISSUE 8

Are the Adverse Effects
of Smoking Exaggerated?

YES: Robert A. Levy and Rosalind B. Marimont, from "Lies, Damned Lies, and 400,000 Smoking-Related Deaths," *Regulation* (vol. 21, no. 4, 1998)

NO: Alicia M. Lukachko and Elizabeth M. Whelan, from "Our 'Damned Lies' Spark Another Exchange," *Regulation* (vol. 23, no. 1, 2000)

ISSUE SUMMARY

YES: Robert A. Levy, a senior fellow at the Cato Institute, and Rosalind B. Marimont, a mathematician and scientist, contend that the government distorts and exaggerates the dangers of cigarette smoking. Levy and Marimont state that factors such as poor nutrition and obesity are overlooked as causes of death among smokers. They argue that cigarette smoking is harmful but that the misapplication of statistics about smoking should be regarded as "junk science."

NO: Alicia M. Lukachko and Elizabeth M. Whelan, assistant director of public health and president, respectively, of the American Council on Science and Health, contend that cigarette smoking has been the leading cause of disease and death over the last four decades. They argue that Levy and Marimont's methodology is haphazard and unscientific.

Most people, including those who smoke, recognize that cigarette smoking is harmful. Because of tobacco's reputation as an addictive substance that jeopardizes people's health, many activists are requesting that more stringent restrictions be placed on it. Currently, cigarette packages are required to carry warnings describing the dangers of tobacco products. In many countries tobacco products cannot be advertised on television or billboards. Laws that prevent minors from purchasing tobacco products are being enforced more vigorously than ever. Many, such as the World Health Organization, feel that global leadership in curtailing the proliferation of cigarette smoking is lacking.

Defenders of the tobacco industry point to benefits associated with nicotine, the mild stimulant that is the chief active chemical in tobacco. In previous centuries, for example, tobacco was used to help people with a variety of ailments, including skin diseases; internal and external disorders; and diseases of the eyes, ears, mouth, and nose. Tobacco and its smoke were employed often by Native Americans for sacramental purposes. For users, nicotine provides a sense of euphoria, and smoking is a source of gratification that does not impair thinking or performance. One can drive a car, socialize, study for a test, and engage in a variety of activities while smoking. Nicotine can relieve anxiety and stress, and it can reduce weight by lessening one's appetite and by increasing metabolic activity. Many smokers assert that smoking cigarettes enables them to concentrate better and that abstaining from smoking impairs their concentration.

Critics paint a very different picture of tobacco products, citing some of the following statistics: Tobacco is responsible for approximately 30 percent of deaths among people between ages 35 and 69, making it the single most prominent cause of premature death in the developed world. The relationship between cigarette smoking and cardiovascular disease, including heart attack, stroke, sudden death, peripheral vascular disease, and aortic aneurysm, is well documented. Even as few as one to four cigarettes daily can increase the risk of fatal coronary heart disease. Cigarettes have also been shown to reduce blood flow and the level of high-density lipoprotein cholesterol, which is the beneficial type of cholesterol.

Cigarette smoking is strongly associated with cancer, accounting for over 85 percent of lung cancer cases and 30 percent of all deaths due to cancer. Cancer of the pharynx, larynx, mouth, esophagus, stomach, pancreas, uterus, cervix, kidney, and bladder have been related to smoking. Studies have shown that smokers have twice the rate of cancer compared to nonsmokers.

According to smokers' rights advocates, the majority of smokers are already aware of the potential harm of tobacco products; in fact, most smokers tend to overestimate the dangers of smoking. Therefore, adults should be allowed to smoke if that is their wish. Many promote the idea that the Food and Drug Administration and a number of politicians are attempting to deny smokers the right to engage in a behavior that they freely choose. On the other hand, tobacco critics maintain that due to the addictiveness of nicotine—the level of which some claim is manipulated by tobacco companies—smokers do not have the ability to stop their behavior. That is, after a certain point, smoking cannot be considered freely chosen behavior.

In the following selections, Robert A. Levy and Rosalind B. Marimont argue that the scientific evidence demonstrating that tobacco use is harmful to smokers is disputable. Levy and Marimont state that smoking has been unfairly demonized and that cigarette smoking is not illegal nor does it cause intoxication, violent behavior, or unemployment. Alicia M. Lukachko and Elizabeth M. Whelan contend that the statistics regarding the effects of cigarette smoking clearly demonstrate a high level of harm.

Robert A. Levy and
Rosalind B. Marimont

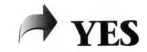 **YES**

Lies, Damned Lies, and 400,000 Smoking-Related Deaths

Truth was an early victim in the battle against tobacco. The big lie, repeated ad nauseam in anti-tobacco circles, is that smoking causes more than 400,000 premature deaths each year in the United States. That mantra is the principal justification for all manner of tobacco regulations and legislation, not to mention lawsuits by dozens of states for Medicaid recovery, class actions by seventy-five to eighty union health funds, similar litigation by thirty-five Blue Cross plans, twenty-four class suits by smokers who are not yet ill, sixty class actions by allegedly ill smokers, five hundred suits for damages from secondhand smoke, and health-related litigation by twelve cities and counties—an explosion of adjudication never before experienced in this country or elsewhere.

The war on smoking started with a kernel of truth—that cigarettes are a high risk factor for lung cancer—but has grown into a monster of deceit and greed, eroding the credibility of government and subverting the rule of law. Junk science has replaced honest science and propaganda parades as fact. Our legislators and judges, in need of dispassionate analysis, are instead smothered by an avalanche of statistics—tendentious, inadequately documented, and unchecked by even rudimentary notions of objectivity. Meanwhile, Americans are indoctrinated by health "professionals" bent on imposing their lifestyle choices on the rest of us and brainwashed by politicians eager to tap the deep pockets of a pariah industry.

The aim of this paper is to dissect the granddaddy of all tobacco lies—that smoking causes 400,000 deaths each year. To set the stage, let's look at two of the many exaggerations, misstatements, and outright fabrications that have dominated the tobacco debate from the outset.

Third-Rate Thinking About Secondhand Smoke

"Passive Smoking Does Cause Lung Cancer, Do Not Let Them Fool You," states the headline of a March 1998 press release from the World Health Organization. The release begins by noting that WHO had been accused of suppressing its own study because it "failed to scientifically prove that there is an association between passive smoking . . . and a number of diseases, lung cancer in particular." Not true, insisted WHO. Smokers themselves are not the only ones who suffer health problems because of their habit; secondhand smoke can be fatal as well.

The press release went on to report that WHO researchers found "an estimated 16 percent increased risk of lung cancer among nonsmoking spouses of smokers. For workplace exposure the estimated increase in risk was 17 percent." Remarkably, the very next line warned: "Due to small sample size, neither increased risk was statistically significant." Contrast that conclusion with the hype in the headline: "Passive Smoking Does Cause Lung Cancer." Spoken often enough, the lie becomes its own evidence.

The full study would not see the light of day for seven more months, until October 1998, when it was finally published in the *Journal of the National Cancer Institute.* News reports omitted any mention of statistical insignificance. Instead, they again trumpeted relative risks of 1.16 and 1.17, corresponding to 16 and 17 percent increases, as if those ratios were meaningful. Somehow lost in WHO's media blitz was the National Cancer Institute's own guideline: "Relative risks of less than 2 [that is, a 100 percent increase] are considered small. . . . Such increases may be due to chance, statistical bias, or effects of confounding factors that are sometimes not evident." To put the WHO results in their proper perspective, note that the relative risk of lung cancer for persons who drink whole milk is 2.4. That is, the increased risk of contracting lung cancer from whole milk is 140 percent—more than eight times the 17 percent increase from secondhand smoke.

What should have mattered most to government officials, the health community and concerned parents is the following pronouncement from the WHO study: After examining 650 lung cancer patients and 1,500 healthy adults in seven European countries, WHO concluded that the "results indicate no association between childhood exposure to environmental tobacco smoke and lung cancer risk."

EPA's Junk Science

Another example of anti-tobacco misinformation is the landmark 1993 report in which the Environmental Protection Agency declared that environmental tobacco smoke (ETS) is a dangerous carcinogen that kills three thousand Americans yearly. Five years later, in July 1998, federal judge William L. Osteen lambasted the EPA for "cherry picking" the data, excluding studies that "demonstrated no association between ETS and cancer," and withholding "significant portions of its findings and reasoning in striving to confirm its *a priori* hypothesis." Both "the record and EPA's explanation," concluded the court, "make it clear that using standard methodology, EPA could not produce statistically significant results." A more damning assessment is difficult to imagine, but here are the court's conclusions at greater length, in its own words.

EPA publicly committed to a conclusion before research had begun; excluded industry [input thereby] violating the [Radon Research] Act's procedural requirements; adjusted established procedure and scientific norms to validate the Agency's public conclusion, and aggressively utilized the Act's authority to disseminate findings to establish a de facto regulatory scheme intended to restrict Plaintiff's products and to influence public opinion. In conducting the ETS Risk Assessment, EPA disregarded information and made findings on selective information; did not disseminate significant epidemiologic information; deviated from its Risk Assessment Guidelines; failed to disclose important findings and reasoning; and left significant questions without answers. EPA's conduct left substantial holes in the administrative record. While so doing, EPA produced limited evidence, then claimed the weight of the Agency's research evidence demonstrated ETS causes Cancer.

—*Flue-Cured Tobacco Coop. Stabilization Corp. v. United States Environmental Protection Agency,* 4 F. Supp. 2d 435, 465–66 (M.D.N.C. 1998)

Hundreds of states, cities, and counties have banned indoor smoking—many in reaction to the EPA report. California even prohibits smoking in bars. According to Matthew L. Myers, general counsel of the Campaign for Tobacco-Free Kids, "the release of the original risk assessment gave an enormous boost to efforts to restrict smoking." Now that the study has been thoroughly debunked, one would think that many of the bans would be lifted. Don't hold your breath. When science is adulterated and debased for political ends, the culprits are unlikely to reverse course merely because they have been unmasked.

In reaction to the federal court's criticism EPA administrator Carol M. Browner said, "It's so widely accepted that secondhand smoke causes very real problems for kids and adults. Protecting people from the health hazards of secondhand smoke should be a national imperative." Like *Alice in Wonderland,* sentence first, evidence afterward. Browner reiterates: "We believe the health threats . . . from breathing secondhand smoke are very real." Never mind science; it is Browner's beliefs that control. The research can be suitably tailored.

For the EPA to alter results, disregard evidence, and adjust its procedures and standards to satisfy agency prejudices is unacceptable behavior, even to a first-year science student. Those criticisms are about honesty, carefulness, and rigor—the very essence of science.

Classifying Diseases as Smoking-Related

With that record of distortion, it should come as no surprise that anti-tobacco crusaders misrepresent the number of deaths due to smoking. Start by considering the diseases that are incorrectly classified as smoking-related. The Centers for Disease Control and Prevention (CDC) prepares and distributes information on smoking-attributable mortality, morbidity and economic costs (SAMMEC). In its *Morbidity and Mortality Weekly Report* for 27 August 1993, the CDC states that 418,690 Americans died in 1990 of various diseases that they contracted because, according to the government, they smoked.

Diseases are categorized as smoking-related if the risk of death for smokers exceeds that for nonsmokers. In the jargon of epidemiology, a relative risk that is greater than 1 indicates a connection between exposure (smoking) and effect (death). Recall, however, the National Cancer Institute's guideline: "Relative risks of less than two are considered small. . . . Such increases may be due to chance, statistical bias, or effects of confounding factors that are sometimes not evident." And the *Federal Reference Manual on Scientific Evidence* confirms that the threshold test for legal significance is a relative risk of two or higher. At any ratio below two, the results are insufficiently reliable to conclude that a particular agent (e.g., tobacco) caused a particular disease.

What would happen if the SAMMEC data were to exclude deaths from those diseases that had a relative risk of less than two for current or former smokers? Table 1 shows that 163,071 deaths reported by CDC were from diseases that should not have been included in the report. Add to that another 1,362 deaths from burn injuries—unless one believes that Philip Morris is responsible when a smoker falls asleep with a lit cigarette. That is a total of 164,433 misreported deaths out of 418,690. When the report is properly limited to diseases that have a significant relationship with smoking, the death total declines to 254,257. Thus, on this count alone, SAMMEC overstates the number of deaths by 65 percent.

Table 1

Disease Category	Relative Risk	Deaths From Smoking
Cancer of pancreas	1.1–1.8	2,931*
Cancer of cervix	1.9	647*
Cancer of bladder	1.9	2,348*
Cancer of kidney, other urinary	1.2–1.4	353
Hypertension	1.2–1.9	5,450
Ischemic heart disease (age 35–64)	1.4–1.8	15,535*
Ischemic heart disease (age 65+)	1.3–1.6	64,789
Other heart disease	1.2–1.9	35,314
Cerebrovascular disease (age 35–64)	1.4	2,681*
Cerebrovascular disease (age 65+)	1.0–1.9	14,610
Atherosclerosis	1.3	1,267*
Aortic aneurysm	1.3	448*
Other arterial disease	1.3	372*
Pneumonia and influenza	1.4–1.6	10,552*
Other respiratory diseases	1.4–1.6	1,063*
Pediatric diseases	1.5–1.8	1,711
Sub-total		160,071
Environmental tobacco smoke	1.2	3,000
Total		163,071

* Number of deaths for this category assumes population deaths distributed between current and former smokers in same proportion as in Cancer Prevention Survey CPS-II, provided by the American Cancer Society.

Calculating Excess Deaths

But there is more. Writing on "Risk Attribution and Tobacco-Related Deaths" in the 1993 *American Journal of Epidemiology,* T. D. Sterling, W. L. Rosenbaum, and J. J. Weinkam expose another overstatement—exceeding 65 percent—that flows from using the American Cancer Society's Cancer Prevention Survey (CPS) as a baseline against which excess deaths are computed. Here is how one government agency, the Office of Technology Assessment (OTA), calculates the number of deaths caused by smoking:

The OTA first determines the death rate for persons who were part of the CPS sample and never smoked. Next, that rate is applied to the total U.S. population in order to estimate the number of Americans who would have died if no one ever smoked. Finally, the hypothetical number of deaths for assumed never-smokers is subtracted from the actual number of U.S. deaths, and the difference is ascribed to smoking. That approach seems reasonable if one important condition is satisfied: The CPS sample must be roughly the same as the overall U.S. population with respect to those factors, other than smoking, that could be associated with the death rate. But as Sterling, Rosenbaum, and Weinkam point out, nothing could be further from the truth.

The American Cancer Society bases its CPS study on a million men and women volunteers, drawn from the ranks of the Society's members, friends, and acquaintances. The persons who participate are more affluent than average, overwhelmingly white, married, college graduates, who generally do not have hazardous jobs. Each of those characteristics tends to reduce the death rate of the CPS sample which, as a result, enjoys an average life expectancy that is substantially longer than the typical American enjoys.

Because OTA starts with an atypically low death rate for never-smokers in the CPS sample, then applies that rate to the whole population, its baseline for determining excess deaths is grossly underestimated. By comparing actual deaths with a baseline that is far too low, OTA creates the illusion that a large number of deaths are due to smoking.

That same illusion pervades the statistics released by the U.S. Surgeon General, who in his 1989 report estimated that 335,600 deaths were caused by smoking. When Sterling, Rosenbaum, and Weinkam recalculated the Surgeon General's numbers, replacing the distorted CPS sample with a more representative baseline from large surveys conducted by the National Center for Health Statistics, they found that the number of smoking-related deaths declined to 203,200. Thus, the Surgeon General's report overstated the number of deaths by more than 65 percent simply by choosing the wrong standard of comparison.

Sterling and his coauthors report that not only is the death rate considerably lower for the CPS sample than for the entire U.S. but, astonishingly, even smokers in the CPS sample have a lower death rate than the national average for both smokers and nonsmokers. As a result, if OTA were to have used the CPS death rate for smokers, applied that rate to the total population, then subtracted the actual number of deaths for all Americans, it would have found that smoking saves 277,621 lives each year. The authors caution, of course, that their calculation is sheer nonsense, not a medical miracle. Those "lives would be saved only if the U.S. population would die with the death rate of smokers in the afflu-ent CPS sample."

Unhappily, the death rate for Americans is considerably higher than that for the CPS sample. Nearly as disturbing, researchers like Sterling, Rosenbaum, and Weinkam identified that statistical predicament many years ago; yet the government persists in publishing data on smoking-related deaths that are known to be greatly inflated.

Controlling for Confounding Variables

Even if actual deaths were compared against an appropriate baseline for non-smokers, the excess deaths could not properly be attributed to smoking alone. It cannot be assumed that the only difference between smokers and nonsmokers is that the former smoke. The two groups are dissimilar in many other respects, some of which affect their propensity to contract diseases that have been identi-fied as smoking-related. For instance, smokers have higher rates of alcoholism, exercise less on average, eat fewer green vegetables, are more likely to be ex-posed to workplace carcinogens, and are poorer than nonsmokers. Each of those factors can be a "cause" of death from a so-called smoking-related disease; and each must be statistically controlled for if the impact of a single factor, like smoking, is to be reliably determined.

Sterling, Rosenbaum, and Weinkam found that adjusting their calcula-tions for just two lifestyle differences—in income and alcohol consumption—between smokers and nonsmokers had the effect of reducing the Surgeon General's smoking-related death count still further, from 203,200 to 150,000. That means the combined effect of using a proper standard of comparison coupled with controls for income and alcohol was to lower the Surgeon Gen-eral's estimate 55 percent—from 335,600 to 150,000. Thus, the original esti-mate was a disquieting 124 percent too high, even without adjustments for important variables like occupation, exercise, and nutritional habits.

What if smokers got plenty of exercise and had healthy diets while non-smokers were couch potatoes who consumed buckets of fast food? Naturally, there are some smokers and nonsmokers who satisfy those criteria. Dr. William E. Wecker, a consulting statistician who has testified for the tobacco industry, scanned the CPS database and found thousands of smokers with relatively low risk factors and thousands of never-smokers with high risk factors. Comparing the mortality rates of the two groups, Dr. Wecker discovered that the smokers were "healthier and die less often by a factor of three than the never-smokers." Obviously, other risk factors matter, and any study that ignores them is utterly worthless.

Yet, if a smoker who is obese; has a family history of high cholesterol, dia-betes, and heart problems; and never exercises dies of a heart attack, the govern-ment attributes his death to smoking alone. That procedure, if applied to the other causal factors identified in the CPS study, would produce more than twice as many "attributed" deaths as there are actual deaths, according to Dr. Wecker. For example, the same calculations that yield 400,000 smoking-related deaths suggest that 504,000 people die each year because they engage in little or no exercise. Employing an identical formula, bad nutritional habits can be shown to account for 649,000 excess deaths annually. That is nearly 1.6 million deaths from only three causes—without considering alcoholism, accidents, poverty, etc.—out of 2.3 million deaths in 1995 from all causes combined. And on it goes—computer-generated phantom deaths, not real deaths—constrained neither by accepted statistical methods, by common sense, nor by the number of people who die each year.

Adjusting for Age at Death

Next and last, we turn to a different sort of deceit—one pertaining not to the number of smoking-related deaths but rather to the misperception that those deaths are somehow associated with kids and young adults. For purposes of this discussion, we will work with the far-fetched statistics published by CDC—an annual average from 1990 through 1994 of 427,743 deaths attributable to tobacco. Is the problem as serious as it sounds?

At first blush, it would seem that more than 400,000 annual deaths is an extremely serious problem. But suppose that all of the people died at age ninety-nine. Surely then, the seriousness of the problem would be tempered by the fact that the decedents would have died soon from some other cause in any event. That is not far from the truth: while tobacco does not kill people at an average age of ninety-nine, it does kill people at an average age of roughly seventy-two—far closer to ninety-nine than to childhood or even young adulthood. Indeed, according to a 1991 RAND study, smoking "reduces the life expectancy of a twenty-year-old by about 4.3 years"—not a trivial concern to be sure, but not the horror that is sometimes portrayed.

Consider Table 2, which shows the number of deaths and age at death for various causes of death: The three nonsmoking categories total nearly 97,000 deaths—probably not much different than the correctly calculated number of smoking-related deaths—but the average age at death is only thirty-nine. As contrasted with a seventy-two-year life expectancy for smokers, each of those nonsmoking deaths snuffs out thirty-three years of life—our most productive years, from both an economic and child-rearing perspective.

Perhaps that is why the Carter Center's "Closing the Gap" project at Emory University examined "years of potential life lost" (YPLL) for selected diseases, to identify those causes of death that were of greatest severity and consequence. The results were reported by R.W. Amler and D.L. Eddins, "Cross-Sectional Analysis: Precursors of Premature Death in the United States," in the 1987 *American Journal of Preventive Medicine*. First, the authors determined for each disease the annual number of deaths by age group. Second, they multiplied for each age group the number of deaths times the average number of years remaining before customary retirement at age sixty-five. Then they computed YPLL by summing the products for each disease across age groups.

Thus, if smoking were deemed to have killed, say, fifty thousand people from age sixty through sixty-four, a total of 150,000 years of life were lost in that age group—i.e., fifty thousand lives times an average of three years remaining

Table 2

Cause of Death	Number of Deaths per Year	Mean Age at Death
Smoking-attributed	427,743	72
Motor vehicle accidents	40,982	39
Suicide	30,484	45
Homicide	25,488	32

Source: Centers for Disease Control and Prevention

Table 3

Cause	Deaths	YPLL
Alcohol-related	99,247	1,795,458
Gaps in primary care*	132,593	1,771,133
Injuries (excluding alcohol-related)	64,169	1,755,720
Tobacco-related	338,022	1,497,161

*Inadequate access, screening and preventive interventions.

to age sixty-five. YPLL for smoking would be the accumulation of lost years for all age groups up to sixty-five.

Amler and Eddins identified nine major precursors of preventable deaths. Measured by YPLL, tobacco was about halfway down the list—ranked four out of nine in terms of years lost—not "the number one killer in America" as alarmists have exclaimed. Table 3 shows the four most destructive causes of death, based on 1980 YPLL statistics. Bear in mind that the starting point for the YPLL calculation is the number of deaths, which for tobacco is grossly magnified for all of the reasons discussed above.

According to Amler and Eddins, even if we were to look at medical treatment—measured by days of hospital care—nonalcohol-related injuries impose a 58 percent greater burden than tobacco, and nutrition-related diseases are more burdensome as well.

Another statistic that more accurately reflects the real health repercussions of smoking is the age distribution of the 427,743 deaths that CDC mistakenly traces to tobacco. No doubt most readers will be surprised to learn that—aside from burn victims and pediatric diseases—*tobacco does not kill a single person below the age of 35.*

Each year from 1990 through 1994, as shown in Table 4, only 1,910 tobacco-related deaths—less than half of 1 percent of the total—were persons below age thirty-five. Of those, 319 were burn victims and the rest were infants whose parents smoked. But the relationship between parental smoking and pediatric diseases carries a risk ratio of less than 2, and thus is statistically insignificant. Unless better evidence is produced, those deaths should not be associated with smoking.

Table 4

U.S. Smoking-Attributable Mortality by Cause and Age of Death
1990–1994 Annual Average

Age at Death	Pediatric Diseases	Burn Victims	All Other Diseases	Total
Under 1	1,591	19	0	1,610
1–34	0	300	0	300
35–49	0	221	21,773	21,994
50–69	0	286	148,936	149,222
70–74	0	96	62,154	62,250
75–84	0	133	120,537	120,670
85 +	0	45	71,652	71,697
Totals	1,591	1,100	425,052	427,743

Source: Private communication from the Centers for Disease Control and Prevention

On the other hand, the National Center for Health Statistics reports that more than twenty-one thousand persons below age thirty-five died from motor vehicle accidents in 1992, more than eleven thousand died from suicide, and nearly seventeen thousand died from homicide. Over half of those deaths were connected with alcohol or drug abuse. That should put smoking-related deaths in a somewhat different light.

Most revealing of all, almost 255,000 of the smoking-related deaths—nearly 60 percent of the total—occurred at age seventy or above. More than 192,000 deaths—nearly 45 per-cent of the total—occurred at age seventy-five or higher. And roughly 72,000 deaths—almost 17 percent of the total—occurred at the age of 85 or above. Still, the public health community disingenuously refers to "premature" deaths from smoking, as if there is no upper age limit to the computation.

The vast overestimate of the dangers of smoking has had disastrous results for the health of young people. Risky behavior does not exist in a vacuum; people compare uncertainties and apportion their time, effort, and money according to the perceived severity of the risk. Each year, alcohol and drug abuse kills tens of thousands of people under the age of thirty-five. Yet according to a 1995 survey by the U.S. Department of Health and Human Services, high school seniors thought smoking a pack a day was more dangerous than daily consumption of four to five alcoholic beverages or using barbiturates. And the CDC reports that the number of pregnant women who drank frequently quadrupled between 1991 and 1995—notwithstanding that fetal alcohol syndrome is the largest cause of preventable mental retardation, occurring in one out of every one thousand births.

Can anyone doubt that the drumbeat of antismoking propaganda from the White House and the health establishment has deluded Americans into thinking that tobacco is the real danger to our children? In truth, alcohol and drug abuse poses an immensely greater risk and antismoking zealots bear a heavy burden for their duplicity.

Conclusion

The unvarnished fact is that children do not die of tobacco-related diseases, correctly determined. If they smoke heavily during their teens, they may die of lung cancer in their old age, fifty or sixty years later, assuming lung cancer is still a threat then.

Meanwhile, do not expect consistency or even common sense from public officials. Alcoholism contributes to crime, violence, spousal abuse, and child neglect. Children are dying by the thousands in accidents, suicides, and homicides. But states go to war against nicotine—which is not an intoxicant, has no causal connection with crime, and poses little danger to young adults or family members.

The campaign against cigarettes is not entirely dishonest. After all, a seasoning of truth makes the lie more digestible. Evidence does suggest that cigarettes substantially increase the risk of lung cancer, bronchitis, and emphysema. The relationship between smoking and other diseases is not nearly so clear, however; and the scare-mongering that has passed for science is appalling. Not only is tobacco far less pernicious than Americans are led to believe, but its destructive effect is amplified by all manner of statistical legerdemain—counting diseases that should not be counted, using the wrong sample as a standard of comparison, and failing to control for obvious confounding variables.

To be blunt, there is no credible evidence that 400,000 deaths per year—or any number remotely close to 400,000—are caused by tobacco. Nor has that estimate been adjusted for the positive effects of smoking—less obesity, colitis, depression, Alzheimer's disease, Parkinson's disease and, for some women, a lower incidence of breast cancer. The actual damage from smoking is neither known nor knowable with precision. Responsible statisticians agree that it is impossible to attribute causation to a single variable, like tobacco, when there are multiple causal factors that are correlated with one another. The damage from cigarettes is far less than it is made out to be.

Most important, the government should stop lying and stop pretending that smoking-related deaths are anything but a statistical artifact. The unifying bond of all science is that truth is its aim. When that goal yields to politics, tainting science in order to advance predetermined ends, we are all at risk. Sadly, that is exactly what has transpired as our public officials fabricate evidence to promote their crusade against big tobacco.

**Alicia M. Lukachko and
Elizabeth M. Whelan**

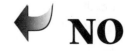 **NO**

Our "Damned Lies" Spark
Another Exchange

A Critical Assessment

In "Lies, Damned Lies, & 400,000 Smoking-Related Deaths" (Regulation, Vol. 21, No. 4), Robert Levy and Rosalind Marimont contend that the government's estimate that cigarette smoking causes 400,000 premature deaths a year is scientifically unsound and substantially inflated. The authors assert: "The war on smoking . . . has grown into a monster of deceit and greed, eroding the credibility of government and subverting the rule of law."

In May 1999, Levy and Marimont's arguments resurfaced in an article by *Boston Globe* columnist Jeff Jacoby. Mr. Jacoby's column has been circulated widely and cited in op-ed pages nationwide.

Levy and Marimont's article also served in the defense of U.S. tobacco companies in the recent Florida "Engle case," the largest class action lawsuit filed against the tobacco industry.

For more than 20 years, the American Council on Science and Health (ACSH) has relied on sound science to educate the public about risks to health. ACSH has paid particular attention to well-established and preventable causes of disease and death, especially cigarette smoking.

In this letter, we evaluate the plausibility of the estimate that smoking causes 400,000 premature deaths a year, review the confirmed health problems caused by smoking, explain the scientific methods used to establish those risks, and evaluate the key arguments used by Levy and Marimont to discount the fatalities caused by cigarette smoking.

The Health Hazards of Smoking

Cigarette smoking has been recognized as a leading cause of disease and death for at least 40 years. Few subjects have received such thorough and extensive scientific scrutiny by both governmental and independent bodies. Thousands of scientific studies have confirmed that smoking is a major health hazard. Besides the relationship between smoking and disease, many studies have found that the overall death rate among smokers is two to three times greater than that of nonsmokers. Cigarettes also contain nicotine, a chemical proven to be highly addictive (which internal tobacco-industry documents have acknowledged).

Despite overwhelming evidence to the contrary, Levy and Marimont state that the hazards of smoking remain largely speculative. They allege that the "war on smoking started with a kernel of truth—that cigarettes are a high risk factor for lung cancer." Ironically, it is Levy and Marimont's article that contains only a kernel of truth about the risks of smoking. In fact, active cigarette smoking has been causally linked to lung cancer and associated with an array of other diseases; specifically:

- Cigarette smoking is a principal cause of cancer of the esophagus, larynx, lip, mouth, pharynx, tongue, kidney, pancreas, urinary bladder, and uterine cervix.
- Cigarette smoking has been identified as a major cause of cardiovascular disease, including atherosclerosis, coronary heart disease (angina and heart attack), stroke, sudden death, and aortic aneurysm.
- Cigarette smoking causes chronic obstructive lung disease (emphysema, chronic bronchitis, and related conditions). Smokers have been found to suffer more respiratory problems (such as colds, pneumonia, influenza, and bronchitis) and their recovery from those illnesses is slower.
- For men under age 65, smoking has been shown to be an independent risk factor for impotence, including erectile dysfunction. For women, smoking can impair fertility, induce premature menopause and spontaneous abortion, and lead to a host of complications of pregnancy and childbirth.
- Cigarette smoking increases the risk for osteoporosis (a reduction in bone mass) and periodontal (gum) disease.
- Smoking precipitates vision problems, including blindness secondary to cataracts and macular degeneration, and premature hearing loss.
- Smokers face a significantly greater chance than do nonsmokers of suffering complications during and after surgery.

Evidence suggests that smoking also increases the risk for other diseases, such as rheumatoid arthritis, and cancers of the prostate and stomach. Those relationships, however, have not yet been scientifically established.

Preliminary research also indicates that cigarette smoking may be associated with reduced risk for endometrial cancer and Parkinson's disease. Yet the harmful effects of cigarette smoking dramatically outweigh any of its potential benefits.

Environmental Tobacco Smoke

A mounting body of scientific research reveals that exposure to environmental tobacco smoke (ETS) also poses health risks. The most common and firmly established adverse health effects associated with exposure to ETS are irritation of the eyes, nose, and respiratory tract; exacerbation of asthma and emphysema; and increased susceptibility to respiratory infections. Furthermore, studies have consistently shown that ETS contributes to lung cancer and heart disease. (See *Environmental Tobacco Smoke, Health Risk or Health Hype?*, a 1999 report by the American Council on Science and Health.)

As Levy and Marimont's article itself illustrates, concerns about second-hand smoke extend far beyond public health. The political implications of finding a causal association between ETS and disease have fueled long and bitter struggles between pro- and anti-tobacco organizations and individuals. In an effort to resist the trend toward indoor-smoking restrictions and to allay public fears, some parties, including the tobacco industry, have argued that ETS does not pose a "meaningful" lung cancer risk—and therefore does not present a threat to public health.

Similarly, authors Levy and Marimont focus their arguments about secondhand smoke exclusively on lung cancer in an attempt to dismiss all of the health effects associated with ETS. Their argument is simplistic, as it ignores ETS-related health risks other than lung cancer—heart disease and respiratory illnesses, for example—that should also be considered when developing public health policy.

Establishing Cause and Effect

Scientists rely on epidemiology—the study of the distribution and determinants of disease frequency—to determine whether a factor, such as cigarette smoking, causes a particular health outcome, that is, disease or death. They begin by suggesting and then establishing an association.

The best way to evaluate the effect of smoking on health is to compare groups of smokers with groups of nonsmokers to assess the differences between them (if any) in health outcomes. Researchers try to ensure that, aside from smoking, the smokers and nonsmokers have similar characteristics, so that differences in health outcomes are more likely attributable to smoking than to other factors. Statistical analysis of the research data can help to explain differences in health outcomes attributable to smoking, even where there are dissimilarities between the groups. ·

When an association is found between smoking and disease or death, researchers must determine whether the apparent association is valid. A valid association is unlikely to be the result of chance, bias on the part of researchers or study participants, or confounders—other factors that caused the disease and are independently associated with smoking.

Statistical tests are routinely applied to research findings to assess the probability that the results are "statistically significant" and not merely coincidental. A test for statistical significance takes into account such factors as the number of persons examined (sample size) and the strength of the association between the exposure and the health outcome. Generally, the larger the sample size and the stronger the association, the more likely it is that the results will be found to be significant.

Even if a result is statistically significant, bias and potential confounders must be addressed to demonstrate a valid association. Furthermore, a statistically significant finding does not alone confirm a causal relationship. To conclude that smoking causes a particular disease, researchers must assess the relationship against five criteria:

Strength of the association found between smoking and disease.   Relative risk is the ratio of disease among smokers to disease among nonsmokers. A relative risk of 1 indicates that there is no association between the exposure and the outcome. The closer relative risk is to 1, the smaller or weaker the association.

A relative risk of 2, for example, would indicate that smokers are twice as likely as nonsmokers to develop the health outcome under study (e.g., death from heart disease). The larger the relative risk, the less likely an association can be attributed solely to bias or confounders. But a small relative risk does not exclude the possibility of a causal relationship, nor does it preclude the possibility that the relative risk is statistically significant.

Consistency of the finding across studies.   If several well-designed studies replicate a finding, the more likely it that the relationship being studied is real. As stated previously, the enormous body of research on the health effects of smoking corroborates the relationship between smoking and disease.

Biological plausibility of the hypothesis.   The relationship between an exposure and a disease must be consistent with what is known about biology and the disease. Much is understood about the biological mechanisms by which smoking causes disease, though more remains to be learned. It is known that cigarette smoke contains approximately 4,000 chemical components, many of which are toxins and some of which are human carcinogens.

Presence of a dose-response relationship.   In a dose-response relationship, risk increases with the degree of exposure. Many studies have shown that increases in the duration of cigarette use and number of cigarettes smoked increase the risk for smoking-related disease and death.

Sequence of cause and effect.   The exposure or hypothesized cause must precede the effect. There is ample research to affirm that cigarette use precedes adverse health outcomes.

We will apply these five principles below, when we assess Levy and Marimont's claims.

Calculating Premature Deaths Caused by Cigarette Smoking

The number of deaths attributable to cigarette smoking may be thought of as the reduction in the number of deaths that would obtain if no one had ever smoked. That reduction is essentially estimated in the following way:

1. Apply death rates for smoking-related diseases among representative nonsmokers to the entire population. That gives the number of deaths expected if everyone were a nonsmoker.

2. Subtract the expected number of deaths from the actual number of deaths.

The calculation is complicated by the fact that the many people who have smoked and quit have a greater risk of smoking-related disease than do people who have never smoked. Therefore, some formulas, such as that used by the Centers for Disease Control and Prevention (CDC), distinguish between current smokers, former smokers, and "never-smokers" in estimating the incidence of smoking-related deaths.

Estimates of the death toll from smoking can vary widely, depending on what diseases are considered smoking-related, the data sources used, the control for confounding variables (e.g., age), and variations in formulas.

For more than two decades, the U.S. government has been estimating the number of Americans who die prematurely from smoking. The government currently estimates that about 430,000 deaths occur each year in the United States as a result of cigarette smoking. (Higher estimates fall in the range of 600,000 to 700,000 annual deaths.)

Assessment of Levy and Marimont's Charges

In "Lies, Damned Lies, & 400,000 Smoking-Related Deaths," Levy and Marimont challenge the reality of the associations found between smoking and disease and, ultimately, the veracity of the estimate that smoking causes 400,000 premature deaths a year. The authors try to minimize smoking's death toll by using largely haphazard and unscientific methods. Here, we assess Levy and Marimont's key arguments.

> *Argument 1. Relative risks less than 2 are "statistically insignificant" and "insufficiently reliable to conclude that a particular agent (e.g., tobacco) caused a particular disease." Based on that claim, Levy and Marimont subtract more than 160,000 of the 400,000 annual deaths caused by smoking.*

A relative risk less than 2, although small, can be statistically significant and can reflect a causal relationship. Given the pervasiveness of a risk factor, such as smoking, and the prevalence of some of the diseases it causes, small relative risks can, and do, represent a serious threat to public health. For example, cigarette smoking is a much greater risk factor for mortality from lung cancer than from heart disease. But because heart disease affects many more people than lung cancer, the number of smoking-related deaths from heart disease rivals those from lung cancer.

Levy and Marimont's assumptions regarding small relative risks violate basic principles of epidemiology. The authors confuse two distinct concepts, that of relative risk and that of statistical significance.

The size of a relative risk, alone, does not signify its statistical significance. Rather, as explained earlier, a research finding must undergo statistical tests to assess its "significance." A small relative risk suggests a weak association (or risk factor), not necessarily an insignificant finding. Again, a small relative risk may have a substantial effect on public health if the exposure affects a large proportion of the population.

Moreover, the value of a relative risk, in itself, does not imply a causal relationship between risk factor and disease. As discussed above, relative risk is one of several factors that must be considered when judging causality. Judged in that light, a small relative risk may reflect a causal relationship.

Levy and Marimont offer a good illustration of this point. In their derision of the risks associated with ETS, Levy and Marimont claim that "the relative risk of lung cancer for persons who drink whole milk is 2.4." Even if we accept this highly dubious association, the other criteria necessary to judge causality (biological plausibility, consistency of findings, etc.) are not fulfilled. Thus, whole milk cannot legitimately be judged a cause of lung cancer on relative risk alone.

The authors mislead readers by misrepresenting a quotation from the National Cancer Institute (NCI), which qualifies relative risks, as the agency's "own guideline." In fact, NCI has no such guideline about relative risks, and the quotation cited is taken from a 1994 NCI press release on abortion and the risk of breast cancer. Taken in context, the so-called guideline makes a much different point than the one suggested by the authors.

In sum, Levy and Marimont arbitrarily, and without scientific justification, reduce CDC's estimate of smoking deaths by 163,071 by asserting that a relative risk less than 2 is statistically insignificant. But, as we have argued, their logic is fundamentally flawed.

Argument 2. The American Cancer Society's Cancer Prevention Survey (CPS)— a widely used data set for the calculation of public health statistics—is unrepresentative of the general population and is therefore "the wrong sample [to use] as a standard of comparison" when estimating smoking-related deaths in the United States.

It is true that the American Cancer Society's CPS has greater proportions of white, older, more educated, married, and middle-class people than the entire U.S. population. That, alone, does not invalidate findings derived from CPS. It has a uniquely strong study design, from which valid estimations have been drawn.

Moreover—and perhaps more important—the relative risks of dying from smoking-related diseases, as estimated from CPS, are within the range of estimates from other studies. That consistency lends credence to CDC's estimate of smoking-related deaths, which is based on relative risks drawn from CPS.

The important issue whether a particular study's results are applicable to other populations should be considered only after determining the study's validity. Levy and Marimont overlook the overriding strengths of CPS: its excellent study design and valid findings. With more than one million participants, CPS is the largest U.S. study that collects data over an extensive period of time on the relationship between smoking and mortality.

After accepting that the results of CPS reflect valid cause and effect relationships, the next important question is how the results for a mostly white, middle-class population would differ, if at all, from those for the entire United States. The answer depends on how the data are used. The absolute mortality rates are lower in CPS than in the general population, but CDC's estimation of smoking-related deaths relies on ratios from CPS—relative risks for smokers and former smokers. Those relative risk estimates are close to relative risk estimates from other studies, which corroborates the reliability of CDC's estimate.

Levy and Marimont advocate substituting data from the National Center for Health Statistics (specifically, the National Mortality Followback Survey and the National Health Interview Survey) for data from CPS, as does long-time tobacco industry consultant T.D. Sterling. However, Sterling's work has been criticized, justly, for its implausible findings (e.g., previous smoking was found to be protective against coronary heart disease and cerebrovascular disease among males over age 65), and for combining data from two surveys with largely dissimilar, and thus incompatible, study designs.

By contrast, CPS uses an appropriate study design to derive valid estimates of relative risk: following large cohorts of smokers and nonsmokers over an appropriate length of time to observe health outcomes.

Argument 3. CDC fails "to control for obvious confounding variables" in its estimation of smoking-related deaths. Levy and Marimont argue that after accounting for other factors that may contribute to deaths among smokers, CDC's estimate should be greatly reduced.

CDC's estimate of annual smoking-related deaths does control for age, the confounding variable that has the greatest effect on the association of smoking with disease and death. Analyses that have controlled for several factors (e.g., exercise and alcohol intake) indicate a minimal effect of potential confounders on the age-adjusted risk of disease or death from smoking.

According to Levy and Marimont, "if a smoker who is obese, has a family history of high cholesterol, diabetes, and heart problems, and never exercises dies of a heart attack, the government attributes his death to smoking alone." What the authors are reasonably questioning here is the effect of potential confounders—other factors that may explain some of the deaths attributed to smoking—on estimates of smoking-related deaths. For some diseases, the influence of confounders is trivial—smoking causes approximately 87 percent of lung cancers, for example. But for diseases that have several significant risk factors, such as cardiovascular disease, the effect of confounders may indeed be significant.

As Levy and Marimont point out, failing to account for confounders can cause inaccurate estimates of smoking-related deaths. But the authors incorrectly assume that CDC's age-adjusted estimate would be reduced significantly by controlling for potential confounders. In fact, it has been shown that controlling for confounders can cause increases in attributable risk, which suggests that CDC's estimate might be conservative.

When assessing the effect of confounding variables on CDC's estimate, it is important to consider the results of studies that have examined the effects of confounders on smoking risk. The Nurses' Health Study (NHS)—a well-designed, prospective cohort study, with 12 years of followup on registered nurses in the United States—controlled for many potential confounders, including hypertension, diabetes, high serum cholesterol, weight, parental history of heart attack before age 60, past use of oral contraceptives, postmenopausal estrogen use, and age at which smoking started. NHS found a multivariate relative risk of 1.87 for death of current smokers compared with "never-smokers," almost the same as their age-adjusted estimate of 1.86. NHS also found a slight strengthening of the association between current smoking and mortality from cardiovascular disease, after adjusting for alcohol and exercise.

In a 1997 analysis of the CPS data used by CDC, Battelle controlled for risk factors—including age, education, alcohol intake, diabetes and hypertension—and found smoking-related mortality estimates for the combined disease categories of lung cancer, ischemic heart disease, bronchitis/emphysema, chronic airway obstruction, and cerebrovascular disease to be 2 percent higher than CDC's age-adjusted estimates.

Thus, contrary to Levy and Marimont's claim, the available data strongly suggest that further adjustment for potential confounders other than age would have little effect on CDC's estimate of roughly 400,000 smoking-related deaths a year.

Argument 4. *Smoking-related mortality is overstated, particularly with respect to children, given that the majority of smoking-related deaths occur late in life.*

In fact, it has been estimated that more than half of all smoking-related deaths occur between ages 35 and 69, which translates into an average loss of roughly 23 years of life. Cigarette smoking also accounts for approximately 30 percent of all deaths among those 35–69 years of age. That the majority of deaths from smoking occur among adults does not mitigate the real risks that cigarettes pose to children.

Levy and Marimont aver that smoking "kill[s] people at an average age of roughly 72—far closer to 99 than to childhood or even young adulthood." This unreferenced assertion is inconsistent with studies suggesting that the average age of death among smokers is much less than 72 years.

It is important to consider that what the authors are reporting is an average age of death. Cigarette smoking kills people at ages much less than 72, as well as at ages much greater than 72. Long-term, follow-up studies have found that smokers are three times more likely to die between the ages of 45 and 64, and two times more likely to die between the ages of 65 and 84, than are non-smokers. Thirty-three percent of nonsmokers live to age 85, while only 12 percent of smokers live that long.

Levy and Marimont insinuate that the deaths of older adults should not be considered premature or preventable. But many adults remain healthy into their eighties and nineties. It is inappropriate to set an arbitrary age limit on premature death. A premature, preventable death is a premature, preventable death at any age. The authors' underlying assumption is that deaths among the elderly are less consequential than deaths among the young, a "modest proposal" that controverts the fundamental, humanitarian principle of medicine and public health: all human lives are valuable.

In an effort to minimize the impact of smoking-related mortality, Levy and Marimont present smoking-related deaths in terms of years of potential life lost (YPLL). The authors, however, rely on an outdated way of calculating YPLL, by considering only those years under age 65. YPLL is more accurately calculated from life expectancy, which extends well beyond age 65.

After inappropriately comparing smoking-attributed mortality with immediate deaths from motor vehicle accidents, suicide, and homicide, the authors state that "measured by YPLL, tobacco was . . . not 'the number one killer in America' as alarmists have exclaimed." Some premature, preventable deaths with causes other than smoking do occur at a much younger age than deaths caused by smoking. But given the vast number of deaths caused by cigarette use, smoking remains the leading cause of preventable death.

It is important to note that YPLL is just one of many measures representing the public health effect of a risk factor. Aside from mortality due to smoking, the authors fail to take into account smoking-related morbidity and the poor quality of life that often accompanies the chronic illnesses caused by cigarette smoking.

The authors assert that the concern about smoking among young people is unfounded because the majority of cigarette-related deaths occur later in life. They suggest that alcohol and drug abuse are more legitimate threats to the young. However, the dangers from alcohol and drug abuse do not preclude the dangers of cigarette smoking.

Cigarettes and cigarette smoke contain nicotine, a powerfully addictive drug. People who begin smoking as children are more likely to become lifetime smokers and, therefore, to die from smoking-caused disease. Smoking at a young age (or any age) causes irreversible genetic and cellular damage that may take years to emerge as disease. Furthermore, studies have found that cigarette smoking is associated with, and tends to precede, alcohol and illicit drug use—the very behaviors Levy and Marimont deem most threatening to children.

Levy and Marimont's arguments obscure the real risks associated with cigarette smoking—effects that may not be immediately observed, but are harmful nonetheless.

Conclusion

Levy and Marimont fail to present a scientifically sound and convincing argument that the estimate of 400,000 annual smoking-related deaths is a specious, statistical gimmick. In an effort to minimize smoking's death toll, they make unsupported assumptions about the effects of potential confounders and inappropriately dismiss relative risks less than 2. Moreover, their criticisms of the CPS data and their disregard for the long-term effects of cigarette smoking are misguided. We conclude that the estimate of 400,000 annual deaths from cigarette smoking is indeed reliable and may even be an underestimate.

"Lies, Damned Lies, & 400,000 Smoking-Related Deaths" does, however, bring to light some reasonable questions that the public may share about the methods used to determine smoking-related deaths. The article clearly illustrates the importance of educating nonscientists about basic epidemiological and biostatistical concepts.

In their conclusion, the authors make further misleading and unscientific claims, stating, for example, that "the actual damage from smoking is neither known nor knowable with precision." But as we have said, smoking and tobacco use is the most-studied health risk factor in the history of human health research. In fact, the first report of diminished life span among smokers appeared in 1938. The pathological effects of chronic tobacco use in individuals are well documented. Using rigorous study designs and analytical methods, scientists have established with a high degree of certainty the causal role of tobacco in disease and death.

Levy and Marimont suggest that the "correctly calculated number of smoking-related deaths" is about 100,000 a year. Even if one were to accept the authors' gross miscalculation, is not the premature, debilitating, and often painful death of "only" 100,000 Americans (of any age) worthy of being addressed as a significant public health problem?

The authors might well heed their own advice when they criticize federal officials for "tainting science to advance predetermined ends." By straying from basic epidemiological principles in their arguments, and by touting opinions that masquerade as facts, the authors have themselves strayed far from science.

POSTSCRIPT

Are the Adverse Effects of Smoking Exaggerated?

Much data indicate that smoking cigarettes is injurious to human health. For example, more than 400,000 people die from tobacco-related illnesses each year in the United States, costing the U.S. health care system billions of dollars annually. Thousands more people develop debilitating conditions such as chronic bronchitis and emphysema. Levy and Marimont, however, question the accuracy of this data. How the data are presented and interpreted may affect how one feels about the issue of placing more restrictions on tobacco products. If cigarette smoking is demonized, as Levy and Marimont suggest, it is not difficult to influence people's positions on regulating tobacco. Currently, they contend, there is a great deal of antismoking sentiment in society because of how the statistics are presented. Although Levy and Marimont do not recommend that people use tobacco products, they do state that the consequences linked to these products are exaggerated.

Despite the reported hazards of tobacco smoking, many proponents of smokers' rights assert that cigarette smoking is a matter of choice. However, many could argue that smoking is not a matter of choice because smokers become addicted to nicotine. Others contend that the decision to start smoking is a matter of choice, but once tobacco dependency occurs, most smokers are in effect deprived of the choice to stop smoking. Contributing to the tobacco dilemma is the expansion of tobacco manufacturers into many developing countries and the proliferation of advertising despite its ban from television and radio.

Nevertheless, tobacco proponents maintain that people make all types of choices, and if the choices that people make are ultimately harmful, then that is their responsibility. A basic question is, Do people have the right to engage in self-destructive behavior?

Several times a year the SmokeFree Educational Services publishes *Smoke-Free Air*, a newsletter describing actions that have been taken to limit smoking in public locations. Also, Mike Mitka's article "Surgeon General's Newest Report on Tobacco," *Journal of the American Medical Association* (September 20, 2000) lists current smoking-related statistics and describes efforts to stem cigarette smoking. Efforts to prevent cigarette smoking are detailed by the U.S. Department of Health and Human Services in *Reducing Tobacco Use: A Report of the Surgeon General* (2000). Finally, in "Prying Open the Door to the Tobacco Industry's Secrets About Nicotine," *Journal of the American Medical Association* (October 7, 1998), Richard D. Hurt and Channing R. Robertson describe actions taken by states to get the tobacco industry to admit that it covered up industry documents revealing that nicotine is an addictive drug and that industry strategies utilized this knowledge to increase cigarette sales.

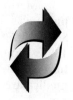

ISSUE 9

Should Marijuana Be Legal for Medicinal Purposes?

YES: Lester Grinspoon, from "Whither Medical Marijuana?" *Contemporary Drug Problems* (Spring 2000)

NO: James R. McDonough, from "Marijuana on the Ballot," *Policy Review* (April/May 2000)

ISSUE SUMMARY

YES: Professor of psychiatry Lester Grinspoon contends that, despite the fact that the majority of Americans support marijuana use for medical purposes, the federal government is suppressing its medical use for fear that it may become more acceptable for recreational use. He believes that pharmaceutical companies may develop commercial alternatives but questions the effectiveness of these alternatives.

NO: James R. McDonough, director of the Florida Office of Drug Control, agrees that compounds in marijuana, such as THC, may have the potential to be medically valuable. However, smoked marijuana has not been proven to be of medicinal value. In addition, there are existing, approved drugs that are more effective for conditions that may be helped by marijuana use.

Since the mid-1990s voters in California, Arizona, Oregon, Colorado, and other states have passed referenda to legalize marijuana for medical purposes. Despite the position of these voters, however, the federal government does not support the medical use of marijuana, and federal laws take precedence over state laws. A major concern of opponents of these referenda is that legalization of marijuana for medicinal purposes will lead to its use for recreational purposes.

Marijuana's medicinal qualities have been recognized for centuries. Marijuana was utilized medically as far back as 2737 B.C., when Chinese emperor Shen Nung recommended marijuana, or cannabis, for medical use. By the 1890s some medical reports had stated that cannabis was useful as a pain reliever. However, despite its historical significance, the use of marijuana for medical treatment is still a widely debated and controversial topic.

Marijuana has been tested in the treatment of glaucoma, asthma, convulsions, epilepsy, and migraine headaches, and in the reduction of nausea, vomiting, and loss of appetite associated with chemotherapy treatments. Many medical professionals and patients believe that marijuana shows promise in the treatment of these disorders and others, including spasticity in amputees and multiple sclerosis. Yet others argue that there are alternative drugs and treatments available that are more specific and effective in treating these disorders than marijuana and that marijuana cannot be considered a medical replacement.

Because of the conflicting viewpoints and what many people argue is an absence of reliable scientific research supporting the medicinal value of marijuana, the drug and its plant materials remain in Schedule I of the Controlled Substances Act of 1970. This act established five categories, or schedules, under which drugs are classified according to their potential for abuse and their medical usefulness, which in turn determines their availability. Drugs classified under Schedule I are those that have a high potential for abuse and no scientifically proven medical use. Many medical marijuana proponents have called for the Drug Enforcement Administration (DEA) to move marijuana from Schedule I to Schedule II, which classifies drugs as having a high potential for abuse but also having an established medical use. A switch to Schedule II would legally allow physicians to utilize marijuana and its components in certain treatment programs. To date, however, the DEA has refused.

Currently, marijuana is used medically but not legally. Most of the controversy surrounds whether or not marijuana and its plant properties are indeed of medical value and whether or not the risks associated with its use outweigh its proposed medical benefits. Research reports and scientific studies have been inconclusive. Some physicians and many cancer patients say that marijuana greatly reduces the side effects of chemotherapy. Many glaucoma patients believe that marijuana use has greatly improved their conditions. In view of these reports by patients and the recommendations by some physicians to allow inclusion of marijuana in treatment, expectations have been raised with regard to marijuana's worth as a medical treatment.

Marijuana opponents argue that the evidence in support of marijuana as medically useful suffers from far too many deficiencies. The DEA, for example, believes that studies supporting the medical value of marijuana are scientifically limited, based on biased testimonies of ill individuals who have used marijuana and their families and friends, and grounded in the unscientific opinions of certain physicians, nurses, and other hospital personnel. Furthermore, marijuana opponents feel that the safety of marijuana has not been established by reliable scientific data weighing marijuana's possible therapeutic benefits against its known negative effects.

In the following selections, Lester Grinspoon asserts that the federal government has set up needless political roadblocks to prevent needy individuals from receiving the medical benefits of marijuana. James R. McDonough argues that marijuana should not be legalized for medical purposes because the current research on marijuana's medicinal benefits is inconclusive and that other drugs are available that preclude the need to use marijuana.

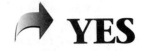
Whither Medical Marijuana?

Cannabis was first admitted to Western pharmacopoeias one and a half centuries ago. In 1839 W. B. O'Shaughnessy at the Medical College of Calcutta observed its use in the indigenous treatment of various disorders and found that tincture of hemp was an effective analgesic, anticonvulsant, and muscle relaxant.[1] Publication of O'Shaughnessy's paper created a stir within a medical establishment which at that time had access to only a few effective medicines. In the next several decades, many papers on cannabis appeared in the Western medical literature. It was widely used until the first decades of the 20th century, especially as an analgesic and hypnotic. Symptoms and conditions for which it was found helpful included tetanus, neuralgia, labor pain, dysmenorrhea, convulsions, asthma, and rheumatism.[2]

Administering a medicine through smoking was unheard of until the late 19th century, when pharmaceutical house, prepared coca leaf cigars and cheroots were occasionally used in lieu of cocaine.[3] If physicians had realized that titration of the dose was easier and relief came faster when marijuana was inhaled, they might have preferred to administer it by smoking. However, in the 19th century it was prepared chiefly as a tincture (alcoholic solution), generally referred to as tincture of hemp, tincture of cannabis, or Cannabis indica. The potency and bioavailability of oral cannabis varied widely, and there were no reliable bioassay techniques. Nevertheless, physicians prescribed cannabis without much concern about overdoses or side effects, because they knew how safe it was. But understandably, they considered it less reliable as an analgesic than opium and opium derivatives. Furthermore, unlike opiates, it could not be used parenterally because it was not water-soluble. Then, at the turn of the century, the first synthetic analgesics and hypnotics (aspirin and barbiturates) became available. Physicians were immediately attracted to these drugs because their potencies were fixed and they were easily dispensed as pills.

Beginning in the 1920s, interest in cannabis as a recreational drug grew, along with a disinformation campaign calculated to discourage that use. In 1937 the first draconian federal legislation against marijuana, the Marijuana Tax Act, was passed. At that time the medical use of cannabis had already declined considerably; the Act made prescription of marijuana so cumbersome that physicians abandoned it. Now physicians themselves became victims of the "Reefer Madness" madness. Beginning with an editorial published in the *Journal of the American Medical Association* in 1945, the medical establishment became one of the most effective agents of cannabis prohibition.[4]

The modern renaissance of medicinal cannabis began in the early 1970s, when several young patients who were being treated with the recently developed cancer chemotherapies discovered that marijuana was much more effective than conventional medicines for the relief of the intense and prolonged nausea and vomiting induced by some of these agents.[5] Word spread rapidly over the cancer treatment grapevine. By mid-decade, the capacity of marijuana to lower intraocular pressure had been observed, and patients suffering from glaucoma began to experiment with it.[6] As the AIDS epidemic gathered momentum, many patients who suffered HIV-associated weight loss learned that marijuana was the most effective and least toxic treatment for this life-threatening symptom. These three new medical uses of cannabis have led to wider folk experimentation. The use of marijuana in the symptomatic treatment of convulsive disorders, migraine, insomnia, and dysmenorrhea has been rediscovered.

We have now identified more than 30 symptoms and syndromes for which patients have found cannabis useful,[7] and others will undoubtedly be discovered. Many patients regard it as more effective than conventional medicines, with fewer or less disturbing side effects. Consider the pain of osteoarthritis, which was often treated in the 19th century with tincture of cannabis. Aspirin, the first of the non-steroidal antiinflammatory drugs (NSAIDs), rapidly displaced cannabis as the treatment of choice for this and many other kinds of mild to moderate pain. But NSAIDs now take more than 7,000 lives annually in the United States alone; cannabis, by contrast, has never killed anyone using it for the relief of pain or any other purpose.[8] It is not surprising that many patients now treat their osteoarthritis with cannabis, asserting that it provides a better quality of pain relief than NSAIDs and also elevates their spirits.

The number of Americans who understand the medical uses of cannabis has grown greatly in the last few years. The passage of initiatives or legislation allowing some restricted legal use of cannabis as a medicine in eight states is the most striking political manifestation of this growing interest. The state laws have led to a battle with federal authorities who, until recently, proclaimed medical marijuana to be a hoax. Under public pressure to acknowledge the medical potential of marijuana, the director of the Office of National Drug Policy, Barry McCaffrey, authorized a review by the Institute of Medicine [IOM] of the National Academy of Science which was published in March of 1999.[9]

The report acknowledged the medical value of marijuana, but grudgingly. One of its most important shortcomings was a failure to put into perspective the vast anecdotal evidence of marijuana's striking medicinal versatility and limited toxicity. The report states that smoking is too dangerous a form of delivery, but this conclusion is based on an exaggerated evaluation of the toxicity of the smoke. The report's Recommendation Six would allow patients with what it calls "debilitating symptoms (such as intractable pain or vomiting)" to use smoked marijuana for only six months, and then only after all other approved medicines have failed. The treatment would have to be monitored with "an oversight strategy comparable to an institutional review board process."[10] This would make legal use of medical cannabis impossible in practice. The IOM would have patients who find cannabis helpful when taken by inhalation wait for years until a means of delivering smoke-free cannabinoids is developed. But there are already prototype devices which take advantage of the fact that cannabinoids vaporize at temperatures below the ignition point of dried cannabis plant material.

The authors of the IOM report discuss marijuana as if it were a drug like thalidomide, with well-established serious toxicity (phocomelia) and limited clinical usefulness (leprosy). This is inappropriate for a drug with a long history, limited toxicity, unusual versatility, and easy availability. But at least the report confirms that even government officials no longer doubt that cannabis has medical uses. Inevitably, cannabinoids will eventually be allowed to compete with other medicines in the treatment of a variety of symptoms and conditions; the only uncertainty involves the form in which they will be delivered.

When I first considered this issue in the early 1970s, I assumed that cannabis as medicine would be identical to the marijuana that is used for other purposes (the dried flowering tops of female Cannabis indica plants); its toxicity is minimal, its dosage is easily titrated and, once freed of the prohibition tariff, it will be inexpensive. I thought the main problem was its classification in Schedule I of the Comprehensive Drug Abuse and Control Act of 1970, which describes it as having a high potential for abuse, no accepted medical use in the United States, and lack of accepted safety for use under medical supervision. At that time I naively believed that a change to Schedule II would overcome a major obstacle to its legal availability as a medicine. I had already come to believe that the greatest harm in recreational use of marijuana came not from the drug itself but from the effects of prohibition. But I saw that as a separate issue; I believed that, like opiates and cocaine, cannabis could be used medically while remaining outlawed for other purposes. I thought that once it was transferred to Schedule II, clinical research on marijuana would be pursued eagerly. A quarter of a century later, I have begun to doubt this. It would be highly desirable if marijuana could be approved as a legitimate medicine within the present federal regulatory system, but it now seems to me unlikely.

Today, transferring marijuana to Schedule II (high potential for abuse, limited medical use) would not be enough to make it available as a prescription drug. Such drugs must undergo rigorous, expensive, and time-consuming tests before they are approved by the FDA [Food and Drug Administration]. This system is designed to regulate the commercial distribution of drug company products and protect the public against false or misleading claims about their efficacy and safety. The drug is generally a single synthetic chemical that a pharmaceutical company has developed and patented. The company submits an application to the FDA and tests it first for safety in animals and then for clinical safety and efficacy. The company must present evidence from double-blind controlled studies showing that the drug is more effective than a placebo and as effective as available drugs. Case reports, expert opinion, and clinical experience are not considered sufficient. The cost of this evaluation exceeds 200 million dollars per drug.

It is unlikely that whole smoked marijuana should or will ever be developed as an officially recognized medicine via this route. Thousands of years of use have demonstrated its medical value; the extensive government-supported effort of the last three decades to establish a sufficient level of toxicity to support the harsh prohibition has instead provided a record of safety that is more compelling than that of most approved medicines. The modern FDA protocol is not necessary to establish a risk-benefit estimate for a drug with such a history. To impose this protocol on cannabis would be like making the same demand of aspirin, which was accepted as a medicine more than 60 years before the advent of the double-blind controlled study. Many years of experience have shown us that aspirin has many uses and limited toxicity, yet today it could not be marshalled through the FDA approval process. The patent has long since expired, and with it the incentive to underwrite the enormous cost of this modern seal of approval. Cannabis too is unpatentable, so the only source of funding for a "start-from-scratch" approval would be the government, which is, to put it mildly, unlikely to be helpful. Other reasons for doubting that marijuana would ever be officially approved are today's anti-smoking climate and, most important, the widespread use of cannabis for purposes disapproved by the government.

To see the importance of this obstacle, consider the effects of granting marijuana legitimacy as a medicine while prohibiting it for any other use. How would the appropriate "labeled" uses be determined and how would "off-label" uses be proscribed? Then there is the question of who will provide the cannabis. The federal government now provides marijuana from its farm in Mississippi to eight patients under a now-discontinued Compassionate IND [investigational new drug] program. But surely the government could not or would not produce marijuana for many thousands of patients receiving prescriptions, any more than it does for other prescription drugs. If production is contracted out, will the farmers have to enclose their fields with security fences and protect them with security guards? How would the marijuana be distributed? If through pharmacies, how would they provide secure facilities capable of keeping fresh supplies? Would the price of pharmaceutical marijuana have to be controlled: not too high, lest patients be tempted to buy it on the street or grow their own; not too low, lest people with marginal or fictitious "medical" conditions besiege their doctors for prescriptions? What about the parallel problems with potency? When urine tests are demanded for workers, how would those who use marijuana legally as a medicine be distinguished from those who use it for other purposes?

To realize the full potential of cannabis as a medicine in the setting of the present prohibition system, we would have to address all these problems and more. A delivery system that successfully navigated this minefield would be cumbersome, inefficient, and bureaucratically top-heavy. Government and medical licensing boards would insist on tight restrictions, challenging physicians as though cannabis were a dangerous drug every time it was used for any new patient or purpose. There would be constant conflict with one of two outcomes: patients would not get all the benefits they should, or they would get the benefits by abandoning the legal system for the black market or their own gardens and closets.

A solution now being proposed, notably in the IOM Report, is what might be called the "pharmaceuticalization" of cannabis: prescription of isolated individual cannabinoids, synthetic cannabinoids, and cannabinoid analogs. The IOM Report states that "if there is any future for marijuana as a medicine, it lies in its isolated components, the cannabinoids, and their synthetic derivatives." It goes on: "Therefore, the purpose of clinical trials of smoked marijuana would not be to develop marijuana as a licensed drug, but such trials could be a first step towards the development of rapid-onset, non-smoked cannabinoid delivery systems."[11] Some cannabinoids and analogs may have advantages over whole smoked or ingested marijuana in limited circumstances. For example, cannabidiol may be more effective as an anti-anxiety medicine and an anticonvulsant when it is not taken along with THC [the chief intoxicant in marijuana], which sometimes generates anxiety. Other cannabinoids and analogs may occasionally prove more useful than marijuana because they can be administered intravenously. For example, 15 to 20 percent of patients lose consciousness after suffering a thrombotic or embolic stroke, and some people who suffer brain syndrome after a severe blow to the head become unconscious. The new analog dexanabinol (HU-211) has been shown to protect brain cells from damage by glutamate excitotoxicity in these circumstances, and it will be possible to give it intravenously to an unconscious person.[12] Presumably other analogs may offer related advantages. Some of these commercial products may also lack the psychoactive effects which make marijuana useful to some for non-medical purposes. Therefore they will not be defined as "abusable" drugs subject to the constraints of the Comprehensive Drug Abuse and Control Act. Nasal sprays, nebulizers, skin patches, pills, and suppositories can be used to avoid exposure of the lungs to the particulate matter in marijuana smoke.

The question is whether these developments will make marijuana itself medically obsolete. Surely many of these new products would be useful and safe enough for commercial development. It is uncertain, however, whether pharmaceutical companies will find them worth the enormous development costs. Some may be (for example, a cannabinoid inverse agonist that reduces appetite might be highly lucrative), but for most specific symptoms, analogs or combinations of analogs are unlikely to be more useful than natural cannabis. Nor are they likely to have a significantly wider spectrum of therapeutic uses, since the natural product contains the compounds (and synergistic combinations of compounds) from which they are derived. THC and cannabidiol, as well as dexanabinol, protect brain cells after a stroke or traumatic injury. Synthetic tetrahydrocannabinol (dronabinol or Marinol) has been available for years, but patients generally find whole smoked marijuana to be more effective.

The cannabinoids in whole marijuana can be separated from the burnt plant products by vaporization devices that will be inexpensive when manufactured in large numbers. Inhalation is a highly effective means of delivery, and faster means will not be available for analogs (except in a few situations such as parenteral injection in a patient who is unconscious or suffering from pulmonary impairment). Furthermore, any new analog will have to have an acceptable therapeutic ratio. The therapeutic ratio of marijuana is not known because it has never caused an overdose death, but it is estimated on the basis of extrapolation from animal data to be 20,000 to 40,000. The therapeutic ratio of a new analog is unlikely to be higher than that; in fact, new analogs may be less safe than smoked marijuana because it will be physically possible to ingest more of them. And there is the problem of classification under the Comprehensive Drug Abuse and Control Act for analogs with psychoactive effects. The more restrictive the classification of a drug, the less likely drug companies are to develop it and physicians to prescribe it. Recognizing this economic fact of life, Unimed, the manufacturer of Marinol, has recently succeeding in getting it reclassified from Schedule II to Schedule III. Nevertheless, many physicians will continue to avoid prescribing it for fear of the drug enforcement authorities.

A somewhat different approach to the pharmaceuticalization of cannabis is being taken by a British company, G. W. Pharmaceuticals. Recognizing the great usefulness of naturally occurring cannabinoids, this firm is developing a seed bank of cannabis strains with particular value in the treatment of various symptoms and disorders. They are also attempting to develop products and delivery systems which will skirt the two primary concerns about the use of marijuana as a medicine: the smoke and the psychoactive effects (the "high").

To avoid the need for smoking, G. W. Pharmaceuticals is exploring the possibility of delivering cannabis extracts sublingually or via nebulizers. The company expects its products to be effective therapeutically at doses too low to produce the psychoactive effects sought by recreational and other users. My clinical experience leads me to question whether this is possible in most or even many cases. Furthermore, the issue is complicated by tolerance. Recreational users soon discover that the more often they use marijuana, the less "high" they feel. A patient who smokes cannabis frequently for the relief of, say, chronic pain or elevated intraocular pressure will not experience a "high" at all. Furthermore, as a clinician who has considerable experience with medical cannabis use, I have to question whether the psychoactive effect is necessarily undesirable. Many patients suffering from serious chronic illnesses say that cannabis generally improves their spirits. If they note psychoactive effects at all, they speak of a slight mood elevation—certainly nothing unwanted or incapacitating.

In principle, administration of cannabis extracts via a nebulizer has the same advantages as smoked marijuana—rapid onset and easy titratability of the effect. But the design of the G. W. Pharmaceutical nebulizer negates this advantage. The device has electronic controls that monitor the dose and halt delivery if the patient tries to take more than the physician or pharmacist has set it to deliver. The proposal to use this cumbersome and expensive device apparently reflects a fear that patients cannot accurately titrate the amount or a concern that they might take more than they need and experience some degree of "high" (always assuming, doubtfully, that the two can easily be separated, especially when cannabis is used infrequently). Because these products will be considerably more expensive than natural marijuana, they will succeed only if patients and physicians take the health risks of smoking very seriously and feel that it is necessary to avoid any hint of a psychoactive effect.

In the end, the commercial success of any cannabinoid product will depend on how vigorously the prohibition against marijuana is enforced. It is safe to predict that new analogs and extracts will cost much more than whole smoked or ingested marijuana even at the inflated prices imposed by the prohibition tariff. I doubt that pharmaceutical companies would be interested in developing cannabinoid products if they had to compete with natural marijuana on a level playing field. The most common reason for using Marinol is the illegality of marijuana, and many patients choose to ignore the law for reasons of efficacy and price. The number of arrests on marijuana charges has been steadily increasing and has now reached nearly 700,000 annually, yet patients continue to use smoked cannabis as a medicine. I wonder whether any level of enforcement would compel enough compliance with the law to embolden drug companies to commit the many millions of dollars it would take to develop new cannabinoid products. Unimed is able to profit from the exorbitantly priced dronabinol only because the United States government underwrote much of the cost of development. Pharmaceutical companies will undoubtedly develop useful cannabinoid products, some of which may not be subject to the constraints of the Comprehensive Drug Abuse and Control Act. But this pharmaceuticalization will never displace natural marijuana for most medical purposes.

Thus two powerful forces are now colliding: the growing acceptance of medical cannabis and the proscription against any use of marijuana, medical or non-medical. There are no signs that we are moving away from absolute prohibition to a regulatory system that would allow responsible use of marijuana. As a result, we are going to have two distribution systems for medical cannabis: the conventional model of pharmacy-filled prescriptions for FDA-approved medicines, and a model closer to the distribution of alternative and herbal medicines. The only difference, an enormous one, will be the continued illegality of whole smoked or ingested cannabis. In any case, increasing medical use by either distribution pathway will inevitably make growing numbers of people familiar with cannabis and its derivatives. As they learn that its harmfulness has been greatly exaggerated and its usefulness underestimated, the pressure will increase for drastic change in the way we as a society deal with this drug.

References

1. W. B. O'Shaughnessy. On the Preparations of the Indian Hemp, or Gunjah (*Cannabis indica*): The Effects on the Animal System in Health, and Their Utility in the Treatment of Tetanus and Other Convulsive Diseases. *Transactions of the Medical and Physical Society of Bengal* (1838–1840), p. 460.

2. L. Grinspoon. *Marihuana Reconsidered*. Cambridge, Mass.: Harvard University Press, 1971, pp. 218–230.

3. L. Grinspoon and J. B. Bakalar. *Cocaine: A Drug and Its Social Evolution*, Revised Edition. New York: Basic Books, 1985, p. 279.

4. Marihuana Problems. Editorial, *Journal of the American Medical Association*, Vol. 127 (1945), p. 1129.

5. L. Grinspoon and J. B. Bakalar. *Marihuana, the Forbidden Medicine*, Revised and Expanded Edition. New Haven: Yale University Press, 1997, pp. 25–27.

6. R. S. Hepler and I. M. Frank. Marihuana Smoking and Intraocular Pressure. *Journal of the American Medical Association*, Vol. 217 (1971), p. 1392.

7. L. Grinspoon and J. B. Bakalar. *Marihuana, the Forbidden Medicine*, Revised and Expanded Edition. New Haven: Yale University Press, 1997.

8. S. Girkipal, D. R. Ramey, D. Morfeld, G. Singh, H. T. Hatoum, and J. F. Fries. Gastrointestinal Tract Complications of Nonsteroidal Anti-inflammatory Drug Treatment in Rheumatoid Arthritis. *Archives of Internal Medicine,* Vol. 156 (July 22, 1996), pp. 1530–1536.
9. *Marijuana and Medicine: Assessing the Science Base.* J. E. Joy, S. J. Watson, Jr., and J. A. Benson, Jr., Editors. Institute of Medicine, Washington, D.C.: National Academy Press (1999).
10. Ibid, pp. 7–8.
11. Ibid, p. 11.
12. R. R. Leker, E. Shohami, O. Abramsky, and H. Ovadia. Dexanabinol; A Novel Neuroprotective Drug in Experimental Focal Cerebral Ischemia. *Journal of Neurological Science,* Vol. 162, No. 2 (January 15, 1999), pp. 114–119; E. Shohami, M. Novikov, and R. Bass. Long-term Effect of HU-211, a Novel Non-competitive NMDA Antagonist, on Motor and Memory Functions after Closed Head Injury in the Rat. *Brain Research,* Vol. 674, No. 1 (March 13, 1995), pp. 55–62.

James R. McDonough 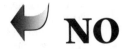 **NO**

Marijuana on the Ballot

While it has long been clear that chemical compounds found in the marijuana plant offer potential for medical use, smoking the raw plant is a method of delivery supported neither by law nor recent scientific evidence. The Food and Drug Administration's approval process, which seeks to ensure the purity of chemical compounds in legitimate drugs, sets the standard for medical validation of prescription drugs as safe and effective. Diametrically opposed to this long-standing safeguard of medical science is the recent spate of state election ballots that have advocated the use of a smoked plant—the marijuana leaf—for "treating" an unspecified number of ailments. It is a tribute to the power of political activism that popular vote has displaced objective science in advancing what would be the only smoked drug in America under the guise of good medicine.

Two recent studies of the potential medical utility of marijuana advocate development of a non-smoked, rapid onset delivery system of the cannabis compounds. But state ballot initiatives that seek legalization of smoking marijuana as medicine threaten to circumvent credible research. Advocates for smoking marijuana appear to want to move ahead at all costs, irrespective of dangers to the user. They make a well-financed, emotional appeal to the voting public claiming that what they demand is humane, useful, and safe. Although they rely largely on anecdote to document their claims, they seize upon partial statements that purport to validate their assertions. At the same time, these partisans—described by Chris Wren, the highly respected journalist for the *New York Times,* as a small coalition of libertarians, liberals, humanitarians, and hedonists—reject the main conclusions of medical science: that there is little future in smoked marijuana as a medically approved medication.

A Dearth of Scientific Support

Compounds found in marijuana may have medical potential, but science does not support smoking the plant in its crude form as an appropriate delivery system. An exploration of two comprehensive inquiries into the medical potential of marijuana indicates the following:

- Science has identified only the *potential* medical benefit of chemical compounds, such as THC, found in marijuana. Ambitious research is necessary to understand fully how these substances affect the human body.
- Experts who have dealt with all available data *do not* recommend that the goal of research should be smoked marijuana for medical conditions. Rather, they support development of a smoke-free, rapid-onset delivery system for compounds found in the plant.

In 1997, the National Institutes of Health (NIH) met "to review the scientific data concerning the potential therapeutic uses of marijuana and the need for and feasibility of additional research." The collection of experts had experience in relevant studies and clinical research, but held no preconceived opinions about the medical use of marijuana. They were asked the following questions: What is the current state of scientific knowledge; what significant questions remain unanswered; what is the medical potential; what possible uses deserve further research; and what issues should be considered if clinical trials are conducted?

Shortly thereafter, the White House Office of National Drug Control Policy (ONDCP) asked the Institute of Medicine (IOM) to execute a similar task: to form a panel that would "conduct a review of the scientific evidence to assess the potential health benefits and risks of marijuana and its constituent cannabinoids." Selected reviewers were among the most accomplished in the disciplines of neuroscience, pharmacology, immunology, drug abuse, drug laws, oncology, infectious diseases, and ophthalmology. Their analysis focused on the effects of isolated cannabinoids, risks associated with medical use of marijuana, and the use of smoked marijuana. Their findings in the IOM study stated:

> "Compared to most drugs, the accumulation of medical knowledge about marijuana has proceeded in reverse. Typically, during the course of drug development, a compound is first found to have some medical benefit. Following this, extensive tests are undertaken to determine the safety and proper dose of the drug for medical use. Marijuana, in contrast, has been widely used in the United States for decades. . . . The data on the adverse effects of marijuana are more extensive than the data on effectiveness. Clinical studies of marijuana are difficult to conduct."

Nevertheless, the IOM report concluded that cannabinoid drugs do have *potential* for therapeutic use. It specifically named pain, nausea and vomiting, and lack of appetite as symptoms for which cannabinoids may be of benefit, stating that cannabinoids are "moderately well suited" for AIDS wasting and nausea resulting from chemotherapy. The report found that cannabinoids "probably have a natural role in pain modulation, control of movement, and memory," but that this role "is likely to be multi-faceted and remains unclear."

In addressing the possible effects of smoked marijuana on pain, the NIH report explained that no clinical trials involving patients with "naturally occurring pain" have ever been conducted but that two credible studies of cancer pain indicated analgesic benefit. Addressing another possible benefit—the reduction of nausea related to chemotherapy—the NIH report described a study comparing oral administration of THC (via a drug called Dronabinol) and smoked marijuana. Of 20 patients, nine expressed no preference between the two, seven preferred the oral THC, and only four preferred smoked marijuana. In summary, the report states, "No scientific questions have been definitively answered about the efficacy of smoked marijuana in chemotherapy-related nausea and vomiting."

In the area of glaucoma, the effect of marijuana on intraocular pressure (the cause of optic nerve damage that typifies glaucoma) was explored, and smoked marijuana was found to reduce this pressure. However, the NIH report failed to find evidence that marijuana can "safely and effectively lower intraocular pressure enough to prevent optic nerve damage." The report concluded that the "mechanism of action" of smoked marijuana or THC in pill form on intraocular pressure is not known and calls for more research.

In addressing appetite stimulation and wasting related to AIDS, the NIH report recognized the potential benefit of marijuana. However, the report also noted the lack of pertinent data. The researchers pointed out that the evidence known to date, although plentiful, is anecdotal, and "no objective data relative to body composition alterations, HIV replication, or immunologic function in HIV patients are available."

Smoking marijuana as medicine was recommended by neither report. The IOM report called smoked marijuana a "crude THC delivery system" that is not recommended because it delivers harmful substances, pointing out that botanical products are susceptible to problems with consistency, contaminations, uncertain potencies, and instabilities. The NIH report reached the same conclusion and explained that eliminating the smoked aspect of marijuana would "remove an important obstacle" from research into the potential medical benefits of the plant.

These studies present a consistent theme: Cannabinoids in marijuana do show potential for symptom management of several conditions, but research is inadequate to explain definitively *how* cannabinoids operate to deliver these potential benefits. Nor did the studies attribute any curative effects to marijuana; at best, only the symptoms of particular medical conditions are affected. The finding most important to the debate is that the studies did not advocate smoked marijuana as medicine. To the contrary, the NIH report called for a non-smoked alternative as a focus of further research. The IOM report recommended smoking marijuana as medicine only in the most extreme circumstances *when all other medication has failed* and then only when administration of marijuana is under strict medical supervision.

These conclusions from two studies, based not on rhetorical conjecture but on credible scientific research, do not support the legalization of smoked marijuana as medicine.

The Scientific Community's Views

The conclusions of the NIH and IOM reports are supported by commentary published in the nation's medical journals. Much of this literature focuses on the problematic aspect of smoke as a delivery system when using cannabinoids for medical purposes. One physician-authored article describes smoking "crude plant material" as "troublesome" to many doctors and "unpleasant" to many patients. Dr. Eric Voth, chairman of the International Drug Strategy Institute, stated in a 1997 article published in the *Journal of the American Medical Association* (JAMA): "To support research on smoked pot does not make sense. We're currently in a huge anti-tobacco thrust in this country, which is appropriate. So why should we waste money on drug delivery that is based on smoking?" Voth recommends non-smoked analogs to THC.

In September, 1998, the editor in chief of the *New England Journal of Medicine*, Dr. Jerome P. Kassirer, in a coauthored piece with Dr. Marcia Angell, wrote:

> "Until the 20th century, most remedies were botanical, a few of which were found through trial and error to be helpful. All of that began to change in the 20th century as a result of rapid advances in medical science. In particular, the evolution of the randomized, controlled clinical trial enabled researchers to study with precision the safety, efficacy, and dose effects of proposed treatments and the indications for them. No longer do we have to rely on trial and error and anecdotes. We have learned to ask and expect statistically reliable evidence before accepting conclusions about remedies."

Dr. Robert DuPont of the Georgetown University Department of Psychiatry points out that those who aggressively advocate smoking marijuana as medicine "undermine" the potentially beneficial roles of the NIH and IOM studies. As does Dr. Voth, DuPont discusses the possibility of nonsmoked delivery methods. He asserts that if the scientific community were to accept smoked marijuana as medicine, the public would likely perceive the decision as influenced by politics rather than science. Dupont concludes that if research is primarily concerned with the needs of the sick, it is unlikely that science will approve of smoked marijuana as medicine.

Even those who advocate smoking marijuana for medicine are occasionally driven to caution. Dr. Lester Grinspoon, a Harvard University professor and advocate of smoking marijuana, warned in a 1994 JAMA article: "The one area we have to be concerned about is pulmonary function. The lungs were not made to inhale anything but fresh air." Other experts have only disdain for the loose medical claims for smoked marijuana. Dr. Janet Lapey, executive director of Concerned Citizens for Drug Prevention, likened research on smoked marijuana to using opium pipes to test morphine. She advocates research on isolated active compounds rather than smoked marijuana.

The findings of the NIH and IOM reports, and other commentary by members of the scientific and medical communities, contradict the idea that plant smoking is an appropriate vehicle for delivering whatever compounds research may find to be of benefit.

Enter the FDA

The mission of the Food and Drug Administration's (FDA) Center for Drug Evaluation and Research is "to assure that safe and effective drugs are available to the American people." Circumvention of the FDA approval process would remove this essential safety mechanism intended to safeguard public health. The FDA approval process is not designed to keep drugs out of the hands of the sick but to offer a system to ensure that drugs prevent, cure, or treat a medical condition. FDA approval can involve testing of hundreds of compounds, which allows scientists to alter them for improved performance. The IOM report addresses this situation explicitly: "Medicines today are expected to be of known composition and quantity. Even in cases where marijuana can provide relief from symptoms, the crude plant mixture does not meet this modern expectation."

For a proposed drug to gain approval by the FDA, a potential manufacturer must produce a new drug application. The application must provide enough information for FDA reviewers to determine (among other criteria) "whether the drug is safe and effective for its proposed use(s), whether the benefits of the drug outweigh its risks [and] whether the methods used in manufacturing the drug and the controls used to maintain the drug's quality are adequate to preserve the drug's integrity, strength, quality, and purity."

On the "benefits" side, the Institute of Medicine found that the therapeutic effects of cannabinoids are "generally modest" and that for the majority of symptoms there are approved drugs that are more effective. For example, superior glaucoma and antinausea medications have already been developed. In addition, the new drug Zofran may provide more relief than THC for chemotherapy patients. Dronabinol, the synthetic THC, offers immunocompromised HIV patients a safe alternative to inhaling marijuana smoke, which contains carcinogens.

On the "risks" side, there is strong evidence that smoking marijuana has detrimental health effects. Unrefined marijuana contains approximately 400 chemicals that become combustible when smoked, producing in turn over 2,000 impure chemicals. These substances, many of which remain unidentified, include carcinogens. The IOM report states that, when used chronically, "marijuana smoking is associated with abnormalities of cells lining the human respiratory tract. Marijuana smoke, like tobacco smoke, is associated with increased risk of cancer, lung damage, and poor pregnancy outcomes." A subsequent study by Dr. Zuo-Feng Zhary of the Jonsson Cancer Center at UCLA determined that the carcinogens in marijuana are much stronger than those in tobacco.

Chronic bronchitis and increased incidence of pulmonary disease are associated with frequent use of smoked marijuana, as are reduced sperm motility and testosterone levels in males. Decreased immune system response, which is likely to increase vulnerability to infection and tumors, is also associated with frequent use. Even a slight decrease in immune response can have major public health ramifications. Because marijuana by-products remain in body fat for several weeks, interference with normal body functioning may continue beyond the time of use. Among the known effects of smoking marijuana is impaired lung function similar to the type caused by cigarette smoking.

In addressing the efficacy of cannabinoid drugs, the IOM report—after recognizing "potential therapeutic value"—added that smoked marijuana is "a crude THC delivery system that also delivers harmful substances." Purified cannabinoid compounds are preferable to plants in crude form, which contain inconsistent chemical composition. The "therapeutic window" between the desirable and adverse effects of marijuana and THC is narrow at best and may not exist at all, in many cases.

The scientific evidence that marijuana's potential therapeutic benefits are modest, that other approved drugs are generally more effective, and that smoking marijuana is unhealthy, indicates that smoked marijuana is not a viable candidate for FDA approval. Without such approval, smoked marijuana cannot achieve legitimate status as an approved drug that patients can readily use. This reality renders the advocacy of smoking marijuana as medicine both misguided and impractical.

Medicine by Ballot Initiative?

While ballot initiatives are an indispensable part of our democracy, they are imprudent in the context of advancing smoked marijuana as medicine because they confound our system of laws, create conflict between state and federal law, and fail to offer a proper substitute for science.

Ballot initiatives to legalize smoking marijuana as medicine have had a tumultuous history. In 1998 alone, initiatives were passed in five states, but any substantive benefits in the aftermath were lacking. For example, a Colorado proposal was ruled invalid before the election. An Ohio bill was passed but subsequently repealed. In the District of Colombia, Congress disallowed the counting of ballot results. Six other states permit patients to smoke marijuana as medicine but only by prescription, and doctors, dubious about the validity of a smoked medicine, wary of liability suits, and concerned about legal and professional risks are reluctant to prescribe it for their patients. Although voters passed Arizona's initiative, the state legislature originally blocked the measure. The version that eventually became Arizona law is problematic because it conflicts with federal statute.

Indeed, legalization at the state level creates a direct conflict between state and federal law in every case, placing patients, doctors, police, prosecutors, and public officials in a difficult position. The fundamental legal problem with prescription of marijuana is that federal law prohibits such use, rendering state law functionally ineffective.

To appreciate fully the legal ramifications of ballot initiatives, consider one specific example. California's is perhaps the most publicized, and illustrates the chaos that can result from such initiatives. Enacted in 1996, the California Compassionate Use Act (also known as Proposition 215) was a ballot initiative intended to afford legal protection to seriously ill patients who use marijuana therapeutically. The act explicitly states that marijuana used by patients must first be recommended by a physician, and refers to such use as a "right" of the people of California. According to the act, physicians and patients are not subject to prosecution if they are compliant with the terms of the legislation. The act names cancer, anorexia, AIDS, chronic pain, spasticity, glaucoma, arthritis, and migraine as conditions that may be appropriately treated by marijuana, but it also includes the proviso: "or any other illness for which marijuana provides relief."

Writing in December 1999, a California doctor, Ryan Thompson, summed up the medical problems with Proposition 215:

> "As it stands, it creates vague, ill-defined guidelines that are obviously subject to abuse. The most glaring areas are as follows:
>
> - A patient does not necessarily need to be seen, evaluated or diagnosed as having any specific medical condition to qualify for the use of marijuana.
> - There is no requirement for a written prescription or even a written recommendation for its medical use.
> - Once 'recommended,' the patient never needs to be seen again to assess the effectiveness of the treatment and potentially could use that 'recommendation' for the rest of his or her life.
> - There is no limitation to the conditions for which it can be used, it can be recommended for virtually any condition, even if it is not believed to be effective."

The doctor concludes by stating: "Certainly as a physician I have witnessed the detrimental effects of marijuana use on patients and their families. It is not a harmless substance."

Passage of Proposition 215 resulted in conflict between California and the federal government. In February 1997, the Executive Office of the President issued its response to the California Compassionate Use Act (as well as Arizona's Proposition 200). The notice stated:

> "[The] Department of Justice's (D.O.J.) position is that a practitioner's practice of recommending or prescribing Schedule I controlled substances is not consistent with the public interest (as that phrase is used in the federal Controlled Substances Act) and will lead to administrative action by the Drug Enforcement Administration (DEA) to revoke the practitioner's registration."

The notice indicated that U.S. attorneys in California and Arizona would consider cases for prosecution using certain criteria. These included lack of a bona fide doctor-patient relationship, a "high volume" of prescriptions (or recommendations) for Schedule I drugs, "significant" profits derived from such prescriptions, prescriptions to minors, and "special circumstances" like impaired driving accidents involving serious injury.

The federal government's reasons for taking such a stance are solid. Dr. Donald Vereen of the Office of National Drug Control Policy explains that "research-based evidence" must be the focus when evaluating the risks and benefits of any drug, the only approach that provides a *rational* basis for making such a determination. He also explains that since testing by the Food and Drug Administration and other government agencies is designed to protect public health, circumvention of the process is unwise.

While the federal government supports FDA approved cannabinoid-based drugs, it maintains that ballot initiatives should not be allowed to remove marijuana evaluation from the realm of science and the drug approval process—a position based on a concern for public health. The Department of Health and Human Services has revised its regulations by making research-grade marijuana more available and intends to facilitate more research of cannabinoids. The department does not, however, intend to lower its standards of scientific proof.

Problems resulting from the California initiative are not isolated to conflict between the state and federal government. California courts themselves limited the distribution of medical marijuana. A 1997 California appellate decision held that the state's Compassionate Use Act only allowed purchase of medical marijuana from a patient's "primary caregiver," not from "drug dealers on street corners" or "sales centers such as the Cannabis Buyers' Club." This decision allowed courts to enjoin marijuana clubs.

The course of California's initiative and those of other states illustrate that such ballot-driven movements are not a legally effective or reliable way to supply the sick with whatever medical benefit the marijuana plant might hold. If the focus were shifted away from smoking the plant and toward a non-smoked alternative based on scientific research, much of this conflict could be avoided.

Filling "Prescriptions"

It is one thing to pass a ballot initiative defining a burning plant as medicine. It is yet another to make available such "medicine" if the plant itself remains—as it should—illegal. Recreational use, after all, cannot be equated with medicinal use, and none of the ballots passed were constructed to do so.

Nonetheless, cannabis buyers' clubs were quick to present the fiction that, for medical benefit, they were now in business to provided relief for the sick. In California, 13 such clubs rapidly went into operation, selling marijuana openly under the guise that doing so had been legitimized at the polls. The problem was that these organizations were selling to people under the flimsiest of facades. One club went so far as to proclaim: "All use of marijuana is medical. It makes you smarter. It touches the right brain and allows you to slow down, to smell the flowers."

Depending on the wording of the specific ballots, legal interpretation of what was allowed became problematic. The buyers' clubs became notorious for liberal interpretations of "prescription," "doctor's recommendation," and "medical." In California, Lucy Mae Tuck obtained a prescription for marijuana to treat hot flashes. Another citizen arrested for possession claimed he was medically entitled to his stash to treat a condition exacerbated by an ingrown toenail. Undercover police in several buyers clubs reported blatant sales to minors and adults with little attention to claims of medical need or a doctor's direction. Eventually, 10 of the 13 clubs in California were closed.

Further exacerbating the confusion over smoked marijuana as medicine are doctors' concerns over medical liability. Without the Food and Drug Administration's approval, marijuana cannot become a pharmaceutical drug to be purchased at local drug stores. Nor can there be any degree of confidence that proper doses can be measured out and chemical impurities eliminated in the marijuana that is obtained. After all, we are talking about a leaf, and a burning one at that. In the meantime, the harmful effects of marijuana have been documented in greater scientific detail than any findings about the medical benefits of smoking the plant.

Given the serious illnesses (for example, cancer and AIDS) of some of those who are purported to be in need of smoked marijuana for medical relief and their vulnerability to impurities and other toxic substances present in the plant, doctors are loath to risk their patients' health and their own financial well-being by prescribing it. As Dr. Peter Byeff, an oncologist at a Connecticut cancer center, points out: "If there's no mechanism for dispensing it, that doesn't help many of my patients. They're not going to go out and grow it in their backyards." Recognizing the availability of effective prescription medications to control nausea and vomiting, Byeff adds: "There's no reason to prescribe or dispense marijuana."

Medical professionals recognize what marijuana-as-medicine advocates seek to obscure. The chemical makeup of any two marijuana plants can differ significantly due to minor variations in cultivation. For example, should one plant receive relative to another as little as four more hours of collective sunlight before cultivation, the two could turn out to be significantly different in chemical composition. Potency also varies according to climate and geographical origin; it can also be affected by the way in which the plant is harvested and stored. Differences can be so profound that under current medical standards, two marijuana plants could be considered completely different drugs. Prescribing unproven, unmeasured, impure burnt leaves to relieve symptoms of a wide range of ailments does not seem to be the high point of American medical practice.

Illegal Because Harmful

Cannabinoids found in the marijuana plant offer the potential for medical use. However, lighting the leaves of the plant on fire and smoking them amount to an impractical delivery system that involves health risks and deleterious legal consequences. There is a profound difference between an approval process that seeks to purify isolated compounds for safe and effective delivery, and legalization of smoking the raw plant material as medicine. To advocate the latter is to bypass the safety and efficacy built into America's medical system. Ballot initiatives for smoked marijuana comprise a dangerous, impractical shortcut that circumvents the drug-approval process. The resulting decriminalization of a dangerous and harmful drug turns out to be counterproductive—legally, politically, and scientifically.

Advocacy for smoked marijuana has been cast in terms of relief from suffering. The Hippocratic oath that doctors take specifies that they must "first, do no harm." Clearly some people supporting medical marijuana are genuinely concerned about the sick. But violating established medical procedure *does* do harm, and it confounds the political, medical, and legal processes that best serve American society. In the single-minded pursuit of an extreme position that harkens back to an era of home medicine and herbal remedies, advocates for smoked marijuana as medicinal therapy not only retard legitimate scientific progress but become easy prey for less noble-minded zealots who seek to promote the acceptance and use of marijuana, an essentially harmful—and, therefore, illegal—drug.

POSTSCRIPT

Should Marijuana Be Legal for Medicinal Purposes?

Grinspoon strongly advocates the legalization of marijuana for medical treatment. He believes that the delay in the medicalization of marijuana stems from arduous and restrictive procedures of the federal government and that the government blocks people in need from receiving medication that is both therapeutic and benign.

From McDonough's perspective, promoting marijuana as a medicinal agent would be a mistake because it has not been proven medically useful or safe. Moreover, he feels that the availability of marijuana should not be predicated on personal accounts of its benefits or on whether or not the public supports its use. Also, McDonough asserts that studies showing that marijuana has medical value suffer from unscientific methodology and other deficiencies. The results of previous research, McDonough contends, do not lend strong credence to marijuana's medicinal value.

Some people have expressed concern about what will happen if marijuana is approved for medicinal use. Would it then become more acceptable for non-medical recreational use? There is also a possibility that some people would misinterpret the government's message and think that marijuana *cures* cancer when, in fact, it would only be used to treat the side effects of the chemotherapy.

A central question is, If physicians feel that marijuana use is justified to properly care for seriously ill patients, should they promote this form of medical treatment even though it falls outside the law? Does the relief of pain and suffering for patients warrant going beyond what federal legislation says is acceptable? Also, should physicians be prosecuted if they recommend marijuana to their patients? What about the unknown risks of using an illegal drug? Is it worthwhile to ignore the possibility that marijuana may produce harmful side effects in order to alleviate pain or to treat other ailments?

Many medical marijuana proponents contend that the effort to prevent the legalization of marijuana for medical use is purely a political battle. Detractors maintain that the issue is purely scientific—that the data supporting marijuana's medical usefulness are inconclusive and scientifically unsubstantiated. And although the chief administrative law judge of the Drug Enforcement Administration (DEA) made a recommendation to change the status of marijuana from Schedule I to Schedule II, the DEA and other federal agencies are not compelled to do so, and they have resisted any change in the law.

Lester Grinspoon and James B. Bakalar's book *Marihuana, the Forbidden Medicine* (Yale University Press, 1997) provides a thorough history and overview of marijuana's medical benefits. Articles that discuss whether or not marijuana should be legalized as a medication include "Marijuana and Medicine: Assessing the Science," by Stanley Watson, John Benson, and Janet Joy, *Archives of General Psychiatry* (June 2000); "The Growing Debate on Medical Marijuana: Federal Power vs. States Rights," by Alreen Hussein, *California Western Law Review* (vol. 37, no. 2, 2001); and "Cannabis Control: Costs Outweigh the Benefits," by Alex Wodak et al., *British Medical Journal* (January 12, 2002). In an often cited study by Richard Doblin and Mark Kleiman, "Marijuana as Medicine: A Survey of Oncologists," in Arnold Trebach and Kevin Zeese, eds., *New Frontiers in Drug Policy* (Drug Policy Foundation, 1991), almost half of the oncologists surveyed recommended marijuana to their patients to help them deal with the side effects of chemotherapy.

ISSUE 10

Do the Advantages of Psychiatric Medicines Outweigh Their Disadvantages?

YES: Bruce M. Cohen, from "Mind and Medicine: Drug Treatments for Psychiatric Illnesses," *Social Research* (Fall 2001)

NO: Ronald W. Dworkin, from "The Medicalization of Unhappiness," *The Public Interest* (Summer 2001)

ISSUE SUMMARY

YES: Physician Bruce M. Cohen maintains that psychiatric medicines are beneficial in that they enable individuals with a variety of illnesses to return to normal aspects of consciousness. He argues that people with conditions such as anxiety, depression, and psychosis respond very well to medications and that these types of drugs have been utilized successfully for hundreds of years.

NO: Physician Ronald W. Dworkin questions whether the increase in the use of psychiatric drugs, especially antidepressant drugs, results from more people needing these drugs or from physicians' becoming more aggressive in diagnosing people as depressed. Dworkin expresses concern that antidepressant drugs are being prescribed for everyday conditions such as unhappiness and boredom.

One of the most common emotional problems in America is depression. It is estimated that approximately 10 percent of Americans experience some type of depression during their lives. Although some of the newer antidepressant drugs, such as Prozac, Paxil, and Zoloft, have not been available that long, they account for billions of dollars in sales. Does this mean that nowadays more people are becoming depressed or that people are more likely to be diagnosed with depression?

Although antidepressant drugs were originally developed to treat depression—for which they are believed to be about 60 percent effective—these drugs are now prescribed for an array of other conditions. Some of these conditions include eating disorders like bulimia and obesity, obsessive-compulsive disorders, panic attacks, and anxiety. An important question about these drugs is currently being debated: Are they prescribed too casually? Some experts feel that physicians are giving antidepressant drugs to patients who do not need chemical treatment to overcome their afflictions. Yale University professor Sherwin Nuland has argued that drugs like Prozac are relatively safe for their approved applications but that they are inappropriate for less severe problems.

As with most drugs, antidepressants produce a number of adverse side effects. These effects include hypotension (low blood pressure), weight gain, and irregular heart rhythms. Other side effects that may be experienced are headaches, fatigue, profuse sweating, anxiety, reduced appetite, jitteriness, dizziness, stomach discomfort, nausea, sexual dysfunction, and insomnia. Because these drugs are relatively new, long-term side effects have yet to be determined.

Soon after Prozac was introduced, several lawsuits were filed against Eli Lilly and Company, the drug's manufacturer, due to Prozac's side effects. The drug was linked to violent and suicidal behavior. Some individuals charged with violent crimes claimed that Prozac made them act violently and that they should not be held accountable for their actions while on the drug. Prozac has also been implicated in a number of suicides, although it is unclear whether Prozac caused these individuals to commit suicide or whether they would have committed suicide anyway. Paxil and Zoloft, which were introduced after Prozac, reportedly have fewer side effects.

Psychiatrist Peter R. Breggin, who feels that antidepressant drugs are prescribed too frequently, has argued that they are being used to replace traditional psychotherapy. Breggin contends that psychiatry has given in to the pharmaceutical companies. In contrast to psychiatry, antidepressant drugs are less expensive and more convenient. However, do these drugs get at the root of the problems that many people have? The United States Public Health Service recommends drug therapy for severe cases of depression but psychotherapy for mild or moderate cases.

One may accept the use of drug therapy when one's medical condition is caused by a chemical imbalance. However, should drugs be employed to alter one's personality, to help one become more confident and less introverted? One could argue that if drugs help people with these personal qualities, then that is a healthy use of these drugs. Are using these drugs any different than people using cigarettes to relax or using alcohol to overcome shyness?

In the following selections, Bruce M. Cohen argues that antidepressant drugs are invaluable because they effectively treat anxiety, depression, and psychosis. The benefits of these drugs, asserts Cohen, outweigh their potential side effects. Ronald W. Dworkin argues that antidepressant drugs are prescribed too quickly for nonmedical conditions like unhappiness and boredom. He maintains that physicians are too aggressive in prescribing these drugs.

Bruce M. Cohen 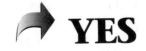 **YES**

Mind and Medicine: Drug Treatments for Psychiatric Illnesses

Psychiatric Disorders as Medical Illnesses

Psychiatric illnesses are conditions of the brain that lead to alternations in thinking, mood, and behavior. These illnesses are observed in cultures throughout the world and are probably at least as old as human beings. Recognizable features of psychiatric disorders are described in the texts of many early societies, including those of ancient Egypt, Israel, Greece, India, and China. Also ancient are attempts to treat people with disorders of cognition and emotion by what today would be called psychosocial therapies (including counseling, asylum, and exploration of thought) and psychopharmacologic therapies (that is, plant products or other drugs).

The most common symptoms experienced by those with psychiatric disorders fall into a few categories. Mood may be abnormally high or low. Irritability and anxiety are often felt. Thinking, and its expression in speech and other behaviors, may be illogical. Delusions, which are patently false beliefs not shared by others, can be present. Obsessions and compulsions may continuously haunt the sufferers. Prominent perceptual abnormalities may occur, the most common being hallucinations, which are false sensory percepts, usually the hearing of voices within one's own head. Finally, psychiatric disorders often are associated with changes of physiologic rhythms and the basic drives of life, with disrupted sleep, appetite, and energy.

Some symptoms of psychiatric disorders, notably depression or anxiety, seem to be extremes of normal states, just as hypertension is an extreme of blood pressure. Others, such as hallucinations, appear more distinct from normal experience, although most of us have occasionally thought we heard a voice when we were alone or saw a person when no one was there. These normal experiences are fleeting, while the symptoms of psychiatric disorders last from months to a lifetime.

Symptoms rarely occur alone. Rather, they tend to occur in recognizable clusters, called syndromes. Common syndromes in internal medicine include the pneumonias or congestive heart failure. The most common psychiatric syndromes include the depressive disorders, the anxiety disorders, and the psychotic disorders, such as bipolar disorders and schizophrenia. It is the latter that are most frequently associated with hallucinations and delusions.

Psychiatric disorders are medical illnesses. Like other medical disorders, they are due to the interaction of inherited and environmental factors that, together, lead to the development of illness. While the specific genes that predispose to psychiatric disorders have not yet been identified, the presence of these genes is thoroughly and convincingly documented from family, twin, and adoption studies. Similarly, subtle but repeatedly observed differences in the brain between those with and without psychiatric disorders are now documented by post mortem studies and observation of the brain during life using technologies such as magnetic resonance imaging (MRI), positron emission tomography (PET), and single photon emission computerized tomography (SPECT).

The explicit causes of most current cases of psychiatric disorder are not yet known, but numerous medical conditions that can cause psychiatric disorders are well documented. Over a century ago, many of the patients in psychiatric hospitals had infectious, nutritional, toxic, and hormonal conditions, such as syphilis, pellagra, lead poisoning, and hyper- and hypothyroidism which affected their thinking and mood. Today these medical disorders have responded well to preventive measures, based on diet and environmental advances, or to treatment with medications.

Psychiatric illnesses of unknown cause also tend to respond well to treatment, with success rates as high as those seen in other branches of medicine. Psychotherapeutic medication can restore to normal aspects of consciousness, including feeling, perception, and cognition. For this reason medication is at the core of treatment for most psychiatric disorders.

Drugs and the Brain

Taking drugs with the intent to change aspects of consciousness is very old and quite common. Alcohol, cocaine, opiates, and peyote have been used for thousands of years. These drugs appear to act on systems built into the brain to modulate behaviors associated with eating, sleeping, sexual activity, or other drives and rewards. Co-opting receptors and processes developed to respond to internal chemical messages, these external agents alter arousal, attention, emotional state, and thinking.

Foods can have effects on mood and cognition as well. Deficiencies of some nutrients, as noted, can lead to psychiatric illness, and the oldest recreational drugs are in essence food products or derivatives. Based on this history, numerous nutritional substances are currently being examined as possible treatments for psychiatric disorders.

Hormones, including thyroid, adrenal, and sex hormones, can have profound effects on brain function, drive, cognition, and feelings, and hormonal abnormalities, as was noted, can cause psychiatric symptoms. Hormone replacement—using hormones as drugs—can restore or, occasionally, disrupt mental function.

Further links between physiology, pharmacology, and psychology are evident from the effects of drugs given for purposes unrelated to brain function, but with unwanted actions there. For example, older antihistamines for allergies, which reached receptors throughout the body (including the brain), affected alertness, concentration, and memory. Newer agents were designed that were not absorbed into brain and, therefore, have few mental side effects.

These examples provide compelling evidence that drugs can change all the aspects of consciousness. This knowledge has been used for religious, recreational, and medicinal purposes for generations. With the revolution in organic chemistry, biochemistry, and molecular biology over the past hundred years, the development of new drugs targeted to specific illnesses, such as psychiatric disorders, has become more sophisticated and more successful.

Medication for Psychiatric Disorders

Medicinal treatments for psychiatric disorders are used throughout the world and have their origins in many ancient societies. The oldest documented of these medicinal preparations, made from the plant *Rauwolfia serpentina*, appears in Ayurmedic texts of India over 2,000 years ago. It was recommended for several medical illnesses including those whose description sounds much like the psychotic disorders: the schizophrenias and bipolar disorders. The active ingredient of this preparation was likely reserpine, which was isolated in the 1930s and used briefly but effectively to treat psychotic disorders in the 1950s. It was superseded by easier to use agents, the neuroleptic antipsychotic drugs (which will be described later), in the same decade.

Another "modern" treatment for psychiatric disorders, lithium, prescribed to patients with bipolar disorders, may also have been used in ancient times. Lithium is an element related to sodium and potassium. Like these elements, it most frequently occurs in nature as a salt, often appearing in spring waters. Between A.D. 100 and 300, during the Roman Empire, Arataeus, a physician from Cappadocia, and Soranus of Ephesus recommended waters from particular alkaline springs, which probably contained lithium, for the treatment of mania. While dose could not have been carefully controlled, their advice accords with the use of lithium today.

Eastern Hemisphere plant preparations containing opium have been used to alleviate pain for centuries, and in the late nineteenth and early twentieth centuries, opiate compounds isolated from these plants were used with limited efficacy for the treatment of psychotic disorders and severe depression. Similarly, coca leaves from the Western Hemisphere, chewed by generations for their energizing effects, yielded cocaine, used by Freud and others around 1900 for its stimulating and short-lived antidepressant effects.

None of these older medicinal preparations had strong and reliable enough therapeutic effects or tolerable toxicity for the routine treatment of patients with psychiatric disorders. Breakthroughs leading to the discovery of drugs currently in use, which have good safety and efficacy, occurred in the 1950s, with the introduction of the so-called tricyclic antidepressants, such as Tofranil (imipramine); neuroleptic antipsychotic drugs, such as Thorazine (chlorpromazine); and benzodiazepine anti-anxiety agents, such as Librium (chlordiazepoxide). These drugs revolutionized the care of people with psychiatric disorders, leading to the release of many patients from institutions and the return of others to productive lives.

These first modern medications were followed by many copies and by newer generations of psychotherapeutic drugs in the 1980s and 1990s. Examples include the serotonin specific re-uptake inhibitors, such as Prozac (fluoxetine), for depression; the atypical antipsychotic agents, such as Zyprex (olanzapine), for psychotic disorders; and the mood-stabilizing anticonvulsants, such as Depakote (valproate), for bipolar disorder.

The efficacy of these medications has been proved in numerous studies, including a large number of double-blind, placebo-controlled trials in which the drug being tested is compared to inactive substances, as well as compounds that have effects on the brain, such as sedation, that are not believed to address the key symptoms of psychiatric disorders. Neither the clinical investigator nor the patient knows which drug the patient is receiving. Few drugs in medicine have ever been as thoroughly tested and proven effective.

The proper use of these drugs leads to the successful treatment of most people with depressive disorders, anxiety disorders, schizophrenias and bipolar disorders, restoring them to their proper state of mind. As with all medications, there are side effects as well as therapeutic effects, but with careful use, beneficial effects far outweigh side effects for most people. The physical mechanisms underlying these drug effects and the return to normal consciousness are beginning to be understood, providing important information on the nature of psychiatric disorders and the relationship between brain and psyche.

Medications for Anxiety

In a lifetime, nearly one in six of us will experience a disorder in which anxiety is a prominent symptom. Current anti-anxiety medications, or anxiolytics, grew out of a recognition that alcohol, prized for the comfort and disinhibition it brought, could ease feelings of anxiety. Alcohol relieves distress or discomfort whether or not these feelings are pathological, as indicated by its common social use to relax couples on an evening out or large groups at a party.

Alcohol can provide some relief for those with disorders whose cardinal symptoms include anxiety. In these illnesses, feelings of anxiety may be nearly constant or may occur in attacks of panic. In either case the degree of anxiety is out of proportion to and may even bear no relationship to life events. Unfortunately, the relief is limited by the fast metabolism of alcohol and the tendency of the body to become tolerant to its effects. In fact, as the immediate action of alcohol fades, and as tolerance develops, those who drink for recreation or to medicate themselves for anxiety can find that a physiologic rebound opposite to the effects of alcohol occurs, and they become even more anxious.

From about 1900 on, recognizing the beneficial and toxic effects of alcohol, repeated attempts have been made to find chemical agents that share the calming or sedative effects of alcohol but lack its addictive qualities and the rebound that follows its use. These efforts have been only partially successful.

Early attempts to find safer and more effective compounds than alcohol for anxiety disorders and sedation led to discovery of the barbiturates. They were successful in producing anxiolytic effects, but toxic doses have tended to be close to therapeutic doses and tolerance and addiction are common. Barbiturates are still used for epilepsy and for sedation, but rarely in psychiatry for anxiety disorders.

In the 1950s, derivatives of mephenesin, chemically related to barbiturates, were developed and marketed under the names Miltown (meprobamate) and Equanil (tybamate). All these medications were superseded by compounds called benzodiazepine anxiolytics, which were developed in the late 1950s. The earliest of these, Librium (chlordiazepoxide) and Valium (diazepam), became exceedingly popular drugs, felt to have low risk of poisoning and to be associated only rarely with tolerance and addiction.

Today, a large number of long- and short-acting benzodiazepines are on the market as anxiolytics and sedatives. They are good and effective drugs that are neither as dangerous as alcohol or barbiturates nor as safe as early hopes and claims suggested. Tolerance is common and addiction not rare.

Like alcohol, benzodiazepines reduce anxiety whether or not an individual has an anxiety disorder. Used continuously, their anxiolytic effect tends to fade. While they often blunt the attacks or nagging presence of pathological anxiety, they rarely eliminate these symptoms entirely when used alone. Nevertheless, their powerful and consistent ability to reduce anxiety soon after they are ingested or injected suggests they may work by altering the very brain mechanisms that mediate anxiety.

Following years of fruitful study, the likely site through which the benzodiazepine anxiolytics have their clinical effects is known. Nerve cells (called neurons in the brain) process signals by both electrical and chemical means. Each cell receives chemical messages from other cells, sends electrical messages down its length, and secretes its own chemical compound or compounds, called neurotransmitters, on the cells it contacts. Neurotransmitters produce their effects by binding to specific proteins, called neurotransmitter receptors, which induce a cascade of chemical reactions in the cell to stimulate or reduce electrical activity each time a chemical signal is received.

Eighty to ninety percent of the neuron to neuron contacts in the brain involve one of two neurotransmitters: gama amino butyric acid (GABA) or glutamate. Glutamate is an excitatory neurotransmitter; its message makes a neuron more likely to fire an electrical signal. GABA is an inhibitory neurotransmitter; it quiets cells, making them less likely to fire a signal.

Benzodiazepines attach to some of the same receptors that bind the neurotransmitter GABA and change their characteristics, making them more sensitive to GABA. In this way, benzodiazepines amplify the GABA signal, shifting the overall balance between excitation and inhibition in the brain toward inhibition. At low doses, benzodiazepines may produce their calming anti-anxiety effect through this shift to inhibition. At high doses, inhibition becomes great enough to induce sleep, or at doses higher still, to cause coma.

GABA is used as a neurotransmitter throughout the brain, and benzodiazepines enhance its inhibitory effects globally in the brain. It is not known if such a widespread effect is needed for relief of anxiety in humans, or if a local effect in specific regions would suffice. Medical technology is not yet ready routinely to deliver drugs solely to where they are needed. This is a common problem in using drugs in patients. Brain cells can deliver chemicals precisely, but medications go throughout the body, both to where they are needed and where they are not.

Medication for Depression

Like anxiety disorders, depressive disorders are quite common, affecting over one in eight of the population, worldwide, in a lifetime. Symptoms of depression and anxiety often occur together, and for many people, so-called antidepressant drugs are a better long-term treatment of anxiety than are the anxiolytic drugs. In chemical structure and mechanism of action, however, the two classes of drugs are unrelated.

One might think that antidepressant drugs would be derived from stimulants, such as the amphetamines. Stimulants can raise mood in almost anyone and can be helpful in some cases of depression. Unfortunately, they are more often not helpful and even when they improve mood, only do so transiently. Like anxiolytics, their short-lived effects can lead to tolerance, craving, and addiction.

The earliest current antidepressants were discovered serendipitously in patients with tuberculosis who were treated with an antibiotic called iproniazide. Some of the patients not only had TB, but were severely depressed, until they received iproniazide. Tests in patients without TB, who suffered from depression, indicated that iproniazide was an effective therapeutic agent in relieving depression and restoring abnormalities of appetite, energy, and sleep that usually accompany this illness.

Pharmacologic studies determined that iproniazide was an inhibitor of an enzyme called monoamine oxidase, which metabolizes, and thereby inactivates, a group of chemical messengers that include norepinephrine (also called noradrenaline), serotonin, and dopamine. Like GABA, these compounds, which chemically are called monoamines, are used in the brain as neurotransmitters. Unlike GABA, the effects of which are rapid, appearing nearly instantaneously and ending as quickly, the effects of the monoamine neurotransmitters are slow by the standards of the brain, lasting seconds or longer once they are released. For this reason, it has been hypothesized that the monoamines set the "tone" of activity by region in the brain.

Inhibiting the breakdown of monoamines leads to a higher concentration of these neurotransmitters in the brain, which might be the means by which iproniazide relieved depression. Evidence supportive of this speculation arises from the mechanisms by which stimulants act to more transiently elevate mood. Specifically, stimulants cause the release of monoamine neurotransmitters in the brain; block the re-uptake of these neurotransmitters back into the cell that released them; or mimic the effects of the monoamine neurotransmitters at the receptor proteins that recognize their presence. Based on the success of iproniazide, more monoamine oxidase inhibitor drugs (all called by the acronym MAOI) like iproniazid were developed, tested, and proved to be effective antidepressants.

Soon after the introduction of MAOIs, a new and different class of antidepressants was independently discovered. These compounds were observed in a search for agents to treat psychotic disorders, such as schizophrenia. In the early 1950s, the first modern drugs for psychosis became available. They had a structure containing three rings of carbon and occasional nitrogen, sulfur, and oxygen atoms. Many such compounds were designed, synthesized, and tested, and a clever observer noted that one compound in particular, while it lacked effects to treat psychosis, seemed to brighten mood substantially in depressed patients. The compound, imipramine, proved to be a greatly successful antidepressant, still on the market over 40 years later. Other compounds structurally similar, with three rings and, therefore, called tricyclic antidepressants, or TCAs, were developed to treat depression. Like the MAOIs, they relieve all the symptoms of depression, not just the dysphoric mood of patients.

Also like MAOIs, TCAs appear to produce their effects through actions on monoamine neurotransmitters. Specifically, they inhibit the uptake of norepinephrine back into the cells that released it. This increases the amount of norepinephrine interacting with neurons and prolongs the time over which norepinephrine acts. They have a similar, but weaker, effect on the re-uptake of serotonin. They have little effect on dopamine, which is the reverse of stimulants, which have their greatest effects on dopamine release and re-uptake.

In the late 1980s, based on the success of the TCAs but searching for a new class of antidepressants, pharmaceutical companies designed drugs that preferentially blocked the re-uptake of serotonin, rather than norepinephrine. The first of these so-called serotonin-specific re-uptake inhibitors, or SSRIs, was Prozac (fluoxetine). It and other SSRIs developed later have been extraordinarily successful, in part because they have different side effects than the TCAs, being safer and seeming to be more comfortable for most people to take. This comfort has led to an increase in the prescription of antidepressants by primary care practitioners as well as psychiatrists, with many newly treated individuals feeling relief from depression and anxiety.

Antidepressants, whether MAOIs, TCAs, or SSRIs, do not seem to benefit those who do not have symptoms of a depressive disorder. The broad use and success of the SSRIs has suggested to some that they have mood-elevating effects in people whether or not the people treated are ill. This is unlikely, as most healthy people only suffer side effects from antidepressants. Rather, as depression is a common illness, like colds in children or high blood pressure in the elderly, and physicians more readily prescribe SSRIs than previous antidepressants, more people with depressive disorders, including milder disorders, are being treated and benefiting from treatment.

Looking to why the brain responds to antidepressants, the available evidence points strongly to drug effects mediated through the monoamine neurotransmitters norepinephrine and serotonin. Two classes of drugs, the MAOIs and the TCAs, discovered independently and serendipitously, have potent actions affecting these chemical signals. A third class of agents, the SSRIs, was developed on the theory that increased serotonin messages would relieve depression. Their success helps confirm the theory. Due to crosstalk, changes in either the serotonin or norepinephrine neurotransmitter system lead to changes in the other system. Furthermore, a role for both norepinephrine and serotonin is suggested by the fact that individual antidepressant drugs whose potency is specific to one or the other monoamine appear equally efficacious in the majority of people.

It is important to note that, while drug effects on serotonin and norepinephrine can relieve depression, this outcome is not direct and immediate. Unlike benzodiazepines for anxiety, or aspirin for headache, the therapeutic effects of antidepressants do not occur in minutes or hours. They require weeks of continued use. Somehow, the brain changes its state in response to the continued presence of drug and the consequent higher levels of monoamine neurotransmitters. Brain-imaging studies suggest that depression fades as regional brain activity changes in response to altered levels of monoamine neurotransmitters induced by antidepressant drugs.

Medications for Psychosis

Psychotic disorders are among the most disabling of illnesses, disturbing thinking, perception, mood, and their interconnections, and diminishing normal human interactions. Fortunately, modern antipsychotic medications are among the more efficacious treatments in medicine today, reversing all or most symptoms in the majority of people with psychotic disorders. The effect is so dramatic that some have called antipsychotic medications the penicillin of psychiatry.

The two most common psychotic illnesses, the schizophrenias and bipolar disorders, affect over one in one hundred people. They often strike the young and can prevent a normal life or reduce successful people to homelessness. Even milder forms or episodes of psychotic illnesses can disrupt relationships among spouses, relatives, and friends. Despite obvious symptoms, including delusions, hallucinations, disrupted speech and thinking, and disorganized behavior, those in the midst of psychosis often do not realize they are ill. This peculiar lack of insight, even in those who have had multiple episodes of illness and been well in between, is another aspect of the unusual state of mind and awareness accompanying these psychotic disorders.

Many patients understand their illnesses and understand the benefits and risks of treatment. In others, lack of insight leads to considerable discussion and debate between the patient and clinicians. When there is an immediate risk of harm to the patient or others due to the symptoms of illness, medication may be started even if the patient does not accept the need for treatment. This is not common. Occasionally, patients who know medications will ameliorate their symptoms choose not to be treated. This, too, is not common, as the symptoms of psychosis are extremely uncomfortable for most people.

Others observe the symptoms of illness, of course, and for many years physicians have tried to help those with psychotic disorders. Reserpine, given in *Rauwolfia serpentina* or as the isolated chemical, had beneficial effects, but at the risk of dangerously low blood pressure and strong sedation. Opiates were used to calm patients, but had minimal effects on the key symptoms of psychosis.

It was not until the early 1950s that the first specific, well-tolerated and effective medication for psychosis, Thorazine (chlorpromazine), was introduced. This medication, and others modeled after it, were so effective that the number of patients with psychotic disorders in hospitals began to drop substantially. With the development of even newer agents that had similar therapeutic effects but fewer side effects, decreases in hospitalization continue, despite a growing population.

The antipsychotic medications were discovered by design, partly from modifying known sedatives, but mostly by looking for agents related to anesthetics, which produced a profound calming effect but not loss of consciousness. The antipsychotic drugs, however, are not all sedatives and are not, as they were once called, major tranquilizers. Some are sedative and some not. Some reduce anxiety, and some can increase it. All work similarly in reducing the symptoms of psychosis, including disrupted thinking, mood, perception, and behavior. Only one, Clozaril (clozapine), may be on average modestly more efficacious than other antipsychotic drugs.

Those without psychotic disorders gain nothing but side effects from these drugs. The drugs have little effect on people with odd or idiosyncratic ideas and behaviors, unless they have the symptoms of schizophrenia or bipolar disorder.

Given that antipsychotic medications all tend to produce a similar therapeutic outcome and were designed to be pharmacologically similar to chlorpromazine, the original antipsychotic drug, it is not surprising that they share common mechanisms of action at a molecular level. Specifically, all antipsychotic drugs block signals at some but not all receptors for the chemical messengers dopamine, norepinephrine, and serotonin.

By blocking signals at these receptors, the antipsychotic drugs produce affects in several key areas of the brain. They change activity in the nucleus accumbens, which is involved, in part, in mediating a sense of reward; the amygdala, which is involved in determining a sense of threat, disquiet, or safety; the thalamus, which appears to be involved in coordinating aspects of thought, perception, and emotion; and the prefrontal cortex, which is the most developed of all areas of the human brain and is involved in attention, decision making, and keeping thoughts in consciousness.

Like the antidepressants, therapeutic effects of antipsychotic drugs can take weeks to develop. How the immediate effects of the antipsychotic drugs become longer term effects is not known. However, there is growing evidence that modulation of signals through the monoamine receptors affected by antipsychotic drugs leads to changes in the activity of GABAergic and glutaminergic cells, which mediate much of the function of the brain.

It is not surprising that even though the antipsychotic drugs have effects on only a few specific receptors in the brain, their use would change activity at many sites. Neurons that employ dopamine, norepinephrine, and serotonin as their chemical messengers are few, but they contact vast numbers of cells throughout the brain. In addition, because cells in the brain are interconnected in a dense network, a limited direct effect can translate into a broad distributed effect.

Most well-described functions of the brain, such as the processing of visual information or the control of movement, are handled by cells distributed across many different, but sometimes overlapping, areas of the brain. It is possible, and even likely, that emotions and thoughts are also a consequence of changes in the activity of specific groups of cells linked to one another but representing different aspects of feeling or cognition and existing in different locations within the brain. The wide distribution of neurons responding to antipsychotic drugs, and mediating their effects, illustrates this point.

Psychiatric Disorders, Psychotherapeutic Medication, and Consciousness

Medications are a key component of the treatment of most psychiatric disorders. They are not, of course, the sole treatment. Proper care requires attention to the psychological and social aspects of illness. These may represent environmental stressors that, unaddressed, can trigger illness in those predisposed. Also, psychological and social problems are frequently consequences of the disruption of mood, thought, and behavior caused by illness. Patients need support in reconstituting their lives and sense of self once their symptoms fade.

It is remarkable, however, just how powerful medications are in relieving the symptoms of psychiatric disorders. Along with genetic, structural, and functional evidence, the effects of drugs are compelling findings suggesting that psychiatric illnesses arise from abnormal activity of the brain; that is, they are medical disorders of the brain.

Arguments can be made for and against the recreational use of drugs. Society accepts some, such as alcohol, and not others, such as marijuana. By comparison, there is little basis for argument about the treatment of psychiatric disorders with medication. For most people, the benefits clearly outweigh the risks.

The effects of psychotherapeutic medications also speak to questions beyond that of the origin and nature of psychiatric disorders. They speak to the nature of consciousness.

Drugs can disturb all aspects of consciousness and drugs can restore aspects of consciousness. As drugs act on the structure, chemistry, and electrical activity of the brain, it is logical to conclude that all aspects of consciousness depend on physical states of the brain.

Evidence is growing as to the precise molecular sites at which drugs act, as well as on the specific changes that occur in cellular metabolism and the state of neural circuits during drug treatment. Pharmacologic studies point to particular regions of the brain or particular distributed groups of nerve cells as being involved in mediating mood, awareness, cognition, or the integration of experience. Studies of the consequences of lesions associated with epilepsy, tumors, strokes, and trauma also suggest that particular parts of the brain are necessary, if not sufficient, to determine aspects of consciousness. Results from pharmacology and pathology agree strongly on which areas are associated with which aspects of consciousness.

No simple connections are likely to exist between a molecule and a thought or a nerve cell and a mood. However, it is reasonable to expect that the state of networks of nerve cells in the brain may be closely related to conscious states of thinking or feeling. Drugs and medications can change the patterns of firing in neural circuits and the tone of neural activity in the brain. By doing so, they can alter those aspects of consciousness that make us most human. The study of drug effects will remain an important tool for designing and testing models of how mind may arise from brain. Equally or more important, the use of currently available drugs and the arrival of new drugs under development will continue to provide good treatments, and some day cures, for the devastating illnesses classified as psychiatric disorders.

NO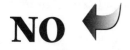

Ronald W. Dworkin

The Medicalization of Unhappiness

The use of psychotropic medication in depressed patients has increased in the United States by more than 40 percent over the last decade, from 32 million office visits resulting in a drug prescription to over 45 million. This is in marked contrast to the period between 1978 and 1987, when the number of office visits resulting in a psychotropic drug prescription remained relatively stable. The bulk of the increase can be accounted for by the aggressive use of SSRIs (selective serotonin reuptake inhibitors) in patients. It is the class of drugs that includes Prozac, Zoloft, and Paxil. The question is: Are more Americans clinically depressed now than in the past, or has medical science started to treat the far more common experience of "everyday unhappiness" with medication, thereby increasing the number of drug prescriptions?

No one knows the answer to this question. We do know that the number of patients diagnosed with depression has doubled over the last 30 years, without any great change in diagnostic criteria. But this simply raises another question: Are doctors more aggressive in diagnosing depression, or are they simply diagnosing "everyday unhappiness" as a variant of depression and reporting it as such?

These questions are at the center of a major debate within the medical community over who the new patients being treated with antidepressants are and what treatment guidelines are being used. There is suspicion among some doctors that it is not the sickest patients who are being given psychotropic drugs but those patients who complain the loudest about being unhappy. Some physicians blame managed care for the problem of over-prescription. Because the office environment under managed care is so rushed and impersonal, many doctors take the path of least resistance by prescribing medication whenever a patient is feeling "blue." Also, managed-care companies save money when depressed patients receive medication rather than an indefinite number of counseling sessions.

This suspicion is well founded, but the origin of the problem does not lie solely in managed care. The sources of over-prescription are much more complex. Physicians are being encouraged to think about everyday unhappiness in ways that make them more likely to treat it with psychotropic medication.

From Ronald W. Dworkin, "The Medicalization of Unhappiness," *The Public Interest,* no. 144 (Summer 2001). Copyright © 2001 by National Affairs, Inc. Reprinted by permission of *The Public Interest* and the author.

It is part of a growing phenomenon in our society: the medicalization of unhappiness.

In the past, medical science cared for the mentally ill, while everyday unhappiness was left to religious, spiritual, or other cultural guides. Now, medical science is moving beyond its traditional border to help people who are bored, sad, or experiencing low self-esteem—in other words, people who are suffering from nothing more than life.

This trend first became widely known with the publication in 1992 of *Listening to Prozac.* Peter Kramer's book, which became a national best-seller, described the positive benefits enjoyed by depressed patients when they were put on Prozac. The drug apparently increased self-esteem and reduced negative feelings when nothing else could. The book led many in the medical community and the broader public to look more favorably on a liberal use of antidepressants.

Medical science should aggressively use drugs like Prozac for patients suffering from clinical depression. This is totally appropriate—and important. But medical science errs when it supposes that a connection exists between everyday unhappiness and clinical depression, something it increasingly does. It is hard to know where everyday unhappiness ends and clinical depression begins, and there is no easy way to distinguish between borderline depression (i.e., low spirits without any physical signs or symptoms) and everyday unhappiness. Traditionally, doctors have relied on their wisdom, intuition, and personal experience to separate the two. Such a method is neither precise nor foolproof, but it is possibly the best we can aspire to. The problem is that medical science has placed everyday unhappiness and depression on a single continuum, thereby interfering with the efforts of doctors to make fine but necessary distinctions.

Medical science has adopted a method of classifying mental disorders that blurs the line between sickness and health. And more radically, it has embraced a theory that explains all mental states in terms of their biochemical origins. Medical science has done this in order to make the problem of unhappiness simpler and more comprehensible to doctors. But the new science actually works against the efforts of doctors to separate everyday unhappiness from depression. The upshot is that physicians are more likely to treat mere unhappiness the way they would treat serious mental illness—with psychotropic drugs.

Categories of Unhappiness

One way that science establishes a link between clinical depression and everyday unhappiness is through a diagnostic instrument called the DSM. First published in 1952 and now in its fifth edition, the DSM (*Diagnostic and Statistical Manual of Mental Disorders*) is the essential diagnostic tool in the psychiatric field. It is a classification scheme for the entire range of human mental pathology. The DSM includes 16 major diagnostic classes (e.g., mood disorders, anxiety disorders, substance-abuse disorders), and these categories are divided up again and again in accordance with certain signs and symptoms. The DSM was originally developed by psychiatrists and psychologists, but even primary-care physicians refer to its nomenclature and categories in determining whether or not a patient has a significant mental illness.

The original purpose of the DSM was to satisfy the psychiatric profession's need for statistical and epidemiological data. But by establishing a relationship between clinical depression and everyday unhappiness when no such relationship existed before, the DSM has led inexorably to a liberal use of psychotropic medication.

Prior to the development of the DSM, feelings of unhappiness were not considered related to any of the authentic disease states that existed in medical science, such as depression or schizophrenia. While clinical depression had an official status in medical science, everyday sadness did not. The DSM changed this by creating large categories of mental illness and then ever-increasing subcategories, replete with subtypes and specifiers. "Major depression," for example, was broken down into a host of subtypes, including "minor depression," which was broken down further into symptoms of everyday unhappiness like pessimism, hopelessness, and despair. With the creation of the DSM, everyday unhappiness suddenly gained a fixed position in medical science, if only as a subcategory of a subcategory of a major mental illness.

The DSM incorporates everyday unhappiness into medicine in another way. It encourages doctors to use its multiaxial system, which allows the mental state of a patient to be assessed in different ways. For example, Axis I is used for reporting any major mental disorders. Axis III is used for reporting a patient's general medical condition. Axis IV is used for assessing a person's psychosocial and environmental problems. It is within Axis IV that everyday unhappiness takes a position within medical science. For example, one can find on Axis IV job dissatisfaction, discord with one's boss, or trouble with one's spouse. Such everyday troubles are given their own special diagnostic code in a companion book called the *ICD-9* (*International Classification of Diseases*). Trouble with one's spouse, for example, is listed as Partner Relational Problem, and is assigned number V61.1. Through the use of this multi-axial system, everyday unhappiness is brought into the orbit of medical science.

By itself, this does not lead to an increased reliance on psychotropic medication. The problem arises because the categories of mental illness in the DSM are so porous as to allow everyday unhappiness to pass into the category of a more significant disease. The diagnosis of "minor depression," for example, requires only a feeling of sadness and a loss of pleasure in daily activities—a mood that may characterize the pain of everyday life as well as any medical pathology. Because "minor depression" often gets treated with medication, so too does everyday unhappiness.

"Adjustment disorder with depressed mood" is another DSM category that has the potential to be confused with everyday emotional trouble. Included in this diagnostic group would be the person who is sad and tearful because of some painful event, like the termination of a romantic relationship or a sudden business difficulty. Distinguishing an adjustment disorder from the despondency that people might feel during one of life's routine downturns can be very difficult. Because adjustment disorders are often treated with medication, everyday unhappiness is too.

Another catch-all category is "Depressive Disorder NOS (Not Otherwise Specified)." An example of a patient with "Depressive Disorder NOS" was described to me by a psychiatrist as someone who says, "Doctor, I'm feeling sad and my sleep is restless. I don't know if I'm depressed or getting depressed, but I'm feeling down. My appetite is fine and I've got plenty of energy, but I'm unhappy." Such a patient may be a candidate for antidepressants.

Doctors have long recognized this deficiency of the DSM, but it was not a serious problem in 1952 when it was created. Psychotropic medications were not as readily available as they are now, so doctors could not use drugs to treat everyday unhappiness even if they had wanted to. With the development of psychotropic medications, doctors now can. The combination of safe, effective drugs like Prozac and a relatively imprecise method of categorizing mental pathology results in a wide use of psychotropic medication in borderline cases of depression.

Many psychiatrists argue that over-prescription is largely the fault of primary-care physicians, who provide the majority of mental-health care in this country. In the view of the psychiatrists, primary-care physicians are not sufficiently well versed in the nuances of the DSM to use it properly. In one study, over 30 percent of the family practitioners interviewed confessed to needing further training to treat emotional disorders, even though it was part of their routine practice to do so. But even though mental-health professionals are more experienced in treating depression, patients do not want to be referred to a psychiatrist or therapist for fear of the stigma attached—the fear of being thought "crazy." For this reason, they insist on being treated in the primary-care setting, where expertise in managing mental illness is not great. Again, the result is an increased use of psychotropic medication in cases of everyday emotional trouble.

The "Laws" of Sadness

While the potential for diagnostic error may cause some doctors to think twice about aggressively writing drug prescriptions, a new medical theory actually justifies the liberal use of psychotropic drugs. Doctors now point to a biochemical mechanism that comes close to uniting serious mental pathology and everyday emotional trouble under a single principle. It is called the "biogenic amine theory."

According to this theory, blocking the reuptake of serotonin or other neurotransmitters in the brain has a positive effect on the human psyche. Chemical compounds like serotonin, dopamine, noradrenalin, and acetylcholine are the means of communication across nerves. Since many of the drugs used to treat depression increase the amount of these neurotransmitters available in nerve spaces (called synapses), it is reasoned that depression might be caused by a deficiency of amines at the level of the nerve junction.

The biogenic amine theory has been in existence for several decades, it was developed through a series of inferences after the first generation of antidepressants, called tricyclics, was created. Because these drugs brought about an improvement in mood, and because they had a specific effect on the amines in nerve terminals, researchers concluded that amines must regulate mood.

While Kramer's *Listening to Prozac* examined the effects of Prozac on patients who were clinically ill, new research focuses on the effects of Prozac and other SSRIs on everyday unhappiness. According to medical science, the normal spectrum of individual differences in mood and social behavior may be tied to the same mechanism of neurotransmission that governs real mental pathology. One study postulates that different components of the human personality may have their own neurochemical substrates. These unique substrates, such as dopamine and serotonin—the same substrates involved in the biochemistry of clinical depression—may modulate the expression of everyday happiness and sadness.

Physicians have this theory in the back of their minds when they see depressed patients. They admit that depression may have many causes, but they still insist that moods are ultimately determined at the neuronal junctions of the brain where antidepressants work. In their view, all unhappiness necessarily leads back to these junctions in the same way that all roads once led to Rome.

This mindset prepares the way for a broad use of antidepressants. Because the DSM is a relatively arbitrary classification scheme, physicians think that even though their depressed patients may not fit the necessary diagnostic criteria for depression, they "almost do." And because the criteria for depression change with virtually every new edition of the DSM, being slightly off should not prevent a patient from receiving drug treatment, especially since his unhappiness, whatever its cause or level of intensity, will find its way back to the neuronal junctions of the brain as readily as all forms of depression.

Patients think in a similar vein. They understand that the classification scheme by which physicians measure the intensity of depression is arbitrary, and that the difference between a DSM-sanctioned depression and a more mild depression is not at all like the difference between being pregnant and not being pregnant. One cannot be a "little pregnant," but one can be a little depressed. In the minds of patients, the various shades of depression merge into a single unity that expresses itself eventually at the brain's neuronal junctions.

The proven value of psychoactive drugs in treating a wide spectrum of depressed patients encourages people who are just unhappy to ask for them. It seems unfair that patients who fit the DSM criteria for depression get to enjoy the quick benefits of drug treatment while those who do not are forced to endure the long, often painful process of talk therapy—a process that seems obscure and confusing and, to some, a bit dubious. Thus symptoms of depression are increasingly treated according to their level of intensity rather than according to their specific cause, which is unknown anyhow.

Is This Happiness?

The neuronal junctions of the brain where psychotropic drugs exert their effect are looked upon by medical science as a kind of corridor between matter and mood. Here at the subcellular level, the mystery of the human mood is believed to play itself out. A quantum of neurotransmitters is released at the neuronal junctions and a person's mood either rises or flags. The feeling of happiness gains an absolute unit of measurement in medical science and becomes, for all practical purposes, a visible phenomenon.

The flaw in this theory can be understood in the following way: Matter and mood are two different phenomena, as different as light and air, and so can have no physical interface. Just as light and air cannot affect one another, since there is no place in the universe where they "meet," neither can matter and mood affect one another, since there is no place in the physical world where they meet. One is finite, the other is infinite; the two are composed of different substances and so can never be joined together in physical reality.

It is true that neuronal junctions exist in the brain and that complex changes occur within these junctions during mental activity. But this does not necessarily make them a place where matter and mood share a common boundary. To say that they do is like watching a person get into a car, then seconds later watching the car move, and from this observation making the deduction that the car moves because someone gets into it. It is a false science to infer from the study of matter a knowledge any deeper than that of knowing the forms of matter and their relationships. It is a false science to say that on the basis of material knowledge, one can pretend to "know" and understand the emotional experience of life.

Kramer suggests that feelings like homesickness or loneliness are mediated through neurotransmitters like serotonin, or possibly encoded in neurons, and the fact that Prozac eases these conditions seems to confirm this view. But the notion that matter and mood can have a direct connection with one another—that somewhere at the neuronal junction, loneliness and serotonin "meet"—is tantamount to saying that the human mood is material, and that it can be touched by matter. Buried within the biogenic amine theory is an illogical belief—that neurotransmitters are shedding their physical existence, becoming even smaller than atoms, and ultimately merging with pure thought or idea.

The error in the biogenic amine theory can be understood in a slightly different way. Augustine once said that the human heart has more moods and emotions than hairs on the head or stars in the sky. What he meant by this is that happiness has an infinite number of shades, reflecting the infinite that is the human soul, which mirrors the infinite that is God. Even if every particle of serotonin crossing the synaptic cleft of a nerve terminal could be measured, along with every particle of noradrenalin and dopamine, the number of particles would still be finite, while the moods of a human being would still be infinite. By definition, there are simply not enough particles to express every conceivable human mood.

Creating Virtual Realities

But what about drugs like alcohol or narcotics? They alter our moods when ingested, producing feelings like euphoria and indifference. Is this not a case of matter affecting mood by way of a common border inside the brain?

No, it is not, and this is key to understanding how drugs like antidepressants really work. Alcohol and narcotics do not produce such feelings by being received directly into the "substance" of human emotions. On the contrary, they simply alter human consciousness in a way that allows the mind to shift its mood. These drugs work by dampening certain aspects of brain function—*they create an altered mental state*—such that true reality becomes concealed from a person's consciousness. The dampened brain functions allow a person to imagine an alternate "reality" that is generally more pleasing.

For example, when a man contrasts his humble circumstances with some ideal of success, tension arises in his psyche. His conscience berates him, and he feels the well-known misery of failure. He might try some diversion, like golf or stamp-collecting, in order to hide from himself what he does not want to face, but sometimes the diversion does not sufficiently block the sight of things that he dislikes. So he starts to drink, and the alcohol alters his consciousness in such a way that he is diverted. After ingesting alcohol, the eye of his mind no longer sees the images that were causing him so much pain. At this point, the man starts to feel better, even "happier."

Drinking is a reliable method of dealing with unhappiness not because it exerts a direct effect on a person's mood but because it helps conceal from view what he does not want to see. It is by dampening or altering brain functions and by affecting consciousness that alcohol transforms how we feel.

It is the same with antidepressants. They are merely another form of stupefaction. True, people who take them because they are unhappy are not like alcoholics or drug addicts—they function at work, they are well mannered, and they do not vomit in the streets. But although their method is "cleaner," they are attempting the same thing as the person who uses alcohol to raise his spirits. Unlike the drunk, their minds remain awake, clear, and lucid, but the drugs have still tampered with their brain functions, hiding from them what they do not want to see.

This point was revealed to me in the case of one friend who was taking Prozac for general unhappiness, though not under my supervision. He said, "I feel a lot better. I don't have to look into the abyss anymore. I see my problems, but they don't seem as daunting as they once did." With the help of a psychoactive drug, he was able to retire further and further from his mind's sight those images that were painful to him. He still saw their visible outlines, but his new mood was based on an altered perception of their image. He was no longer menaced by them because they had grown distant to him.

The same phenomenon can account for what Kramer calls "cosmetic psychopharmacology." Kramer reports with amazement how one of his female patients, after taking Prozac, changed from a social misfit into an accomplished coquette, capable of maneuvering smoothly from one man to the next, even of securing three dates in a single weekend. But is this any different from what alcohol might do for someone with similar hesitations? Is this really a "new self" courtesy of Prozac? Of course not. A woman wants to flirt with men, but her self-doubt tells her not to do so. The result is tension and unhappiness. So she takes alcohol in order to silence the critic within and feel "liberated." This is nothing new.

Prozac Nation

Yet despite the rather obvious nature of antidepressants, medical science studiously avoids putting antidepressants in the same category as alcohol and narcotics. It struggles to preserve the deceit of a special mood-matter link at the level of the neuronal junctions. Why is this so? Why does it bother to support the irrational notion that mood and matter share a common interface? To the degree that it is a conspiracy, it is one enjoined by our entire culture: People desperately want to believe in such a link; they want to believe that the cause of happiness is located in the physical world, and that happiness somehow comes about scientifically in the form of a pill. The promise of such a view is security and comfort.

First, to admit one's dependence on psychoactive drugs is to shield oneself from life's imponderables and unpredictability. If happiness is serotonin, and serotonin is happiness, then these drugs guarantee happiness, for one can take psychoactive drugs for years. It is with this attitude that people with mild depression might substitute the chance of real happiness with some semblance of happiness achieved through medication.

Second, to declare happiness a law of necessity allows science to emphasize the subcellular processes inside the brain at the expense of everything else. Science can say: "It is man's basic nature to want happiness, but if the natural desire for happiness is linked to the physical nature of his brain, it cannot be linked to culture, which varies from society to society. The search for happiness begins and ends in nature, and so there is no reason to go beyond science." By believing this to be true, people can put aside other approaches to coping with daily troubles—which is convenient, since these remedies, whether they involve talking to a friend or asking for divine guidance, are never a sure thing.

Third, the notion that happiness is a law of science appeals to human pride. If unhappiness is chemical or biological, along with its treatment, a person need not ask, "Why am I unhappy?" In the past, this question provoked serious introspection and self-examination, as the effort to cope with unhappiness merged with larger questions about life and existence. Religion and philosophy demanded that people see themselves as part of a larger whole and taught that happiness depended on more than self-satisfaction. But if happiness is a law of science, then one does not have to go through this humbling experience. Through drugs, one can find happiness as a single, isolated individual.

Fourth, and perhaps most crucial, depressed persons equate the pleasant mood evoked by psychoactive drugs with happiness, even though, in the depths of their hearts, they are not sure exactly what they feel. Still, people do not want to live a lie, and so they will accept their drug-induced "happiness" as the real thing only if they believe that science has truly uncovered the biology of happiness. And this is what the biogenic amine theory of matter and mood represents. It reassures people who take medication that their good feeling is indeed happiness.

For people suffering from clinical depression, the mental state produced by these drugs must be considered an improvement, and often, a necessary one. But for those people who suffer from unhappiness, perhaps because of stress or because they are in bad relationships, these drugs are nothing more than a shortcut to a particular mental state that they believe to be happiness but is not.

Your Mind on Drugs

What exactly do people feel when they take antidepressants? It is difficult to say because each person expresses the feelings aroused by medications like Prozac differently. There is simply no universal feeling. Nevertheless, a broad understanding of the phenomenon is possible, and what emerges among medicated patients is a definite change in consciousness.

In most of the testimonies published, patients note that the good feeling arising from the influence of mood-modifying drugs does not come about immediately. It often takes several weeks, and this delayed effect is considered to be so predictable that doctors warn their patients about it. The slow onset of the drug causes the change in people's attitude to be barely perceptible. There is generally no minute or hour that marks the onset of their improved mood.

And so it is not surprising that after people start taking medication, life continues by virtue of its own momentum. If, before taking the drug, people biked for recreation or shopped because it was their favorite pastime, they generally do so afterward. Except in rare cases of "cosmetic psychopharmacology," described by Kramer, the tastes and interests of a person do not change; the person on medication remains the same person.

For this reason, however, it cannot be a change in life that causes the uplift in spirit, since for the people taking these drugs, life does not change. Generally, most people calculate their happiness by external circumstances. But psychotropic drugs enable people to feel better even though their external circumstances are unchanged. The cause and effect relationship that has dominated their lives is not working properly, and while they feel better, they are confused.

Patients on psychotropic drugs still react to specific external events in an appropriate manner. Their mood goes up or down according to what happens in their environment. But while these patients may smile at a party or laugh at another's jokes, I have often observed a general lack of congruence between outside circumstances and a medicated patient's good feeling, and this observation is commensurate with the amazement expressed by these people at feeling well despite the lack of change in their outside circumstances. The outside world becomes, in a way, detached from their inner life. Its influence decreases.

Casual conversation with hundreds of patients taking psychotropic medication serves as the basis for this opinion. One patient of mine who was asked on a pre-operative evaluation how medication helped him replied, "I see the same things as before, but I don't care so much. I still feel good no matter what happens." Another patient in the same situation said, "I don't know why. I just feel really good about myself." For such people, the relationship between their outer life and their inner life becomes like two wheels that once rotated in tandem, and continue to do so, but are now ever so slightly off, with barely different speeds, such that while they appear to be connected by an axle, it is impossible for them to be so.

People medicated for depression often talk about enjoying activities that they did not enjoy prior to starting medication. But again, there is something suspicious in their pleasure. For example, two friends of mine told me that they "felt better" on medication, which enabled them to play tennis and feel good again while doing so. Yet it was not so much that they extracted pleasure from playing tennis but, rather, brought the pleasure they enjoyed through medication into this activity. It was a pleasure that they experienced for no discernible reason, and it mildly confused them since, deep down, they were the type of people who felt good only when external circumstances were going their way. Yet nothing in their lives had changed but a pill.

It has been observed that people who are not depressed and who take psychoactive drugs sometimes feel uncomfortable. The above observation might explain this phenomenon. The mood of such people is altered by drugs, but in a way that they cannot understand. They become like the traveler in a boat who feels confused by the imperceptible changes beneath his feet, and worse, has no beacon on the horizon on which to fix his gaze. He cannot establish a connection between what he is feeling and what he is seeing, so he starts to feel queasy. Nothing in the outer world seems to move, and so he cannot ascribe his inner feeling to an outside event. And if he does find a beacon sitting on the horizon, he cannot readily admit to himself, "Yes, I feel this way because of what I see," since what he sees never produced a feeling like this before. The whole thing makes no sense, and so he starts to feel seasick.

Know Thy Self

Psychoactive medication, much like alcohol and narcotics, causes a disconnect between the inner and outer life. This is the problem with using it to treat everyday unhappiness. The disconnect caused by medication is very different from the state of thoughtful detachment encouraged by many cultures for the purpose of insulating people from everyday disappointment. The latter contributes to wisdom, stability, and maturity; the former creates a state of mind that is stuporous and purposely unknowing.

Medical science should confine itself to the treatment of clinical depression, rather than extend itself into the realm of everyday unhappiness. Medical science "helps" unhappy people by clouding their thoughts, by making them less aware of the world, and by sapping their urge to see themselves in a true light. People medicated for everyday unhappiness gain inner peace, but they do so through a real decrement in consciousness.

POSTSCRIPT

Do the Advantages of Psychiatric Medicines Outweigh Their Disadvantages?

Mental health practitioners agree that antidepressant drugs can be effective in treating the majority of people with less severe forms of depression. However, there is a sharp disagreement as to whether or not these drugs are prescribed too readily and whether or not they are taking the place of traditional talk therapy. Of course, this debate does not need to focus on which type of treatment is best. Many people receive both drug therapy and psychotherapy. In addition, it has been shown that drug therapy and psychotherapy work best in conjunction with each other.

The pursuit of happiness seems to be of paramount importance in society. Yet should one turn to pills to find happiness? Do antidepressants represent a quick and easy fix? Is it ethical to chemically alter an individual's mood and personality in order for that person to be happy? Will psychopharmacology replace traditional psychotherapy? In a society that values solving problems quickly and easily, these drugs seem to effectively fulfill a need. However, do their advantages outweigh their disadvantages?

A popular slogan many years ago referred to "better living through chemistry." If a drug is available that will make people happier, more confident, and more socially adept, shouldn't that drug be available to people who would derive some degree of benefit from it? One concern is that some individuals might rely on drugs to remedy many of their problems rather than work through the issues that caused the problems in the first place. It is much easier to take a pill than to engage in self-exploration. Is there an analogy that could be made between antidepressant drugs and other drugs—legal or illegal? For example, people are increasingly using alcohol, tobacco, over-the-counter medicines, and illegal drugs to cope with life's daily problems.

In "Is It Really Our Chemicals That Need Balancing?" *Journal of American College Health* (July 2002), Christopher Bailey argues that society is falling into the trap of making minor problems into mental illnesses. The article "Generation Rx: The Risk of Raising Our Kids on Pharmaceuticals," by Rob Waters, *Psychotherapy Networker* (March/April 2000) maintains that children are being put on drugs like stimulants and antidepressants at too early an age. Carl Elliott, in "Pursued by Happiness and Beaten Senseless: Prozac and the American," *Hastings Center Report* (March/April 2000), asserts that too many people are using antidepressant drugs simply because they feel alienated. The side effects of antidepressant drugs are described in "The Darker Side of SSRIs," by Cathy Weitzel and Shiloh Jiwanlal, *RN* (August 2001).

ISSUE 11

Do the Consequences of Caffeine Outweigh the Benefits?

YES: Nell Boyce, from "Storm in a Coffee Cup," *New Scientist* (January 29, 2000)

NO: Edith Howard Hogan, Betsy A. Hornick, and Ann Bouchoux, from "Communicating the Message: Clarifying the Controversies About Caffeine," *Nutrition Today* (January–February 2002)

ISSUE SUMMARY

YES: Writer Nell Boyce states that caffeine is more addictive than most people realize. Boyce maintains that caffeine not only causes dependency but also has a myriad of other effects. Caffeine raises blood pressure, a factor leading to heart disease, and there is also evidence that caffeine consumption during pregnancy involves some risk for the fetus.

NO: Registered dietitians Edith Howard Hogan and Betsy A. Hornick and social worker Ann Bouchoux contend that there are numerous misconceptions related to caffeine. They maintain that caffeine has not been proven to cause heart disease, fibrocystic breast disease, nor some forms of cancer. They conclude that mental alertness and physical performance may be improved by caffeine use.

Caffeine is one of the most widely consumed legal drugs in the world. In the United States, more than 9 out of every 10 people drink some type of caffeinated beverage, mostly for its stimulating effects. Caffeine elevates mood, reduces fatigue, increases work capacity, and stimulates respiration. Caffeine often provides the lift that people need to start the day. Although many people associate caffeine primarily with coffee, caffeine is also found in numerous soft drinks, over-the-counter medications, chocolate, and tea. Because caffeinated drinks are common in society and there are very few legal controls regarding the use of caffeine, its physical and psychological effects are frequently overlooked, ignored, or minimized.

In recent years coffee consumption has declined; however, the amount of caffeine being consumed has not declined appreciably because of the increase in caffeinated soft drink consumption. To reduce their levels of caffeine intake, many people have switched to decaffeinated drinks and coffee. Although this results in less caffeine intake, decaffeinated coffee still contains small amounts of caffeine.

Research studies evaluating the effects of caffeine consumption on personal health date back to the 1960s. In particular, the medical community has conducted numerous studies to determine whether or not there is a relationship between caffeine consumption and cardiovascular disease because heart disease is the leading cause of death in many countries, including the United States. However, studies have yielded conflicting results. Rather than clarifying the debate regarding the consequences of caffeine, the research only adds to the confusion. As a result, studies suggesting that there is a connection between caffeine consumption and adverse physical and psychological effects have come under scrutiny by both the general public and health professions.

One serious limitation of previous research indicating that caffeine does have deleterious effects is that the research focused primarily on coffee use. There may be other ingredients in coffee besides caffeine that produce harmful effects. Moreover, an increasing percentage of the caffeine being consumed comes from other sources, such as soft drinks, tea, chocolate, antihistamines, and diet pills. Therefore, caffeine studies involving only coffee are not truly representative of the amount of caffeine that people ingest.

Another criticism of caffeine research, especially studies linking caffeine use and heart disease, is gender bias. Until recently, research has focused primarily on the caffeine consumption of men. The bias in medical research is not limited to caffeine studies; men have traditionally been the primary group studied with regard to many facets of health, although research into the potential consequences of caffeine use on the fetus and nursing mothers is currently being examined.

People who believe that drinking caffeine in moderation does not pose a significant health threat are critical of previous and current studies. This is particularly true of those studies that demonstrate a relationship between caffeine and heart disease. Critics contend that it is difficult to establish a definitive relationship between caffeine and heart disease due to a myriad of confounding variables. For example, cardiovascular disease has been linked to family history, a sedentary lifestyle, cigarette smoking, obesity, fat intake, and stress. Many individuals who consume large amounts of coffee also smoke cigarettes, drink alcohol, and are hard-driven. Several factors also affect caffeine's excretion from the body. Cigarette smoking increases caffeine metabolization, while the use of oral contraceptives and pregnancy slow down metabolization. Therefore, determining the extent to which caffeine use causes heart disease while adjusting for the influence of these other factors is difficult.

In the following selections, Nell Boyce cautions readers about the use of caffeine, even in moderate amounts. In contrast, Edith Howard Hogan, Betsy A. Hornick, and Ann Bouchoux cast doubt on the negative effects associated with caffeine intake.

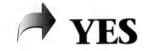

Storm in a Coffee Cup

The situation was very troubling. Counsellors at the Hazelden Foundation in Center City, Minnesota, a leading drug treatment clinic, had learned that some of the residents were smuggling in an addictive stimulant and sharing it with their friends. This was a clear violation of the rules, but the clinic's staff concluded that they would fight no longer, and rescinded the unpopular ban on coffee.

Some of the staff felt relieved. Why withhold a harmless substance that helped the patients stay off alcohol or crack cocaine? After all, the founder of Alcoholics Anonymous famously drank vast amounts of coffee, and almost all AA meetings take place around a coffee pot. But others were concerned that some patients were drinking so much coffee they weren't getting enough sleep. And there was a principle at stake. They felt that the caffeine in coffee was, quite frankly, an addictive drug.

If that's the case, the whole world is cheerfully addicted. In the US, almost everyone drinks coffee. In Britain and Australia people drink coffee and tea. And for Nigerians there's the cola nut to chew on. People consume vast quantities of caffeine in chocolate and soft drinks, and even in a pure pill form. But is it truly a drug of abuse like cocaine or heroin? And if so, should we kick the habit?

These are remarkably tricky questions. Headlines around the world last year proclaimed that French researchers had proved that caffeine wasn't really addictive. In July, Astrid Nehlig from the Strasbourg laboratory of INSERM, the French National Health and Medical Research Institute, announced that giving rats moderate amounts of caffeine does not promote activity in a brain region called the nucleus accumbens, thought to play a role in addiction (*ChemTech*, vol 29, p 30). Even low doses of cocaine, amphetamines, nicotine and morphine all activate this part of the brain. "The activation of the shell of the nucleus accumbens seems to be one of the key mechanisms of addiction of psychostimulants," Nehlig says.

But what of the other mechanisms and brain structures thought to be involved in drug addiction, such as the dopamine system? Caffeine makes us feel alert because it blocks the receptors for a brain chemical called adenosine, which normally dampens the activity of other neurotransmitters. Blocking adenosine boosts brain activity, and may indirectly boost dopamine levels. Cocaine, alcohol, nicotine and heroin also raise dopamine levels. "Obviously caffeine shares some properties with the drugs of abuse," Nehlig admits.

But she rejects the notion that caffeine could be considered an abused drug. Some scientists think that rises in dopamine levels may be a general pleasure response, not anything specifically linked to addiction. The main mechanisms of action of caffeine and the other drugs are different, Nehlig insists. She points out that with caffeine, "the extent of tolerance, withdrawal, or reinforcement is never as dramatic as those observed with the drugs of abuse."

Other researchers don't dismiss these shared properties so lightly. "I usually steer clear of the word addiction because it's loaded with additional baggage," says Roland Griffiths, an expert on caffeine at the Johns Hopkins Medical Institutions in Baltimore, Maryland. But he points to the behavioural changes that caffeine can bring about. "Over the last ten years there has been a greater appreciation in the general public that caffeine is a drug and produces withdrawal, but I would guess that caffeine users are unaware of the extent to which their behaviour is controlled by caffeine."

Take, for example, a simple study in which Griffiths gave moderate caffeine users red or blue capsules containing either a dose of caffeine or an inert powder. On one day everybody got a caffeine pill of one colour, and on the next day they got an inert pill that was the other colour. The following day they got to choose whichever colour they preferred, and 80 per cent of the time they chose the caffeine pill, regardless of whether this was red or blue. He told the participants that they were testing the effects of compounds found in common foods, so they had no idea what they were taking.

People clearly seek out caffeine, and when they can't get it they're not happy. This fact should be obvious to anyone who has ever tried to function in the morning without their usual cuppa, but until recently most researchers assumed that caffeine withdrawal was mild and transient. "There seemed to be an almost flat-out denial on the part of many that this is of any relevance and/or importance," says Griffiths. "Caffeine withdrawal occurs at much lower doses than we had previously recognised."

Withdrawal can occur in people who have as little as 100 milligrams of caffeine a day, about the amount in two cups of tea or one cup of instant coffee. Symptoms include headache, fatigue, difficulty concentrating and drowsiness. The ill effects peak after a day or two without caffeine, and can continue for more than a week. Surprisingly, Griffiths says, withdrawal can be suppressed by rather low levels of caffeine. If you usually imbibe three cups of coffee a day, or around 300 milligrams of caffeine, you can alleviate withdrawal symptoms with as little as 25 milligrams. "There may be lots of people who are dependent who think they are immune to withdrawal," notes Griffiths. Someone who skips their morning coffee and then has a cola with lunch won't suffer as badly.

Slow Reactions

Some researchers worry that children are especially vulnerable to withdrawal, as they often don't have steady access to caffeine. Gail Bernstein at the University of Minnesota in Minneapolis studied 30 children at times when they were drinking caffeine regularly and during withdrawal periods. She showed that they had slower reactions in tests that required them to watch a computer screen and click a mouse in response to certain images during periods of withdrawal (*Journal of the American Academy of Child & Adolescent Psychiatry*, vol 37, p 858). "It's maybe hard to say what you can transfer from the lab to the real world," she admits, but thinks the issue deserves more study, given the aggressive promotion of soft drinks to children.

Although adults tend to drink the same amount of caffeine from day to day, Griffiths says there is no convincing evidence that people can monitor and regulate their caffeine intake. But in one study he did show that if people are given coffee containing different doses of caffeine, they tend to drink more when the dose is low. He notes that "if you put someone in withdrawal, they're going to head towards caffeinated foods."

Researchers have also found that as people get used to drinking coffee, they acquire tolerance to its effects. In one study, people given 400 milligrams of caffeine a day initially experienced sleep problems. But after a week, their total sleep time, and the number of times they awoke, returned to normal. In another study, people got either caffeine or a placebo for 18 days. The two groups did not differ significantly in ratings of mood, until they were given a 300-milligram dose of caffeine: this made people in the placebo group nervous and jittery, but had no such effect on the group that was chronically exposed to caffeine.

At a biochemical level, caffeine increases levels of catecholamines, the neurotransmitters involved in the fight-or-flight response. So your body reacts in the way it would if you were facing down a lion: your pupils dilate, your breathing tubes open up, and your muscles get ready for action. Individuals differ in their reaction to caffeine. Part of this is down to genes, but there are other influences too. The half-life of caffeine is normally four to six hours, but this doubles in women taking oral contraceptives and is halved in smokers. Smokers are more likely than non-smokers to be coffee drinkers, and ex-smokers consume more coffee than non-smokers but less than smokers. If someone quits smoking but keeps drinking their usual amount of coffee or tea, their caffeine levels can suddenly rise to levels that make most people feel jittery, complicating efforts to stay off the cigarettes.

We all know why people should quit smoking. But does continually drinking coffee or tea have any health risks that might make it worth giving up? Large quantities of caffeine are deadly: tea or coffee could kill you, if you managed to drink between 50 and 100 cups in one go. Your liver treats caffeine like any other poison, and plants produce it to keep pests at bay. Yet evidence for coffee's contribution to common diseases remains far from clear. "You'll find that most people go into hyperbole on one side or the other," says Griffiths.

Health worries have been around since at least 1674, when women in London claimed it made their men impotent, according to Mark Pendergrast's 500-page opus on coffee, *Uncommon Grounds*. The most recent coffee concerns began in the 1970s, when epidemiologists linked coffee consumption to heart disease, pancreatic cancer and reproductive problems. More than twenty years later, these links remain controversial, and scientists have yet to confirm any of them. Several large epidemiological studies have failed to find any association between coffee consumption and heart disease.

James Lane of Duke University Medical Center in Durham, North Carolina, is convinced that there are risks, however. Caffeine raises blood pressure, and so could contribute to heart disease later in life, he says. Over the past ten years Lane has shown that the caffeine in four or five cups of coffee can raise blood pressure by about five points and increase production stress hormones such as cortisol and catecholamines. "People in high-stress jobs become dependent on caffeine. But the caffeine is making the stress in their life worse," says Lane.

Lane believes that we haven't picked up this increase in risk because people don't report their caffeine intake accurately. They just don't realise how much they take in, he says, especially when one cup doesn't always equal another. A large coffee from Starbucks, for example, can contain a whopping half-gram of caffeine, while a small cup of instant may contain less than 100 milligrams (see Figure 1). And consumption isn't necessarily consistent over the years.

There are further complications, too. Coffee and tea are a soup of many chemicals, not just a vehicle for caffeine, says Peter Martin, of Vanderbilt University's new Institute for Coffee Studies in Nashville, Tennessee. Studies by Lane and others that use pure caffeine miss the point, Martin says, because substances such as chlorogenic acids are more abundant in coffee than caffeine. "There may be pharmacological interactions that counteract the effects of caffeine," Martin says. He notes that chlorogenic acids have been shown to affect opiate receptors in the same way as naltrexone, a medication that blocks the "high" feeling that makes people want to use narcotics and alcohol.

Even the way coffee is prepared can create different compounds with effects of their own. In 1996, Dutch investigators reported that unfiltered coffee made in a cafetière or "French press" raised levels of harmful cholesterol by 9 to 14 per cent, while the same amounts of filtered coffee had no effect. The researchers attributed the effect to cafestol and kahweol, alcohols found in coffee oils (*British Medical Journal*, vol 313, p 8). It's perhaps not surprising that there is no clear picture of the effects of caffeine on health.

Mark Klebanoff of the National Institute of Child Health and Human Development near Washington DC decided that rather than relying on his volunteers to report their own caffeine intake, he would look for a metabolite of caffeine called paraxanthine in blood samples to test whether caffeine has any effect on rates of miscarriage. "It's not perfect, but at least it's looking at the issues in another way," says Klebanoff. The study found an increased risk of miscarriage only in women with the very highest levels of paraxanthine, corresponding to more than five cups of coffee a day. Klebanoff views the results as "at least reasonably reassuring for women." Many pregnant women say they quit drinking coffee anyway, because they lose the taste for it.

Brenda Eskenazi of the University of California School of Public Health in Berkeley thinks that women should minimise their caffeine intake during

Figure 1

What's Your Dose?

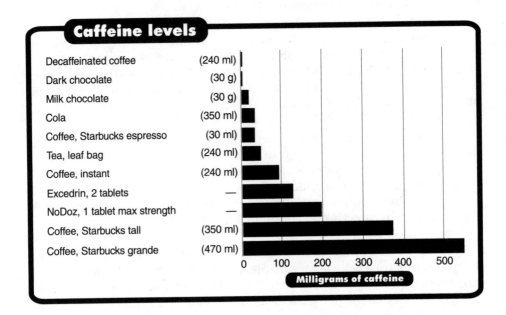

Many people have no idea how much caffeine they consume every day. So the Center for Science in the Public Interest in Washington DC petitioned the US Food and Drug Administration in 1997 to label the caffeine content of various foods. The FDA never took the recommended action, but here are some typical caffeine quantities found in various foods and beverages, according to the CSPI.

pregnancy just to be safe. She notes that caffeine can cross the placenta, is present in breast milk, and has a longer half-life in a pregnant woman's body (11 hours compared to 6). Studies have shown that low doses of caffeine can change a fetal heart rate even when the caffeine has no apparent effect on the mother.

The debate over health effects is likely to continue for as long as people keep drinking coffee and tea. But Klebanoff doesn't think we should worry too much about caffeine. "It didn't take us long to figure out that cigarettes were bad for you," he points out. "If there was something terrible that it does to us, we would have found it by now." But caffeine consumption is so widespread that even small risks for individuals could add up to major problems for society as a whole. "It's such a popular drug," says Lane. "I think we really need to have more people investigating it, just for peace of mind."

Most people who come to work in Griffiths's lab decide that they want to give up caffeine, once they see the evidence of their dependence and how it influences their daily life. If you want to quit, Griffiths suggests that you first spend a week keeping a careful log of your intake. Then taper off slowly, rather than quitting cold turkey, to minimise withdrawal symptoms. But be warned: caffeine has a powerful allure. "Without exception, people in time have decided to go back," says Griffiths, who admits to drinking an occasional caffeinated beverage. "If I have a message it's that people should know that caffeine is a drug and that they should treat it with respect."

Edith Howard Hogan, Betsy A. Hornick, and Ann Bouchoux

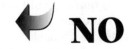

Communicating the Message: Clarifying the Controversies About Caffeine

Abstract

Today's "coffee culture" and the widespread availability of caffeine-containing foods and beverages fuel the ongoing study of caffeine and its subsequent coverage by the media. Although the media has become influential in communicating health and nutrition information to the public, coverage of emerging science, such as the study of caffeine, does not necessarily bring clarity or improved understanding for consumers. This article highlights the current knowledge of caffeine's effects on health, with emphasis on the most common areas of interest and confusion. To address persistent misperceptions about caffeine, this article also accentuates the need for nutrition professionals to help put the findings of caffeine research into perspective and suggests practical ways to do this.

Caffeine-containing foods and beverages have a long history of use. The first pot of tea was believed to have been brewed nearly 5,000 years ago. As early as 575 AD, coffee beans were consumed as food and used as currency in Africa. Interest in caffeine's effects on health only began to heat up during the past century. In 1958, the US Food and Drug Administration (FDA) classified caffeine as Generally Recognized as Safe (GRAS). Since then, thousands of studies have explored the connection between caffeine and health. In fact, caffeine is one of the most well-studied ingredients in our food supply. Despite our considerable knowledge of caffeine and centuries of safe consumption, questions and misperceptions about caffeine's potential health effects persist. Media coverage of research studying caffeine's effect on health may be partially responsible for this confusion.

In recent years, the public's appetite for information on food and health has grown considerably—and the media has attempted to satisfy it. An analysis of nutrition in the news commissioned by the International Food Information Council revealed that media coverage of food news is at an all time high. (1) In some instances, the media's interpretation and presentation of emerging research, especially studies that seem to contradict previous findings, serve to confuse rather than clarify. Moreover, competition for broadcast time, print space, and, ultimately, consumers' attention may mean that careful, deliberate reporting of research findings is sacrificed to achieve quick turnarounds and eye-catching headlines.

An informal survey was conducted to gauge the current media environment surrounding caffeine and health. Survey respondents were 35 American Dietetic Association (ADA) media spokespersons and approximately 115 key media journalists. The respondents were asked to report areas of interest and confusion related to caffeine that they encounter, along with the types of questions they receive from contacts with media, clients, and consumers. . . .

Filtering the Facts

Health professionals are in a position to help clarify the controversies about caffeine—for both consumers and news reporters. Communicating food and nutrition science to any audience involves providing the facts, putting them into perspective, and translating how research findings may affect the public's health and behaviors. To do this, health professionals must be familiar with the science behind an issue. The following section summarizes current knowledge related to caffeine and its effects on health for key areas of interest and confusion reported by ADA spokespeople and media journalists.

Sources and Amounts of Caffeine

Caffeine is a naturally occurring substance found in the leaves, seeds, or fruits of more than 60 plant species, including coffee and cocoa beans, kola nuts, and tea leaves. The most common sources of caffeine for Americans are coffee, tea, soft drinks, and chocolate. Average daily caffeine intake for adults in the United States is estimated at about 2 mg/kg, with more than 80% of the caffeine supplied by coffee. (2)

As a food additive, caffeine is used in various foods for its flavor contribution. The amount of caffeine in food products varies depending on the serving size, type of product, and preparation method. The plant variety also affects caffeine content of teas and coffees.

Consumers often want to know a "safe" amount of caffeine for daily consumption. Most experts agree that the prudent approach for consuming caffeine-containing foods and beverages is moderation and common sense. Moderate caffeine consumption is generally considered to be about 300 mg per day, which is equivalent to approximately 3 cups of coffee. However, people differ greatly in their sensitivity to caffeine so a "moderate" amount can vary depending on the individual. Caffeine sensitivity is influenced by various factors, including the amount and frequency of caffeine consumption, individual metabolism, body weight, and physical condition. (3) Individuals often find their own acceptable level of daily caffeine intake by assessing their reactions to caffeine. Those who feel unwanted effects tend to limit their caffeine consumption, whereas those who do not feel the unwanted effects continue to consume caffeine at their preferred level.

Effects on Children

Children (5–18 years) consume an average of about 38 mg of caffeine daily, primarily from soft drinks and tea. (2) A common concern of parents is whether caffeine has an effect on their children's behavior. No evidence suggests that caffeine is associated with hyperactivity or attention deficit disorder. Children metabolize and excrete caffeine more rapidly than adults, making the effects, if any, shorter lived. Despite their smaller size, children are no more sensitive to the effects of caffeine than adults, and most children don't react adversely to caffeine in the smaller portions they typically consume. However, common sense should prevail in recommending that parents monitor their children's caffeine intake because of the possibility that caffeine-containing foods and beverages may take the place of more healthful choices.

Women who are breast-feeding often question the safety of consuming caffeine-containing foods and beverages. Although a very small amount of caffeine is passed to the infant through breast milk, moderate caffeine consumption ($<$ 300 mg daily) does not change breast milk composition and has no adverse effect on the infant. The American Academy of Pediatrics confirms that moderate caffeine consumption is compatible with breast-feeding. (4)

Fertility and Pregnancy

Women planning to get pregnant often question whether they should eliminate caffeine. Studies of the association between caffeine and probability of conception are equivocal. Although some have found delayed conception associated with caffeine consumption, (5,6) others have shown no association. (7,8) Women who reported drinking more than 300 mg/day of caffeine had a 27% lower chance of conceiving for each cycle in a cross-sectional study of 1,909 women. (5) In contrast, a study that involved more than 2,800 women who had recently given birth and 1,800 women with a medical diagnosis of primary infertility found that caffeine consumption had no appreciable effect on the reported time to conceive in those women who had given birth. (7) In the women who were being treated for infertility, caffeine was not a risk factor for continued infertility. In a recent study of 2,607 planned pregnancies, caffeine consumption was not associated with delayed conception, even at higher levels of $>$ 500 mg/day. (8) A study of the relation between caffeine intake and menstrual function found no effect on menstrual cycles or anovulation. (9)

The safety of consuming caffeine during pregnancy continues to be debated. Although the FDA states that caffeine does not adversely affect reproduction, the agency advises pregnant women to consume caffeine in moderation. Evidence is convincing that women who consume caffeine, even at higher levels, are not at increased risk of bearing children with birth defects. (10,11) Mixed data exist on caffeine's effects on spontaneous miscarriage. When the effects of nausea, smoking, alcohol intake, and age were controlled for, two studies found no association between caffeine intake up to 300 mg/day and spontaneous miscarriage. (12,13) More recently, very high intakes of caffeine ($>$ 6 cups of coffee/day) were associated with increased risk for spontaneous miscarriage. (14) Whereas previous studies estimated caffeine intake from the women's reports, this study used a biologic marker of caffeine intake, the level of the caffeine metabolite paraxanthine in serum, to estimate caffeine exposure. Caffeine has not been linked to premature labor.

In studies on infant outcome, there appears to be no long-term effects on the fetus. A 7-year prospective study found no relationship between caffeine intake during pregnancy and birth weight, length, or head circumference. (15) Follow-up evaluation at ages 8 months, 4 years, and 7 years also revealed no connection between caffeine intake during pregnancy and early childhood development measures of motor skills or intelligence. A recent meta-analysis of 32 studies suggests that caffeine may be associated with a small reduction in birth weight (3–6 g) in women who consume more than 150 mg of caffeine daily. (16) However, factors such as maternal age, smoking, alcohol use, and other confounders were not excluded in this study and may have influenced these results.

Benign Breast Disease

Caffeine was first associated with breast disease in the late 1970s, when one study suggested that abstinence might alleviate the symptoms of fibrocystic breast disease (FBD), a condition of benign fibrous lumps in the breast. Although the study did not find a link between caffeine and development of the disease, some women with FBD reported feeling less breast tenderness when they eliminated caffeine from their diets. However, the findings were based on anecdotal reports from a small number of women, making the conclusions unreliable. The National Cancer Institute (NCI) examined this potential connection in a large case-control study involving more than 3,000 women. (17) No connection was found between caffeine and benign tumors, FBD, or breast tenderness. Both the NCI and the American Medical Association (AMA) Council on Scientific Affairs support the conclusion that there is no association between caffeine intake and FBD.

Cancer

The potential connection between caffeine, and cancer has been studied extensively. Because caffeine comes in direct contact with the gastrointestinal tract, studies have examined whether caffeine may increase the risk of oral, esophageal, stomach, pancreatic, liver, colon, and rectal cancers. Cancers that may be linked to the excretion of caffeine, including cancer of the kidney, bladder, and prostate, have also been studied. The concern raised about caffeine and FBD led to studies that investigated caffeine's possible association with breast cancer. The evidence to date suggests no association between caffeine consumption and the development of cancer. The American Cancer Society's Guidelines on Diet, Nutrition, and Cancer affirm that drinking coffee is not a risk factor in human cancer. (18)

Bone Health

Increased awareness of osteoporosis coupled with contradictory results generated by several studies in recent years has created more interest in the potential effects of caffeine on bone health. Adding fuel to the fire is caffeine's propensity, albeit small, to promote calcium excretion. In observational studies on caffeine's effect on bone density, the confounding factors known to affect bone loss, such as smoking, alcohol use, body weight, physical activity, and hormone replacement therapy (HRT), have been controlled for statistically rather than by experimental design, which may produce results that do not fully account for the complex relationships that exist among confounding factors. For instance, heavy caffeine consumers (> 5 cups coffee/day) are more likely to smoke, less likely to take vitamin supplements, and less likely to consume a "healthy" diet. (19) These interrelated factors can all influence bone health to varying degrees.

A recent study was designed specifically to minimize the effects of confounding factors, including smoking, body weight, and use of HRT. (20) This study evaluated the relationship between long-term caffeine intake and bone status among postmenopausal women and found no association between dietary caffeine intake and bone loss. To explore the possibility that caffeine might have an effect on individuals with lower daily calcium intakes, another study measured total body bone density and compared it with varying levels of caffeine consumption. (21) At none of the calcium intake levels was there a correlation between caffeine consumption and bone density change. In regard to calcium metabolism, the amount of caffeine in a single cup of brewed coffee causes a reduction in calcium absorption of about 4 mg. (22) This amount is readily offset by a tablespoon or two of milk.

Heart Disease

In studies of the effects of caffeine on the cardiovascular system, no association has been found between caffeine consumption and increased risk for heart disease, high blood pressure, or cardiac arrhythmia. Although boiled unfiltered coffee has been associated with increased homocysteine concentrations and elevated blood cholesterol levels, this Scandinavian preparation method is rarely used in the United States. (23) Studies that examined the effects of caffeine and regular coffee on serum lipids found no unfavorable changes. (24,25)

Caffeine intake has not been shown to cause chronic hypertension or any persistent increase in blood pressure. A slight rise in blood pressure, usually not lasting more than several hours, is observed in some individuals, such as older adults with hypertension. (26) However, this temporary rise in blood pressure is modest and is less than that normally experienced with normal daily activities, such as climbing stairs. Hypertensive individuals who consume caffeine regularly are not at increased risk of death due to coronary artery disease or stroke.

A review of studies on caffeine and cardiac arrhythmias concluded that moderate caffeine consumption does not increase the frequency or severity of cardiac arrhythmias. (27) Likewise, abstaining from caffeine does not reduce the occurrence of cardiac arrhythmias and plays no role in the management of this disorder. (28)

Cognitive and Physical Performance

The effects of caffeine, especially caffeinated coffee, on human performance have been studied extensively. Individuals who consume caffeine may experience increased mental alertness, better memory and mood, and improved reasoning powers. As little as 32 mg of caffeine, typical of the amount found in a single serving of a cola beverage, has been shown to improve auditory vigilance and visual reaction time. (29) A recent study demonstrated that caffeine consumption throughout the day may help to maintain aspects of cognitive and psychomotor performance. (30) Older adults may be more sensitive to the effects of caffeine, showing small but significant improvements in vigilance and psychomotor performance after caffeine intake. (31) However, individuals vary widely with respect to sensitivity to caffeine; the amount that can improve alertness in some may make others feel uncomfortable.

Athletes may use caffeine as an ergogenic aid to increase energy, promote fat loss, and improve endurance. The feeling of increased energy is likely related to a decreased perception of fatigue associated with caffeine's action as a central nervous system stimulant. In studies of the performance effects of caffeine, improvements in endurance are believed to be associated with caffeine's effect on increasing use of fat and sparing muscle glycogen. Research has established that caffeine can improve endurance at levels of 3–6 mg/kg. (32) Although higher amounts also may improve performance, athletes are more likely to experience unpleasant side effects, such as nausea, headaches, muscle tremors, and palpitations. Additionally, at doses of 9–13 mg/kg, competitive athletes may experience urinary caffeine levels that exceed the established limits of the International Olympic Committee and the National Collegiate Athletic Association. (32)

Addiction

Depending on the amount consumed, caffeine can act as a mild central nervous system stimulant. Any pharmacologic effects of caffeine are brief because caffeine is normally excreted within several hours of consumption. Although caffeine is sometimes characterized as "addictive," it does not meet important criteria used by the American Psychiatric Association to classify a substance as addictive. These criteria include reinforcing effects, tolerance, withdrawal symptoms, antisocial seeking behavior, and alterations in brain chemistry.

The desirable effects that contribute to caffeine's appeal and the motive to prevent withdrawal symptoms are considered reinforcing effects. With regular use, tolerance develops to some of the effects of caffeine. However, increasing amounts of caffeine are not needed to achieve a stimulant effect. When regular caffeine consumption is abruptly stopped, some people report unpleasant "withdrawal" symptoms, including headache, nausea, fatigue, and reduced concentration. In a recent study of the frequency and range of severity of caffeine withdrawal symptoms, participants were blinded to the study's focus on caffeine withdrawal. (33) Interestingly, adverse effects associated with caffeine cessation were inconsistent and less than expected, suggesting that withdrawal symptoms may be less likely than once thought. Furthermore, there is no evidence that caffeine has comparable physical and social consequences, which are often seen with drugs of abuse. Consumers of caffeine do not demonstrate compulsive antisocial behavior, and there is no alteration of brain chemistry as seen with addicting drugs such as cocaine or heroin.

References

1. Food for Thought III. Executive Summary International Food Information Council Foundation; February 2000. Available at: http://ific.org/relatives/17042.html. Accessed May 25, 2000.

2. Barone JJ, Roberts H. Caffeine consumption. Food Chem Toxicol. 1996; 24:119–129.

3. Hughes JR, Higgins ST, Bickel WK. Caffeine self-administration, withdrawal, and adverse effects among coffee drinkers. Arch Gen Psych. 1988; 48:611–617.

4. American Academy of Pediatrics Committee on Drugs. The transfer of drugs and other chemicals into human milk. Pediatrics. 1994; 93:137–150.

5. Hatch EE, Bracken MB. Association of delayed conception with caffeine consumption. Am J Epidemiol. 1993; 138:1082–1092.

6. Wilcox A, Weinberg C, Baird D. Caffeinated beverages and decreased fertility. Lancet. 1988; 2:1453–1456.

7. Joesoef MF, Beral V, Rolls RT. Are caffeinated beverages risk factors for delayed conception? Lancet. 1990; 335:136–137.

8. Curtis KM, Savitz DA, Arbuckle TE. Effects of cigarette smoking, caffeine consumption, and alcohol intake on fecundability. Am J Epidemiol. 1997; 146:32–41.

9. Fenster L, Quale C, Waller K, et al. Caffeine consumption and menstrual function. Am J Epidemiol. 1999; 149:550–557.

10. Olsen J, Overvad K, Frische G. Coffee consumption, birth weight, and reproductive failures. Epidemiology. 1991; 2:370–374.

11. McDonald AD, Armstrong BG, Sloan M. Cigarette, alcohol, and coffee consumption and congenital defects. Am J Public Health. 1992; 82:91–93.

12. Fenster L, Hubbard AE, Swan SH, et al. Caffeinated beverages, decaffeinated coffee, and spontaneous abortion. Epidemiology. 1997; 8:515–522.

13. Mills JL, Holmes LB, Aarons JH, et al. Moderate caffeine use and the risk of spontaneous abortion and intrauterine growth retardation. JAMA. 1993; 269:593–597.

14. Klebanoff MA, Levine RD, DerSimonian R, Clemens JD, Wilkins DG. Maternal serum paraxanthine, a caffeine metabolite, and the risk of spontaneous abortion. N Engl J Med. 1999; 341:1639–1644.

15. Barr HM, Streissguth AP. Caffeine use during pregnancy and child outcome: a 7-year prospective study. Neurotoxicol Teratol. 1991; 13:441–448.

16. Fernandes O, Sabharwal M, Smiley T, Pastuszak A, Koren G, Einarson T. Moderate to heavy caffeine consumption during pregnancy and relationship to spontaneous abortion and abnormal fetal growth: a meta-analysis. Reprod Toxicol. 1998; 12:435–444.

17. Boyle CA, Berkowitz GS, LiVolsi VA, et al. Caffeine consumption and fibrocystic breast disease: a case-control epidemiologic study. J Natl Cancer Inst. 1984; 72:1015–1019.

18. American Cancer Society 1996 Advisory Committee on Diet, Nutrition, and Cancer Prevention. Guidelines on diet, nutrition, and cancer prevention: reducing the risk of cancer with healthy food choices and physical activity. CA Cancer J Clin. 1996; 46:325–341.

19. Leviton A, Pagano M, Allred EN, el Lozy M. Why those who drink the most coffee appear to be at increased risk of disease: a modest proposal. Ecol Food Nutr. 1994; 31:285–293.

20. Lloyd T, Johnson-Rollings N, Eggli DF, Kieselhorst K, Mauger EA, Cusatis DC. Bone status among postmenopausal women with different habitual caffeine intakes: a longitudinal investigation. J Am Coll Nutr. 2000; 19:256–261.

21. Lloyd T, Rollings N. Dietary caffeine intake and bone status of postmenopausal women. Am J Clin Nutr. 1997; 65:1826–1830.

22. Barger-Lux MJ, Heaney RP. Caffeine and the calcium economy revisited. Osteop Int. 1995; 5:97–102.

23. Grubben MJ, Boers GH, Blom HJ, et al. Unfiltered coffee increases plasma homocysteine concentrations in healthy volunteers: a randomized trial. Am J Clin Nutr. 2000; 71:480–484.

24. Lewis CE, Caan B, Funkhouser E, et al. Inconsistent associations of caffeine-containing beverages with blood pressure and with lipoproteins. The CARDIA Study. Coronary Artery Risk Development in Young Adults. Am J Epidemiol. 1993; 138:502–507.

25. Bak AA, Grobbee DE. Caffeine, blood pressure, and serum lipids. Am J Clin Nutr. 1991; 53:971–975.

26. Rakic V, Burke V, Beilin LJ. Effects of coffee on ambulatory blood pressure in older men and women: a randomized controlled trial. Hypertension. 1999; 33:869–873.

27. Myers MG. Caffeine and cardiac arrhythmias. Ann Int Med. 1991; 114:147–150.

28. Newby DE, Neilson JM, Jarvie DR, Boon NA. Caffeine restriction has no role in the management of patients with symptomatic idiopathic ventricular premature beats. Heart. 1996; 76:355–357.

29. Lieberman HR, Wurtman RJ, Emde GG, Roberts C, Coviella IL. The effects of low doses of caffeine on human performance and mood. Psychopharmacology. 1987; 92:308–312.

30. Hindmarch I, Rigney U, Stanley N, Quinlan P, Rycroft J, Lane J. A naturalistic investigation of the effects of day-long consumption of tea, coffee, and water on alertness, sleep onset, and sleep quality. Psychopharmacology. 2000; 149:203–216.

31. Rees K, Allen D, Lader M. The influence of age and caffeine on psychomotor and cognitive function. Psychopharmacology. 1999; 145:181–188.

32. Graham TE, Spriet LL. Caffeine and exercise performance. Sport Sci Exch. 1996; 9(1).

33. Dews PB, Curtis GL, Hanford KJ, O'Brien CP. The frequency of caffeine withdrawal in a population-based survey and in a controlled, blinded pilot experiment. J Clin Pharmacol. 1999; 39:1221–1232.

34. Improving public understanding: guidelines for communicating emerging science on nutrition, food safety, and health. J Nat Can Inst. 1998; 90:194–199.

35. Ross GW, Abbott RD, Petrovitch H, et al. Association of coffee and caffeine intake with risk of Parkinson disease. JAMA. 2000; 283:2674–2679.

POSTSCRIPT

Do the Consequences of Caffeine Outweigh the Benefits?

Although caffeine is commonly consumed by millions of people without much regard to its physical and psychological effects, many studies have questioned its safety. However, other studies have reported very few hazards. The basic question is whether or not people who drink several cups of coffee or other caffeinated beverages daily should be more concerned than they are. Are claims of caffeine's benefits or hazards exaggerated?

Determining if certain foods or beverages promote disease or have health benefits can be trying. Many people become frustrated because quite a few of the things that we eat or drink are suspected of being unhealthy. For example, various reports indicate that the fat in beef is unhealthy, that we should consume less salt and sugar, that processed foods should be avoided, and that whole milk, butter, and margarine should be reduced or eliminated from our diets. If people paid attention to every report about the harmful effects of the foods and beverages that they consume, then they would not be able to eat much at all. What is the average consumer supposed to do?

A legitimate question is whether or not food studies are worth pursuing because so many of the products that are reportedly bad are enjoyed by millions of people. Caffeine is simply one more example of a commonly used product that has come under scrutiny. In addition, although the research is vast, it is inconclusive and contradictory. One study, for instance, linked caffeine to pancreatic cancer; later it was found that the culprit was not caffeine but cigarette smoking. Research on caffeine's effects on cancers of the bladder, urinary tract, and kidney has also proven to be inconsistent and inconclusive. If professional researchers cannot agree as to whether a product is safe or harmful, how can the average person know what to believe?

Boyce contends that caffeine may cause dependence and that it shares some of the same characteristics of cocaine, alcohol, and nicotine. Hogan et al. counter that caffeine's adverse effects are overstated.

Other articles that examine caffeine's psychological and physical effects are Eric Metcalf's "Coffee to Go: Research Shows That Caffeine, in the Right Amount, Can Boost Performance Without Harming Your Health," *Runner's World* (January 2002); Jeff Novick's "Waking Up to the Effects of Caffeine: How Important Is That Morning Cup of Coffee?" *Health Science* (Spring 2002); Linda Mooney's "Should You Decaf Your Life?" *Prevention* (July 2000); and Laura Goldstein's "Good News About Coffee," *Prevention* (December 2000). An article that addresses caffeine's impact during pregnancy is "Caffeine and Miscarriage Risk," *Family Practice News* (February 1, 2000).

ISSUE 12

Are Too Many Children Receiving Ritalin?

YES: Jonathan Leo, from "Attention Deficit Disorder: Good Science or Good Marketing?" *Skeptic* (June 21, 2000)

NO: Michael Fumento, from "Trick Question," *The New Republic* (February 3, 2003)

ISSUE SUMMARY

YES: Writer Jonathan Leo contends that the tremendous increase in the number of prescriptions written for Ritalin is due to the millions of dollars spent by pharmaceutical companies on promoting the drug. Leo contends that the basis for prescribing Ritalin to children is based on bad science. He argues that the evidence does not support a biological foundation for attention deficit/hyperactivity disorder (ADHD).

NO: Writer Michael Fumento disputes the idea that Ritalin is overprescribed and asserts that there are many myths associated with Ritalin. He maintains that Ritalin does not lead to abuse and addiction, and he concludes that Ritalin is an excellent medication for ADHD.

The number one childhood psychiatric disorder in the United States is attention deficit/hyperactivity disorder (ADHD), which affects approximately 6 million American schoolchildren. ADHD is characterized by inattentiveness, hyperactivity, and impulsivity. Many children are diagnosed as having only attention deficit disorder (ADD), which is ADHD without the hyperactivity. The most commonly prescribed drug for ADHD is the stimulant Ritalin (generic name methylphenidate). American children consume 90 percent of all Ritalin produced worldwide. Only a very small percentage of European children are diagnosed with ADHD; Ritalin is therefore much less likely to be prescribed in Europe.

The use of stimulants to treat such behavioral disorders dates back to 1937. The practice of prescribing stimulants for behavioral problems increased dramatically beginning in 1970, when it was estimated that 150,000 American children were taking stimulant medications. It seems paradoxical for physicians to be prescribing a stimulant such as Ritalin for a behavioral disorder that already involves hyperactivity. However, Ritalin appears to be effective in treating many children, as well as many adults, who suffer from this condition. Looking at this issue from a broader perspective, one needs to ask whether or not behavioral problems should be treated as a disease. Also, does Ritalin really address the problem? Or could it be covering up other maladies that otherwise should be treated?

Ritalin enhances the functioning of the brain's reticular activating system, which helps one to focus attention and to filter out extraneous stimuli. The drug has been shown to improve short-term learning. Ritalin also produces adverse effects, such as insomnia, headaches, irritability, nausea, dizziness, weight loss, and growth retardation. Psychological dependence may develop, but physical dependence is unlikely. The effects of long-term Ritalin use are unknown.

Since 1990 the number of children receiving Ritalin has increased 500 percent. This large increase in the number of children being diagnosed with ADHD may be attributed to a broader application of the criteria for diagnosing ADHD, heightened public awareness, and changes in American educational policy regarding schools' identifying children with the disorder. Some people feel that the increase in prescriptions for Ritalin reflects an increased effort to satisfy the needs of parents whose children exhibit behavioral problems. Ritalin has been referred to as "mother's little helper." Regardless of the reasons for the increase, many people question whether Ritalin is overprescribed and children are overmedicated or whether Ritalin is a miracle drug.

One problem with the increased prevalence of Ritalin prescriptions is that illegal use of the drug has also risen. There are accounts of some parents getting prescriptions for their children and then selling the drugs illegally. On a number of college campuses there are reports of students using Ritalin to get high or to stay awake in order to study. Historically, illegal use of Ritalin has been minimal, although officials of the Drug Enforcement Administration (DEA) are now concerned that its illegal use is proliferating. Problems with its use are unlikely to rival those of cocaine because Ritalin's effects are more moderate than those of cocaine or amphetamines.

The fact is that children now receive prescriptions for Ritalin rather readily. Frequently, parents will pressure their pediatricians into writing the prescriptions. One survey found that almost one-half of all pediatricians spent less than an hour assessing children before prescribing Ritalin. On the other hand, if there is a medication available that can remedy a problem, shouldn't it be prescribed? If a child's academic performance can improve through the use of Ritalin, should that child be denied the drug?

In the following selections, Jonathon Leo argues that too many children are being given Ritalin too hastily. He maintains that the process of diagnosing ADHD is inexact and that the scientific evidence establishing the validity of this syndrome is questionable. Michael Fumento maintains that ADHD is underdiagnosed in many instances. He asserts that Ritalin's bad reputation arises from many misconceptions regarding the drug.

Jonathan Leo

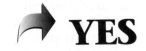

Attention Deficit Disorder: Good Science or Good Marketing?

In the 1960s, Americans discovered illegal mind-altering drugs for themselves. In the 1990s, Americans discovered a legal mind-altering drug for their children. Although it is illegal drugs that draw the attention of the media and law enforcement agencies, over the past decade there has been a meteoric rise in the number of children, under the guidance of a physician, taking mind-altering drugs.

The drug? Ritalin. The most recent estimate is that somewhere between three to five million children in this country are taking Ritalin or a similar type of drug.(1) Furthermore, American children consume 90% of all the Ritalin produced worldwide, making this a unique aspect of American culture.(2) Ritalin is the drug of choice for children who have been diagnosed with Attention Deficit Hyperactivity Disorder or ADHD. It has now become acceptable to give children a drug to alter their personality and behavioral patterns in a specific situation, usually school. The acceptance of this practice, however, has more to do with marketing than science. In the past 10 years, millions of dollars have been spent by scientists to investigate the biological basis of ADHD. Likewise, millions of dollars have been spent by the marketing departments of pharmaceutical companies to promote the use of drugs such as Ritalin.

By comparing the success rate of the scientists on one hand and the marketing departments on the other, it is clear why medicating children has more to do with marketing than science. The scientific basis of ADHD is on shaky ground and very little progress has been made in the last decade. It is hard to pin down the ADHD experts on what they think is the most convincing scientific proof of this disorder. Instead of one very good study that proves their case, there are numerous marginal studies that individually have little significance. However, when these little pieces are piled high it appears to some that significant understanding is at hand.

The phrase "this is one of the most studied pediatric conditions" appears frequently in the ADHD literature, but the major scientific evidence for ADHD is that hyperactive children can be helped, at least in the short run, by taking

Ritalin, a pill that increases a neurotransmitter called dopamine. So, the argument goes, if we know that Ritalin both increases dopamine levels and subdues hyperactive children, then the original hyperactivity must have been due to a dearth of dopamine. This line of reasoning is flawed. We do not use a parallel argument to explain the effects of other drugs such as aspirin. Aspirin relieves headaches but that doesn't mean that a shortage of aspirin caused the headache.(3,4) ADHD may be one of the most extensively studied pediatric conditions, yet there is still no proof of any underlying neuropathology.

Ask a psychiatrist to explain ADHD and Ritalin, and he will most likely recite the diabetes analogy, which goes something like this: ADHD is like diabetes in that both are due to a shortage of a chemical in the body. Diabetics are short of insulin, a condition that causes their blood sugar level to increase. This condition is helped by administering insulin, which brings the blood sugar level down. The child with ADHD has a shortage of dopamine, which leads to impulsive behavior. By administering Ritalin we can increase the dopamine levels and normalize the child.

The problem with this analogy is that, while for diabetes a blood test can be implemented to detect abnormal glucose levels, for ADHD no such biological test exists to detect decreased dopamine levels. For diabetes, too, insulin can be administered, the blood test repeated, and the effect of the drug measured. We cannot measure the effect of Ritalin in this way. Recently, parents who have been concerned with Ritalin affecting their child's growth have withheld the drug on vacations and during summer holidays. This is even referred to as a "drug holiday."(5) Clearly, there is no room in the diabetes analogy for a drug holiday, because diabetics cannot stop taking their insulin whenever they feel like it. Any scientist with a modicum of critical thinking skills can see that the diabetes analogy is not valid.

Psychiatrists frequently use the diabetes analogy to explain any mental illness.(6,7) The ADHD proponents also have their own unique analogy—eyeglasses. According to the National Institutes of Mental Health [NIMH], "Parents and teachers can help children view their medication in a positive way: Compare the pills to eyeglasses. Explain that their medicine is simply a tool to help them focus and pay attention."(8) The problem with the eyeglass analogy is that comparing Ritalin to eyeglasses is like comparing a lightning bolt to a flashlight.

Brain Scans or Scams?

The Holy Grail for ADHD research is to find a diagnostic test that a physician could use to determine if a patient actually has ADHD. For years scientists have sought a legitimate biological marker to lend credence to the ADHD diagnosis. The current trend is to use PET (Positron Emission Tomography) scans to compare the brains of ADHD children with the brains of normal children. Dr. Alan Zametkin, a leader in the effort to show some biological abnormality in the brains of ADHD children, is often cited in Ritalin advertising literature. He has conducted two major brain scan studies in which he compares ADHD patients to controls. The first study was in 1990 when he examined adult brains.(9) This study received considerable press attention because, in the words of Zametkin himself, "Zametkin et al. published a study showing, for the first time, definite and quantifiable central neurophysiological differences between ADHD adults and normal adults."(10) One problem with the Zametkin study was that, while there was an 8% difference in glucose metabolism, there was no difference in outcome on a continuous performance test.

The other (and major) problem is that Zametkin's study included both females and males, but when ADHD males are compared to control males there is no significant difference. The only way to get a statistically significant difference is to group the males and females together. In a subsequent study independent researchers analyzed Zametkin's data and compared the male controls to the female controls and found that there was a significant difference between normal males and normal females.(11) Based on Zametkin's logic that a difference in metabolism leads to medication, then either the normal males or normal females should be medicated. Again, just because there is a difference does not mean there is a disease. Based on the "success" of his first study, Zametkin published a second in 1993 that compared ADHD adolescents to control adolescents.(12) In this study, however, he found no differences in global brain metabolism.

In a review article Zametkin discusses these results: "Several reasons could have accounted for the overall lack of brain metabolism difference between ADHD and normal teenagers. First, the adolescent control group was not as pure as the control group used in the adult study, because 63% of the normal adolescents had a first-degree relative with ADHD, in contrast to the absence of ADHD pathology in families of normal adults. Second, 75% of the adolescents with ADHD had been previously exposed to treatment with stimulants, compared to no history of stimulant treatment in the ADHD adults. Third, an age effect in the development of brain abnormalities in ADHD individuals cannot be ruled out."(10) One of the possibilities that Zametkin seems to ignore is that his findings actually show that there is no biological difference between ADHD and control brains.

It is astonishing that he does not even consider this possibility (at least in print). Despite the negative findings of this second study, the ADHD marketing forces have taken the PET scan research and presented it to the general public as if there were evidence of a neurobiological disorder. CHADD (Children and Adults with Attention Deficit Disorders) is a national organization that promotes the concept that ADHD is a neurobiological disorder, and it has received close to a million dollars from the drug companies that manufacture Ritalin.(9) They use the brain scan picture to show that ADHD is a neurobiological disorder. To the non-scientist it seems as if the brain scan research has revealed some underlying biological deficit. But this is misleading. The advertisement could also be used to describe the difference between the sexes.

The brain scan literature is probably the best example of the very weak science but the very strong marketing forces behind the push to medicate children. Compare two publications. If literature on ADHD is requested from the National Institute of Mental Health, they will send a pamphlet entitled *Attention Deficit Hyperactivity Disorder* (NIMH publication No 94-3572). This pamphlet is clearly designed for parents who are considering putting their child on Ritalin. Under the causes of ADHD there is the following statement:

> They are finding more and more evidence that ADHD does not stem from the home environment, but from biological causes. When you think about it there is no clear relationship between home life and ADHD. Not all children from unstable or dysfunctional homes have ADHD.(8)

The ADHD marketing literature is filled with statements like this, but the ADHD professional literature is considerably more equivocating. In 1998, for example, there was a NIMH consensus conference on ADHD. Its final report contained these cautionary statements: "We don't have an independent valid test for ADHD; further research is necessary to firmly establish ADHD as a brain disorder; existing studies come to conflicting conclusions as to whether the use of psychostimulants increases or decreases the risk of abuse; and finally after years of clinical research and experience with ADHD, our knowledge about the cause or causes of ADHD remain largely speculative."(13) How many parents who are considering putting their children on Ritalin have seen this paper? I suspect the answer is close to zero.

Show Me the Evidence

The superficiality of the scientific evidence for ADHD is most obvious in the writings of the ADHD experts themselves. As an example, consider Russell Barkley, who wrote a major review article in *Scientific American* entitled "Attention Deficit Hyperactivity Disorder."(14) One would think that a review article in such a highly regarded popular journal of science would present the most powerful data available, yet Barkley's evidence in support of a biological link to ADHD is minimal. In fact, the author admits: "No one knows the direct and immediate causes of the difficulties experienced by children with ADHD, although advances in neurological imaging techniques and genetics promise to clarify this issue over the next five years." We are still waiting.

Barkley's statement sums up both the science and the philosophy of the ADHD movement, and should be quoted on the front of every NIMH brochure describing ADHD. Here is a bald admission that we do not understand the scientific basis for this so-called disease. It is also interesting that Barkley is one of the biggest proponents of Ritalin. His resolution to this paradox is to speculate that science will catch up with the drug. Peter Breggin, a doctor and author who does not believe in medicating children with Ritalin,(15) has been accused by Barkley of violating the Hippocratic oath.(16) The fact that a leader of the push to medicate children, who admits we do not understand this disease, accuses a skeptical doctor of ethical impropriety says more about the Ritalin movement than Barkley's review article.

In the past 10 years, while scientists have made very little progress in understanding ADHD, their partners down the hall in the marketing department have been extremely successful. The ADHD marketing forces have taken the decision to medicate children out of the ethical arena, and reshaped the decision to medicate based on three flawed beliefs: 1) Diagnosis equals disease; 2) ADHD is due to biology and not the environment; and 3) a disease can be treated with a pill.

1. Does diagnosis equal disease?   Every human trait falls into a range of values. Some people are tall, some are short, some are dark skinned, some are light skinned, some are outgoing, and some are shy. With height, for example, if we measure the general population we see a bell-shaped curve with the very tall and very short at either end of the spectrum. Regardless of a person's height, or what factors cause a person to be tall or short, we do not label the people in the upper 10% as diseased. We recognize these people as merely being at the upper end of normal biological variability. They don't have faulty genes, just different genes.

The ADHD experts have convinced the American public that the description of a personality trait is actually a disease. This is perhaps the biggest flaw and mistake of the ADHD proponents. They do not understand normal human variation. Where do you draw the line on the scale of children's activity level that demarcates normal children from ADHD children? Even the ADHD experts cannot agree. Some estimate that from 3 to 4% of American children have ADHD, while others go as high as 10, 17, or even 20%.(17,18) Since there is no diagnostic test to determine if a child has this condition, such percentages are arbitrary. Dr. Lawrence Diller addresses the problems of diagnosis in a book chapter titled, "Attention Deficit Disorder: In the Eye of the Beholder."(3) Dr. Diller points out that if we adhere to Dr. Joseph Biederman's estimates that 10% of American children have ADHD,(19) and that we take into account that it is four to five times more common in males than females, then approximately one out of every six boys between the ages of five and twelve years old would be diagnosed with ADHD.

The problem is that in one school, family, or doctor's office these children would have a disease but in another school, family, or doctor's office these children would not have a disease. Of all the variables that go into making a diagnosis of ADHD, "science" is the least important. It should strike the skeptical reader as odd that 5–10% of American children have ADHD, whereas in England only 0.03% of their children have the disease.(2) This discrepancy highlights the shortcomings of the science of ADHD.

Even if scientists are successful in developing a diagnostic test that shows 10% of the children in this country have a different biochemical makeup, or different activity levels in the brain, or even a genetic difference, how do we as a society respond to this? Do we say that they have a disease or do we change the environment? ADHD proponents opt for the former and prescribe Ritalin as a treatment.

2. Genes or environment?   In the past decade research on ADHD has leaned toward a possible genetic component. One hears in the media talk of finding "the gene" for ADHD. This is a grand oversimplification of the interplay between genes and the environment, but administering mind-altering drugs to children is easier to rationalize if the pill is nothing more than a way to correct a neurotransmitter deficit caused by faulty genes. In Dr. Alan Zametkin's paper in the *Journal of the American Medical Association,* for example, he states: "Is there a particular gene linked to the disorder?"(20) To even seriously consider that ADHD is due to a single gene goes against everything that science knows about genes and behavior. As Caltech geneticist Seymour Benzer has shown with fruit flies, even a behavior as simple as moving toward a light involves hundreds of genes.(21,22)

A child's brain is enormously more complicated than the brain of a fruit fly, so to postulate that the ability to sit still in a classroom is due to a single gene, or even a small cohort of genes, seems preposterous. If ADHD is genetic then it must have something to do with the Y chromosome because it is much more prevalent in boys than girls.(17) Also, if ADHD is genetically caused, why is it so much more common in this country and why does ADHD vary among states and school districts?(23) In one school district in Virginia, for example, 20% of the children are diagnosed with ADHD.(24) Is this due to an overabundance of ADHD genes in Virginia, or overzealous school psychiatrists?

Despite such speculations, at this point the only way to diagnose ADHD is by examining the relationship of a child to his environment. A physician does not discover ADHD at an annual check up; it is the teacher observing the child in the school environment who makes the initial diagnosis. The parent and child then go to a specialist, but [in] the office the child might even seem normal, so the expert then relies on the testimony of the teachers and parents. They then go through a checklist to determine if medication is appropriate. Given the level of subjective evaluation involved in such a checklist, it is not unusual for parents to walk out of the office with a prescription for Ritalin.

3. From diagnosis to medication   Whether ADHD has a predominantly genetic or environmental cause, intervention through drugs is ethically problematic. Even the proponents of Ritalin, for example, acknowledge that the drug is an easy substitute for good parenting and good schools. Consider the following statement in the *New England Journal of Medicine,* in an article titled "Treatment of Attention Deficit Hyperactivity Disorder" by Dr. Judith Rapoport. "Training and supporting parents and teachers in techniques of contingency reinforcement (e.g., the point-token reward system, 'time out,' and earning or losing privileges) has substantial beneficial effects on disruptive behavior. The value of these strategies is limited because they are labor intensive (and therefore expensive), are effective only at the time they are administered, cannot be generalized to non-targeted behavior or across settings, and are dependent on the compliance and motivation of teachers and parents."(25)

Here Rapoport is acknowledging that the environment matters, that good parenting does have an effect on behavior, and that teachers and parents can improve their teaching and parenting skills. The problem is time, effort, and money. Ritalin is quick, easy, and cheap. But as Rapoport notes: "Behavior management combined with methylphenidate (Ritalin) is substantially more effective than behavior management alone, but usually no more effective than methylphenidate alone. However, behavior management implemented in a highly structured setting may permit the use of a lower dose of methylphenidate." In other words, there is an inverse relationship between a highly structured environment and the dose of Ritalin. Perhaps the national push to reduce class size will also result in a reduction of the number of children on Ritalin.

The difference between good science and bad science does not depend on where the grants came from but funding certainly should be taken into account Dr. Rapoport's article was mentioned in an editorial in the *New England Journal of Medicine* as one of 19 articles that should not have been published because it violated the journal's conflict of interest policy.(37) One of the authors (Elia) of the article received a grant from Celgene, a company that is developing a drug to treat ADHD.

Who Cares About Science?

When you talk to the parents of children taking Ritalin they typically rave about the success of the drug. To put it simply, this stuff works. Who cares about all the scientific arguments concerning etiology, neurochemistry, and the pharmacological mechanisms of treatment? If school performance is enhanced, who cares about science? Of course, since amphetamines were first discovered it has been known that they increase performance.(26,27)

The marketing of Ritalin has made it hard for physicians who do not believe in it to withhold prescriptions. What is a doctor's response to a parent, who says, "My little boy is a monster without his Ritalin. We've tried everything and nothing works. Our lives are in complete disarray. He's about to get kicked out of school. I can't afford private tutors and home schooling. Our family life is in turmoil. But when we put him on Ritalin I'm telling you it is a miracle. He calms down, he does well in school, and our home life is blissful. If you don't believe in Ritalin show me what I can do to replace Ritalin and still have a relatively normal life."

This is a very real cry of anguish and a sympathetic doctor is going to want to assist the family. But, a concerned and knowledgeable doctor also knows that: 1) parents have faced this dilemma for years; 2) a Ritalin Band-Aid would help only in the short run; 3) it would be more appropriate to recommend a family counselor for the long run; 4) in the world of managed care a pill is easier and cheaper; and 5) if the parents don't get a prescription here they will get it someplace else.

The fact that Ritalin is a uniquely American response to this dilemma raises several questions about the direction our society is going. It is very hard for an individual doctor who does not believe in medicating children to go against the grain. What needs to happen is that the American medical community needs to address a tough question: "Are we treating a disease, or are we handing out a performance enhancing pill to put a temporary patch over other problems in our society?" If we are just handing out a temporary patch then let's call it that, and not a "neurobiological deficit." This is especially problematic because we do not know the long-term effects of the drug. In her review article in 1999 Judith Rapoport says, "Important questions regarding the occurrence of tics, drug doses, and the effects of long-term therapy remain unanswered."(25) Again, Rapoport is considered one of the ADHD experts and she said this only [recently].

There is also the dilemma for parents who do not want their children labeled with ADHD, yet are under pressure from the school district to have the children evaluated. No one disagrees that a child on Ritalin is easier to control. This is about the only fact that the ADHD scientists have proved. However, there are other ways to make it easier for teachers to control children, the most obvious being fewer children in the classroom. For instance, Dr. Howard Gardner believes that schools today are too dependent on numbers and words and need to spend more time on the arts, music, and physical education.(28) Multiple intelligences is one answer to the ADHD dilemma: these kids are smart and creative in their own ways and those talents should be exploited, not drugged.

One of the many alternative views to medication is summed up by John Holt: "We consider it a disease because it makes it difficult to run our schools as we do, like maximum security prisons, for the comfort and convenience of the teachers and administrators who work in them. . . . Given the fact that some children are more energetic and active than others, might it not be easier, more healthy, and more humane to deal with this fact by giving them more time and scope to make use of and work off their energy? . . . Everyone is taken care of, except, of course, the child himself, who wears a label which to him reads clearly enough 'freak,' and who is denied from those closest to him, however much sympathy he may get, what he and all children most need—respect, faith, hope, and trust."(29)

Most readers of *Skeptic* are probably familiar with Dr. Dean Edell, who openly shares the fact that he had ADHD as a child. "I had an attention disorder as a kid and consider myself to be a very successful person. It wasn't easy, but when I needed to go back to medical school, I understood that I needed to buckle down and learn the material. Because of my situation, I have led a very creative life and have found it to be very valuable." He continues, "We just can't drug all the kids who won't fit into the mold. Our culture needs people who think and act differently and there is nothing more frightening to me than looking into a classroom in America where every little kid is the same, all paying attention, all doing their homework and marching to the same drummer."(30) What would have happened to the voice of science and reason in medicine if he had been medicated as a child?

If the medical community is not treating a disease but handing out a performance enhancing drug, then, if anything, Ritalin is underprescribed, because the drug will help almost anyone. College students, for example, have discovered that Ritalin will give them extra focus.(31) Can we fault these students when they are seeking to improve their performance, and then turn around and use the performance enhancing aspect of the drug as the major reason for prescribing it? Clearly we have a disconnect between the science of ADHD and the art of behavioral modification with drugs.

Berkeley or Jail?

As we approach the next presidential election, one of the issues facing our country is how to increase the number of children who go into higher education and decrease the number of children in our jails. The Democrats have one agenda and the Republicans have another, but according to Ritalin proponents the cure for society's problems can be found in a pill. ADHD expert Dr. James Swanson summed it up this way: "Treatment can mean the difference between a kid ending up at Berkeley or ending up in prison. This is a disorder where we can really make a difference."(32) Of course, the world would be a better place if more adolescents went to Berkeley instead of prison, but to suggest that the answer to our country's sociological problems is as easy as taking more drugs is simplistic. It shows a lack of understanding, or at least blissful ignorance, of politics, race relations, sociology, ethics, and child development in this country. America has one of the highest incarceration rates on the planet, marginal race relations, a breakdown of the family, problems with schools, and the list goes on and on. Is the answer to our social problems as easy as taking a pill?

While believing that more Ritalin will keep kids out of jail might not show a very good understanding of science and sociology it does show a good understanding of parental vulnerability. Everyone wants the best for their kids, but if there is ever a time for healthy skepticism it is when someone claims that they have a magic pill that is the difference between failure and success.

Disease or Growing Pains?

Since there are no diagnostic tests to determine who has ADHD, the diagnosis is based on observing the child in the classroom. How do doctors tell the difference between normal childhood behavioral growing pains and actual ADHD? From what I have presented thus far it should not surprise you to learn that there is no rigorous scientific basis for ADHD diagnosis. The following case studies are from an educator's in-service training program on ADHD presented in a seminar format to teachers and other educators. The program includes overheads and a pamphlet for the presenter to use for the presentation. The pamphlet is titled, "A Comprehensive Presentation to Inform Educators about Attention Deficit Disorders" and is produced by CHADD (Children and Adults with Attention Deficit Disorder).(33,34) Keep in mind this is a pamphlet that is distributed to teachers all over our country. CHADD is a strong proponent of the view that ADHD is a neurobiological disease.

Case #1   John, a third grade student, is often noncompliant and does not begin tasks when asked. During a two-week observation period he exhibited the following behaviors on a routine basis: John sharpened his pencil three times before sitting down and working. John fell out of his chair when given an assignment with 50 problems. He pretended to be a clown. The class laughed. After leaving his reading group, on the way back to his seat for independent work, John tripped Sally. He was sent to the corner of the room.

Case #2   Sally is a middle school or senior high student who never gets from class A to class B on time. Often, she doesn't have the materials necessary for the next class. Her tardiness interferes with the class routine. Sally often misses class directions because she is busy trying to make up for lost time. The class has already started working while she is looking for yesterday's homework, which she has left in her locker.

In defense of CHADD, these two case studies are presented in conjunction with behavioral management techniques which are actually very appropriate.

Medication is not at first discussed, but it is clear in CHADD's view that these two children have a neurobiological deficit. The overall theme of CHADD's presentation is that these children have a disease, and later in the presentation the wonders of medication are presented: "Medications can have a strong positive effect for a high percentage (70% or more) of children with ADHD."

Is little John a diseased child, or is he the class clown? Is little Sally sick, or is she just at one end of a spectrum of behavioral variability? Do these kids need medication or social structure and intellectual stimuli? Of course, there is in the literature no mention of PET scans, blood work, or any other diagnostic test on John and Sally, just behavioral observations. So what it comes down to is this: should these children be medicated to control their behavior? Since scientific evidence is lacking, this is a practical and ethical question.

More and more physicians and scientists have publicly questioned whether the Ritalin proponents have misused science and overlooked ethics in the marketing of ADHD.(3,15,35) It is time for the bioethical departments of medical schools to participate in this debate. So far, the idea of "normalizing" children with medication has eluded their radar. The pro-Ritalin advocates are considering gene manipulation in the womb for children who fall in the upper 10% of activity levels, yet the bio-ethicists seem more concerned with the ethics of genetically altering tomatoes and fruit flies. They ignore this problem at their peril. We can only hope that the groundswell for a more rational view of childhood will gain ascendancy before the technology of genetically altering John, Sally and 10% of the next generation is available.

The Future for Children With ADHD

It will be interesting to see what happens in the next millennium if we follow the Ritalin movement's philosophy and its view of child development. Continuing the diabetes analogy, currently diabetics need to take a drug, but in the future these patients will probably be treated with gene therapy. By altering diabetics' genetic makeup they will be disease-free and never need to take medication again.

If we believe that ADHD is a disease like diabetes, what will we do with the 5–10% of the children in this country who have been diagnosed with ADHD? If one agrees with the Ritalin proponents, then gene therapy for a large portion of the children in this country would be a viable option. Consider Alan Zametkin's closing remark in his previously mentioned article, in a discussion on the future of ADHD research: "Can pharmacological or gene manipulations lead to a cure?"(20)

Contemplating gene therapy for children by people who cannot agree on how many children have the disease is alarming. Nobel laureate Sir Peter Medawar addresses the question of genetic engineering for humans: "The moral-political answer is that no such regimen of genetic improvement could be practiced within the framework of a society that respects the rights of individuals." He also notes: "It is the great glory as it is also the great threat of science that everything which is in principle possible can be done if the intention to do it is sufficiently resolute. Scientists may exult in the glory, but in the middle of the 20th century the reaction of ordinary people is more often to cower at the threat."(36)

Even if science does show a mechanistic or a biological basis for this variable personality trait, as a society we still face an important value judgement. If our schools are like pegboards designed for round holes, and 10% of the pegs are square, then we have two choices. Either we must change the peg board (the environment), which requires time and money to accommodate more of the pegs. Or, we can chisel away at the 10% of square pegs (children with problems sitting still) so that they fit into the round holes.

In the past several years pro-Ritalin advocates have had nothing but disregard at best, and contempt at worst, for anybody who is skeptical or concerned about the rising use of Ritalin in this country. In 1996 Dr. Lawrence Stone, the head of the American Academy of Child and Adolescent Psychiatry, said, "The media in general tend to take the particular issues of drugs and also ADHD out of the domain of science and clinical judgment where it really belongs." Judith Rapoport stated, "Most of the media coverage on Ritalin has been overblown."(38) Since these statements the use of Ritalin has been documented to exceed most people's fears, or expectations. The *Journal of the American Medical Association (JAMA)* recently confirmed that Ritalin use in this country has skyrocketed (about 12 out of 1,000 preschoolers in one mid-western population).(39) I would expect that the pro-Ritalin advocates would say that this is a step forward. After all, they have been saying for several years that 10% of our children have a neurobiological disease. I think this is a step backward and that our expectations of childhood have become distorted. I also think the majority of Americans, including many scientists, are seeing that in retrospect the media coverage has not been overblown but that the "science" has been overblown. For a drug addict the first step on the road to recovery is to admit to having a drug problem. For our country the first step on the road to recovery would be for the National Institutes of Health to acknowledge the reality of the current situation in this country—we have a drug problem. If we don't face the reality do not be surprised if 10 years from now even more of our children are taking Ritalin.

References

1.   DEA. 1995. "Methylphenidate (A background paper)." Drug and Chemical Evaluation Section, Office of Diversion Control: Washington D.C.

2. UN. 1995. *Report of the United Nations International Narcotics Control Board.* New York: UN Publications.

3. Diller, L.H. 1998. *Running on Ritalin.* New York Bantam.

4. Pam, A. 1995. "Biological Psychiatry Science or Pseudoscience?" in *Pseudoscience in Biological Psychiatry* (CA. Ross, and Pam, A., Eds.) New York: John Wiley, 7–35.

5. Garber, S.G., M.D. 1996. *Beyond Ritalin.* New York Harper Collins.

6. Andreasen, N.C. 1984. *The Broken Brain.* New York: Harper and Row.

7. Valenstein, E.S. 1998. *Blaming the Brain.* New York: Simon and Schuster Inc.

8. NIMH. 1994. *Attention Deficit Hyperactivity Disorder.* Washington DC: US Government Printing Office. 1–42.

9. Zametkin, A.J., Nordahl, T.E., Gross, M., King, A.C., Semple, W.E., Rumsey, J., Hamburger, M.S., and Cohen, R.M. 1990. "Cerebral Glucose Metabolism in Adults with Hyperactivity of Childhood Onset." *The New England Journal of Medicine,* 323(20): 1361–1367.

10. Ernst, M., and Zametkin, A. 1995. "The Interface of Genetics, Neuroimaging, and Neurochemistry in Attention-Deficit Disorder," in *Psychopharmacology* (F.E. Bloom, and Kupfer, D.J., Eds.) Raven Press, 1643–1652.

11. Reid, R.T., Maag, J.W, and Vasa, S.F. 1993. "Attention Deficit Hyperactivity Disorder as a Disability Category: A Critique." *Exceptional Children,* 60(3): 198–214.

12. Zametkin, A.J., Liebenauer, L.L., Fitzgerald, G.A., King, A.C., Minkunas, D.V., Herscovith, P., Yamada, E.M., and Cohen, R.M. 1993. "Brain Metabolism in Teenagers with Attention Deficit Hyperactivity Disorder." *Arch Psychiatry,* 50: 333–340.

13. NIH. 1998. "Diagnosis and Treatment of Attention Deficit Hyperactivity Disorder," in Consensus Development Conference.

14. Barkley, R.A. 1998. "Attention Deficit Hyperactivity Disorder." *Scientific American,* September.

15. Breggin, P. 1998. *Talking Back to Ritalin.* Maine: Common Courage Press.

16. Barkley, R. 1999. *ADHD, Ritalin, and Conspiracies: Talking Back to Peter Breggin,* CHADD.

17. Cantwell, D.P. 1996. "Attention Deficit Disorder: A Review of the Past 10 Years." *Journal of American Academy of Child and Adolescent Psychiatry,* 358: 978–987.

18. Goldman, L.S. 1998. "Diagnosis and Treatment of Attention Deficit/Hyperactivity Disorder in Children and Adolescents." *Journal of the American Medical Association,* 279: 1100–1107.

19. Biederman, J. 1996. "Are Stimulants Overprescribed for Children with Behavioral Problems?" *Pediatric News,* August: 26.

20. Zametkin, A.J. 1995. "Attention-Deficit Disorder: Born to be Hyperactive." *Journal of the American Medical Association,* 273(23): 1871–1874.

21. Benzer, S. 1991. *Development of the Visual System.* Cambridge: MIT Press.

22. Weiner, J. 1999. "Lord of the Flies: What One of the Century's Great Unsung Scientists Has Discovered about Bugs, Genes, and Us." *The New Yorker,* April: 44–51.

23. Spanos, B. 1996. *Conference Report: Stimulant Use in the Treatment of ADHD.* Washington DC: Drug Enforcement Administration.

24. LeFever, G.B., Dawson, K.V., and Morrow, A.L. 1999. "The Extent of Drug Therapy for Attention Deficit-Hyperactivity Disorder Among Children in Public Schools." *American Journal of Public Health,* 89: 1359–1364.

25. Elia, J., Ambrosini, P.J., and Rapoport, J.L. 1999. "Treatment of Attention-Deficit Hyperactivity Disorder." *New England Journal of Medicine,* 340(10): 780–788.

26. Hughes, A.L. 1944. "Epidemiology of Amphetamine Use in the United States," in *Amphetamine and Its Analogs: Psychopharmacology, Toxicology; and Its Abuse* (A.K. Cho and Segal, D.S., Eds.) San Diego: Academic Press, 439–57.

27. Weiss, B. and G. Laties. 1962. "The Enhancement of Human Performance by Caffeine and the Amphetamines." *Pharmacological Review,* 1962. 14: 1–36.

28. Gardner, H. 1993. *Multiple Intelligences.* New York Basic Books.

29.   Holt, J. 1970. "Federal Involvement in the Use of Behavior Modification Drugs on Grammar School Children." In Committee on Government Operations of the US House of Representatives.

30.   Edell, D. 1999. Radio show. Healthcentral.com.

31.   Tennant, C. 1999. *The Ritalin Racket.* Student.com.correspondent

32.   AP. 1998. "Studies Show Why Ritalin Helps Children with Attention Deficit Disorder." Healthcentral.com.

33.   CHADD. 1993. The Educator's Inservice Program on Attention Deficit Disorders, Version 2.

34.   Fowler, M. 1992. *Attention Deficit Disorders.* Virginia: Caset Associates.

35.   Degrandpre, R. 1999. *Ritalin Nation.* New York: W.W. Norton.

36.   Medawar, P. 1991. *The Threat and the Glory.* Oxford: Oxford University Press.

37.   Angell, M., Utiger, R.D., and Wood, A.J., Disclosure of Author's Conflict of Interest: A Follow Up. *New England Journal of Medicine,* 2000. 342(8).

38.   Ginther, C., Is There a Ritalin Controversy? *Psychiatric Times,* 1996. 13(7).

39.   Zito, J., M., Safer, D.J., dosReis, S., Gardner, J.F., Boles, M., and Lynch, F., 2000. "Trends in Prescribing of Psychotropic Medications to Preschoolers." *Journal of the American Medical Association,* 283(8).

NO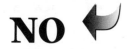

Michael Fumento

Trick Question

It's both right-wing and vast, but it's not a conspiracy. Actually, it's more of an anti-conspiracy. The subject is Attention Deficit Disorder (ADD) and Attention Deficit Hyperactivity Disorder (ADHD), closely related ailments (henceforth referred to in this article simply as ADHD). Rush Limbaugh declares it "may all be a hoax." Francis Fukuyama devotes much of one chapter in his latest book, *Our Posthuman Future,* to attacking Ritalin, the top-selling drug used to treat ADHD. Columnist Thomas Sowell writes, "The motto used to be: 'Boys will be boys.' Today, the motto seems to be: 'Boys will be medicated.'" And Phyllis Schlafly explains, "The old excuse of 'my dog ate my homework' has been replaced by 'I got an ADHD diagnosis.'" A March 2002 article in *The Weekly Standard* summed up the conservative line on ADHD with this rhetorical question: "Are we really prepared to redefine childhood as an ailment, and medicate it until it goes away?"

Many conservative writers, myself included, have criticized the growing tendency to pathologize every undesirable behavior—especially where children are concerned. But, when it comes to ADHD, this skepticism is misplaced. As even a cursory examination of the existing literature or, for that matter, simply talking to the parents and teachers of children with ADHD reveals, the condition is real, and it is treatable. And, if you don't believe me, you can ask conservatives who've come face to face with it themselves.

Myth: ADHD Isn't a Real Disorder

The most common argument against ADHD on the right is also the simplest: It doesn't exist. Conservative columnist Jonah Goldberg thus reduces ADHD to "ants in the pants." Sowell equates it with "being bored and restless." Fukuyama protests, "No one has been able to identify a cause of ADD/ADHD. It is a pathology recognized only by its symptoms." And a conservative columnist approvingly quotes Thomas Armstrong, Ritalin opponent and author, when he declares, "ADD is a disorder that cannot be authoritatively identified in the same way as polio, heart disease or other legitimate illnesses."

From Michael Fumento, "Trick Question," *The New Republic,* vol. 228, no. 4 (February 3, 2003). Copyright © 2003 by The New Republic, LLC. Reprinted by permission.

The Armstrong and Fukuyama observations are as correct as they are worthless. "Half of all medical disorders are diagnosed without benefit of a lab procedure," notes Dr. Russell Barkley, professor of psychology at the College of Health Professionals at the Medical University of South Carolina. "Where are the lab tests for headaches and multiple sclerosis and Alzheimer's?" he asks. "Such a standard would virtually eliminate all mental disorders."

Often the best diagnostic test for an ailment is how it responds to treatment. And, by that standard, it doesn't get much more real than ADHD. The beneficial effects of administering stimulants to treat the disorder were first reported in 1937. And today medication for the disorder is reported to be 75 to 90 percent successful. "In our trials it was close to ninety percent," says Dr. Judith Rapoport, director of the National Institute of Mental Health's Child Psychiatry Branch, who has published about 100 papers on ADHD. "This means there was a significant difference in the children's ability to function in the classroom or at home."

Additionally, epidemiological evidence indicates that ADHD has a powerful genetic component. University of Colorado researchers have found that a child whose identical twin has the disorder is between eleven and 18 times more likely to also have it than is a non-twin sibling. For these reasons, the American Psychiatric Association (APA), American Medical Association, American Academy of Pediatrics, American Academy of Child Adolescent Psychiatry, the surgeon general's office, and other major medical bodies all acknowledge ADHD as both real and treatable.

Myth: ADHD Is Part of a Feminist Conspiracy to Make Little Boys More Like Little Girls

Many conservatives observe that boys receive ADHD diagnoses in much higher numbers than girls and find in this evidence of a feminist conspiracy. (This, despite the fact that genetic diseases are often heavily weighted more toward one gender or the other.) Sowell refers to "a growing tendency to treat boyhood as a pathological condition that requires a new three R's—repression, re-education and Ritalin." Fukuyama claims Prozac is being used to give women "more of the alpha-male feeling," while Ritalin is making boys act more like girls. "Together, the two sexes are gently nudged toward that androgynous median personality . . . that is the current politically correct outcome in American society." George Will, while acknowledging that Ritalin can be helpful, nonetheless writes of the "androgyny agenda" of "drugging children because they are behaving like children, especially boy children." Anti-Ritalin conservatives frequently invoke Christina Hoff Sommers's best-selling 2000 book, *The War Against Boys*. You'd never know that the drug isn't mentioned in her book—or why.

"Originally I was going to have a chapter on it," Sommers tells me. "It seemed to fit the thesis." What stopped her was both her survey of the medical literature and her own empirical findings. Of one child she personally came to know she says, "He was utterly miserable, as was everybody around him. The drugs saved his life."

Myth: ADHD Is Part of the Public School System's Efforts to Warehouse Kids Rather Than to Discipline and Teach Them

"No doubt life is easier for teachers when everyone sits around quietly," writes Sowell. Use of ADHD drugs is "in the school's interest to deal with behavioral and discipline problems [because] it's so easy to use Ritalin to make kids compliant: to get them to sit down, shut up, and do what they're told," declares Schlafly. The word "zombies" to describe children under the effects of Ritalin is tossed around more than in a B-grade voodoo movie.

Kerri Houston, national field director for the American Conservative Union and the mother of two ADHD children on medication, agrees with much of the criticism of public schools. "But don't blame ADHD on crummy curricula and lazy teachers," she says. "If you've worked with these children, you know they have a serious neurological problem." In any case, Ritalin, when taken as prescribed, hardly stupefies children. To the extent the medicine works, it simply turns ADHD children into normal children. "ADHD is like having thirty televisions on at one time, and the medicine turns off twenty-nine so you can concentrate on the one," Houston describes. "This zombie stuff drives me nuts! My kids are both as lively and as fun as can be."

Myth: Parents Who Give Their Kids Anti-ADHD Drugs Are Merely Doping Up Problem Children

Limbaugh calls ADHD "the perfect way to explain the inattention, incompetence, and inability of adults to control their kids." Addressing parents directly, he lectures, "It helped you mask your own failings by doping up your children to calm them down."

Such charges blast the parents of ADHD kids into high orbit. That includes my Hudson Institute colleague (and fellow conservative) Mona Charen, the mother of an eleven-year-old with the disorder. "I have two non-ADHD children, so it's not a matter of parenting technique," says Charen. "People without such children have no idea what it's like. I can tell the difference between boyish high spirits and pathological hyperactivity. . . . These kids bounce off the walls. Their lives are chaos; their rooms are chaos. And nothing replaces the drugs."

Barkley and Rapoport say research backs her up. Randomized, controlled studies in both the United States and Sweden have tried combining medication with behavioral interventions and then dropped either one or the other. For those trying to go on without medicine, "the behavioral interventions maintained nothing," Barkley says. Rapoport concurs: "Unfortunately, behavior modification doesn't seem to help with ADHD." (Both doctors are quick to add that ADHD is often accompanied by other disorders that are treatable through behavior modification in tandem with medicine.)

Myth: Ritalin Is "Kiddie Cocaine"

One of the paradoxes of conservative attacks on Ritalin is that the drug is alternately accused of turning children into brain-dead zombies and of making them Mach-speed cocaine junkies. Indeed, Ritalin is widely disparaged as "kiddie cocaine." Writers who have sought to lump the two drugs together include Schlafly, talk-show host and columnist Armstrong Williams, and others whom I hesitate to name because of my long-standing personal relationships with them.

Mary Eberstadt wrote the "authoritative" Ritalin-cocaine piece for the April 1999 issue of *Policy Review,* then owned by the Heritage Foundation. The article, "Why Ritalin Rules," employs the word "cocaine" no fewer than twelve times. Eberstadt quotes from a 1995 Drug Enforcement Agency (DEA) background paper declaring methylphenidate, the active ingredient in Ritalin, "a central nervous system (CNS) stimulant [that] shares many of the pharmacological effects of amphetamine, methamphetamine, and cocaine." Further, it "produces behavioral, psychological, subjective, and reinforcing effects similar to those of d-amphetamine including increases in rating of euphoria, drug liking and activity, and decreases in sedation." Add to this the fact that the Controlled Substances Act lists it as a Schedule II drug, imposing on it the same tight prescription controls as morphine, and Ritalin starts to sound spooky indeed.

What Eberstadt fails to tell readers is that the DEA description concerns methylphenidate *abuse.* It's tautological to say abuse is harmful. According to the DEA, the drugs in question are comparable when "administered the same way at comparable doses." But ADHD stimulants, when taken as prescribed, are neither administered in the same way as cocaine nor at comparable doses. "What really counts," says Barkley, "is the speed with which the drugs enter and clear the brain. With cocaine, because it's snorted, this happens tremendously quickly, giving users the characteristic addictive high." (Ever seen anyone pop a cocaine tablet?) Further, he says, "There's no evidence anywhere in literature of [Ritalin's] addictiveness when taken as prescribed." As to the Schedule II listing, again this is because of the potential for it to fall into the hands of abusers, not because of its effects on persons for whom it is prescribed. Ritalin and the other anti-ADHD drugs, says Barkley, "are the safest drugs in all of psychiatry." (And they may be getting even safer: A new medicine just released called Strattera represents the first true non-stimulant ADHD treatment.)

Indeed, a study just released in the journal *Pediatrics* found that children who take Ritalin or other stimulants to control ADHD cut their risk of future substance abuse by 50 percent compared with untreated ADHD children. The lead author speculated that "by treating ADHD you're reducing the demoralization that accompanies this disorder, and you're improving the academic functioning and well-being of adolescents and young adults during the critical times when substance abuse starts."

Myth: Ritalin Is Overprescribed Across the Country

Some call it "the Ritalin craze." In *The Weekly Standard,* Melana Zyla Vickers informs us that "Ritalin use has exploded," while Eberstadt writes that "Ritalin use more than doubled in the first half of the decade alone, [and] the number of schoolchildren taking the drug may now, by some estimates, be approaching the *4 million mark.*"

A report in the January 2003 issue of *Archives of Pediatrics and Adolescent Medicine* did find a large increase in the use of ADHD medicines from 1987 to 1996, an increase that doesn't appear to be slowing. Yet nobody thinks it's a problem that routine screening for high blood pressure has produced a big increase in the use of hypertension medicine. "Today, children suffering from ADHD are simply less likely to slip through the cracks," says Dr. Sally Satel, a psychiatrist, AEI fellow, and author of *PC, M.D.: How Political Correctness Is Corrupting Medicine.*

Satel agrees that some community studies, by the standards laid down in the APA's *Diagnostic and Statistical Manual of Mental Disorders (DSM),* indicate that ADHD may often be over-diagnosed. On the other hand, she says, additional evidence shows that in some communities ADHD is *under*-diagnosed and *under*-treated. "I'm quite concerned with children who need the medication and aren't getting it," she says.

There *are* tremendous disparities in the percentage of children taking ADHD drugs when comparing small geographical areas. Psychologist Gretchen LeFever, for example, has compared the number of prescriptions in mostly white Virginia Beach, Virginia, with other, more heavily African American areas in the southeastern part of the state. Conservatives have latched onto her higher numbers—20 percent of white fifth-grade boys in Virginia Beach are being treated for ADHD—as evidence that something is horribly wrong. But others, such as Barkley, worry about the lower numbers. According to LeFever's study, black children are only half as likely to get medication as white children. "Black people don't get the care of white people; children of well-off parents get far better care than those of poorer parents," says Barkley.

Myth: States Should Pass Laws That Restrict Schools From Recommending Ritalin

Conservative writers have expressed delight that several states, led by Connecticut, have passed or are considering laws ostensibly protecting students from schools that allegedly pass out Ritalin like candy. Representative Lenny Winkler, lead sponsor of the Connecticut measure, told *Reuters Health,* "If the diagnosis is made, and it's an appropriate diagnosis that Ritalin be used, that's fine. But I have also heard of many families approached by the school system [who are told] that their child cannot attend school if they're not put on Ritalin."

Two attorneys I interviewed who specialize in child-disability issues, including one from the liberal Bazelon Center for Mental Health Law in Washington, D.C., acknowledge that school personnel have in some cases stepped over the line. But legislation can go too far in the other direction by declaring, as Connecticut's law does, that "any school personnel [shall be prohibited] from recommending the use of psychotropic drugs for any child." The law appears to offer an exemption by declaring, "The provisions of this section shall not prohibit *school medical staff* from recommending that a child be evaluated by an appropriate medical practitioner, or prohibit school personnel from consulting with such practitioner, with the consent of the parent or guardian of such child." [Emphasis added.] But of course many, if not most, schools have perhaps one nurse on regular "staff." That nurse will have limited contact with children in the classroom situations where ADHD is likely to be most evident. And, given the wording of the statute, a teacher who believed a student was suffering from ADHD would arguably be prohibited from referring that student to the nurse. Such ambiguity is sure to have a chilling effect on any form of intervention or recommendation by school personnel. Moreover, 20-year special-education veteran Sandra Rief said in an interview with the National Education Association that "recommending medical intervention for a student's behavior could lead to personal liability issues." Teachers, in other words, could be forced to choose between what they think is best for the health of their students and the possible risk of losing not only their jobs but their personal assets as well.

"Certainly it's not within the purview of a school to say kids can't attend if they don't take drugs," says Houston. "On the other hand, certainly teachers should be able to advise parents as to problems and potential solutions. . . . [T]hey may see things parents don't. My own son is an angel at home but was a demon at school."

If the real worry is "take the medicine or take a hike" ultimatums, legislation can be narrowly tailored to prevent them; broad-based gag orders, such as Connecticut's, are a solution that's worse than the problem.

The Conservative Case for ADHD Drugs

There are kernels of truth to every conservative suspicion about ADHD. Who among us has not had lapses of attention? And isn't hyperactivity a normal condition of childhood when compared with deskbound adults? Certainly there *are* lazy teachers, warehousing schools, androgyny-pushing feminists, and far too many parents unwilling or unable to expend the time and effort to raise their children properly, even by their own standards. Where conservatives go wrong is in making ADHD a scapegoat for frustration over what we perceive as a breakdown in the order of society and family. In a column in *The Boston Herald*, Boston University Chancellor John Silber rails that Ritalin is "a classic example of a cheap fix: low-cost, simple and purely superficial."

Exactly. Like most headaches, ADHD is a neurological problem that can usually be successfully treated with a chemical. Those who recommend or prescribe ADHD medicines do not, as *The Weekly Standard* put it, see them as "discipline in pill-form." They see them as pills.

In fact, it can be argued that the use of those pills, far from being liable for or symptomatic of the Decline of the West, reflects and reinforces conservative values. For one thing, they increase personal responsibility by removing an excuse that children (and their parents) can fall back on to explain misbehavior and poor performance. "Too many psychologists and psychiatrists focus on allowing patients to justify to themselves their troubling behavior," says Satel. "But something like Ritalin actually encourages greater autonomy because you're treating a compulsion to behave in a certain way. Also, by treating ADHD, you remove an opportunity to explain away bad behavior."

Moreover, unlike liberals, who tend to downplay differences between the sexes, conservatives are inclined to believe that there are substantial physiological differences—differences such as boys' greater tendency to suffer ADHD. "Conservatives celebrate the physiological differences between boys and girls and eschew the radical-feminist notion that gender differences are created by societal pressures," says Houston regarding the fuss over the boy-girl disparity among ADHD diagnoses. "ADHD is no exception."

But, however compatible conservatism may be with taking ADHD seriously, the truth is that most conservatives remain skeptics. "I'm sure I would have been one of those smug conservatives saying it's a made-up disease," admits Charen, "if I hadn't found out the hard way." Here's hoping other conservatives find an easier route to accepting the truth.

POSTSCRIPT

Are Too Many Children Receiving Ritalin?

To satisfy their own emotional needs, many parents push their physicians into diagnosing their children with ADHD. These parents believe that their children will benefit if they are labeled ADHD. The pressure for children to do well academically in order to get into the right college and graduate school is intense. Some parents feel that if their children are diagnosed with ADHD, then they may be provided special circumstances or allowances such as additional time when taking college entrance examinations. Some parents also realize that if their children are identified as having ADHD, then their children will be eligible for extra services in school. In some instances, the only way to receive such extra help is to be labeled with a disorder. Also, some teachers favor the use of Ritalin to control students' behavior. During the last few years, there has been increasing emphasis on controlling school budgets. The result has been larger class sizes and higher student-to-teacher ratios. Thus, it should not be surprising that many teachers welcome the calming effect of Ritalin on students whose hyperactivity is disruptive to the class.

Whether or not drug therapy should be applied to behaviors raises another concern. What is the message that children are receiving about the role of drugs in society? Perhaps children will generalize the benefits of using legal drugs like Ritalin to remedy life's problems to using illegal drugs to deal with other problems that they may be experiencing. Children may find that it is easier to ingest a pill rather than to put the time and effort into resolving personal problems.

When to prescribe Ritalin for children also places physicians in a quandary. They may see the benefit of helping students function more effectively in school. However, are physicians who readily prescribe Ritalin unintentionally promoting an antihumanistic, competitive environment in which performance matters regardless of the cost? On the other hand, is it the place of physicians to dictate to parents what is best for their children? In the final analysis, will the increase in prescriptions for Ritalin result in benefits for the child, for the parents, and for society?

Two articles that question the validity of ADHD are "Problems in Diagnosing and Treating ADD/ADHD," by Richard E. Vatz and Lee S. Weinberg, *USA Today* (March 2001) and John Breeding's "Does ADHD Even Exist?" *Mothering* (July/August 2000). An article that examines the role of Ritalin is "Ritalin—Better Living Through Chemistry?" by Leonard Sax, *The World & I* (November 2000). An article that addresses concerns of parents and teachers is "What Teachers and Parents Should Know About Ritalin," by Christina Pancheri and Mary Anne Prater, *Teaching Exceptional Children* (March/April 1999).

ISSUE 13

Do Consumers Benefit When Prescription Drugs Are Advertised?

YES: Merrill Matthews, Jr., from "Advertising Drugs Is Good for Patients," *Consumers' Research Magazine* (August 2001)

NO: Anne B. Brown, from "The Direct-to-Consumer Advertising Dilemma," *Patient Care* (March 30, 2001)

ISSUE SUMMARY

YES: Merrill Matthews, Jr., a health policy adviser with the American Legislative Exchange Council, argues that the advertising of prescription drugs directly to consumers will result in better-informed consumers. He contends that concerns that the cost of prescription drugs will rise due to the cost of advertising are unfounded; instead, advertising creates competition among drug manufacturers, resulting in lower costs. Additionally, communication between doctors and patients may improve because advertising increases patients' knowledge about drugs.

NO: Writer Anne B. Brown asserts that drug advertising has resulted in an increase in the number of visits by patients to their physicians. She also contends that a patient may lose trust in his or her physician if the physician's advice contradicts information in drug advertisements. Brown also expresses concern that many consumers may not have the clinical or pharmacological background to adequately comprehend information in drug advertisements.

One of the most lucrative businesses in the world today is the prescription drug business. Billions of dollars are spent every year for prescription drugs in the United States alone. But the *only* way for consumers to obtain a prescribed drug is through a physician. In the early 1980s drug companies in the United States began to advertise directly to the consumer. It is logical for drug companies to advertise to physicians because they are responsible for writing prescriptions. However, is it logical for pharmaceutical manufacturers to advertise their drugs directly to consumers? Are consumers capable of making informed, rational decisions regarding their pharmaceutical needs? Do consumers derive any benefits when prescription drugs are advertised to them directly?

An increasing number of individuals are assuming more responsibility for their own health care. In the United States, over one-third of all prescriptions are written at the request of patients. Also, many patients do not take their doctors' prescriptions to pharmacies to be filled. Both of these scenarios raise the question of whether or not consumers are adequately educated to make decisions pertaining to their pharmaceutical needs or to assess risks associated with prescription drugs. Evidence suggests that many are not. Prescription drugs, for example, cause more worksite accidents than illegal drugs do. Some commentators, however, argue that there are several advantages to directly advertising drugs to consumers. One advantage is that direct advertisements make consumers better informed about the benefits and risks of certain drugs. For example, it is not unusual for a person to experience side effects from a drug without knowing that the drug is responsible for the side effects. Advertisements can provide this information. Another advantage is that consumers can learn about medications that they might not have known existed. Furthermore, advertising lowers the cost of prescription drugs because consumers are able to ask their physicians to prescribe less expensive drugs than the physician might be inclined to recommend. Finally, prescription drug advertising allows consumers to become more involved in choosing the medications that they need or want.

Critics argue that there are a number of risks associated with the direct advertising of prescription drugs. One concern is with the content of drug advertisements. For example, consumers may not pay enough attention to information detailing a drug's adverse effects. Also, sometimes a drug's benefits are exaggerated. Another problem is that there are many instances in which drugs that have been approved by the Food and Drug Administration (FDA) for one purpose have been promoted for other purposes. Is the average consumer capable of understanding the purposes of the drugs that are being advertised?

Opponents of direct-to-consumer drug advertisements express concern over the way in which the information in advertisements is presented. Promotions for drugs that appear as objective reports are often actually slick publicity material. In such promotions, medical experts are shown providing testimony regarding a particular drug. Many consumers may not be aware that these physicians have financial ties to the pharmaceutical companies. Celebrities—in whom the public often places its trust despite their lack of medical expertise—are also used to promote drugs. Finally, the cost of the drugs advertised, a major concern to most consumers, is seldom mentioned in the advertisements.

In the following selections, Merrill Matthews, Jr., argues that the marketing of prescription drugs helps consumers because they lower the cost of drugs and effectively inform consumers about the benefits of new drugs. Anne B. Brown maintains that consumers do not gain from prescription drug advertising because many people lack clinical and pharmacological expertise. As a result, some patients spend more money because they schedule more visits with their physicians in order to acquire the advertised drugs.

Merrill Matthews, Jr.

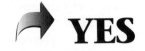 **YES**

Advertising Drugs Is Good for Patients

Many health policy experts believe that direct-to-consumer (DTC) advertising by pharmaceutical companies misinforms gullible consumers, encourages drug overconsumption, increases health care costs, strains doctor-patient relationships and undermines the quality of patient care. For example:

- The American College of Physicians and the American Society of Internal Medicine, in a joint policy statement, wrote: "We are concerned that advertising will result in increased consumption of these highly advertised drugs; though their use may be neither appropriate nor necessary." The organizations also wrote: "Many times, physicians will give in to the demand and when they don't, often patients will 'doctor shop' until they find a physician who will prescribe the medication."

- Sen. Tim Johnson (D-S.D.) also questioned the growth of DTC. "Is the information value worth the yearly increases in drug costs that advertising inevitably causes? Are patients getting the best individual choices of medicines or just the best advertised ones? Are generic drugs, often an excellent cost-effective alternative, getting equal consideration?"

- Finally, members of the Committee on Bioethical Issues of the Medical Society of the State of New York wrote: "Direct drug advertising provides no real benefit to patients, is potentially harmful, and is costly. We therefore urge the U.S. Food and Drug Administration to review and strengthen its policies concerning this practice."

Are these criticisms accurate? In some cases, yes. For example, DTC advertising does encourage more drug consumption—which can lower some health care costs when drug therapy precludes the need for other, more expensive therapies.

However, the above-mentioned concerns largely are misdirected. They focus on the evolving pharmaceutical marketplace when in fact the whole health care system is in transition. And direct-to-consumer pharmaceutical ads are a response to the transitional process, not the cause of it.

From Merrill Matthews, Jr., "Advertising Drugs Is Good for Patients," *Consumers' Research Magazine*, vol. 84, no. 8 (August 2001). Copyright © 2001 by The Institute for Policy Innovation. Reprinted by permission.

The U.S. health care system has reached a cross-roads, and the direction the country takes will determine the type, availability and quality of care for years to come. Pharmaceutical advertising pre-supposes that health care consumers can make choices for themselves—and that's the type of health care system people want. Those who have no choice in health care have no need of advertising.

A health care system in transition   America is in the forefront of the information economy. One of the hallmarks of this new economy is access to much more information by many more people. Patients have much greater access to health care information, especially through the Internet and through advertising. Indeed, the most important change occurring in the health care system is this access to information. According to health care consultant Lyn Siegel:

- About 25% of on-line information is related to health;
- More than 50% of adults who go on the Web use it for health care information; and
- More than 26% of people who go to disease-oriented Web sites ask their doctors for a specific brand of medication. Thus information is driving the transition to a patient-directed health care system.

A generation ago physicians were the possessors of all medical information. Patients went to physicians and accepted evaluations and diagnoses almost without question. Patients who want second opinions and physicians who gracefully accede to their wishes are relatively new phenomena.

In a physician-directed health care system:

- Physicians have all the extant medical knowledge and skills;
- Physicians perform all patient examinations;
- Patients accept their physicians' diagnoses and insurers pay for the care;
- Hospitals admit patients based on physicians' orders and pharmacists fill the prescriptions; and,
- Drug and medical device companies market to the physicians who control all access to patients.

In this model, no one reaches patients without a physician's consent. The physician-directed system worked well for several decades. The vast majority of working Americans had good health insurance benefits that protected them, their families and their assets from catastrophic losses due to a major accident or illness. Third-party payers were generous in their reimbursement policies while doctors and hospitals could do only so much. Whatever doctors recommended, insurers covered.

Once the amazing medical advances of the 1970s and 1980s began to appear, health care costs began to soar. Insured workers and seniors on Medicare were insulated from the cost of care, and so had little incentive to control health care spending. Employers and the government, who paid most health care bills, desperately sought cost-control mechanisms. That's when managed care came in. Its proponents claimed that managed care could lower the cost of comprehensive health care coverage, in part by controlling utilization. While the arguments continue over how well managed care controlled costs and whether it sacrificed quality to achieve savings, the growth in health care spending did slow during the 1990s. Recently, though, the rate of growth has escalated and engendered fears of more double-digit increases in health care spending.

Meanwhile, the expansion of managed care helped to undermine the physician-directed health care system. Insurers and employers gained the power to question and even override doctors' decisions, which put doctors in an uncomfortable and unsatisfactory position.

Patients also reacted negatively. Many believed their doctors were willing or able to give them only the level of care their insurers would cover. This distrust undermined the doctor-patient relationship and spurred patients to seek health care information directly, rather than from their doctor or insurer. Thus health care consumers began to exploit the information economy.

Increasingly, patients are entering the health care system armed with information—and sometimes misinformation. They may not know how to practice medicine, but many know something about their medical condition and the options available to them. And they raise questions if the doctor follows a different path from the one they expect.

As Dr. Thomas R. Reardon, past president of the American Medical Association, has insightfully noted: "Patients themselves are also creating a strong impetus for change. Disillusioned by restrictions on coverage and care, they are increasingly demanding choice of physician, hospital, and even type of health plan. More than ever, patients see physicians as the essential point of trust in a changing system, and demand choice and stability in their vital relationships with their doctors. . . . At the same time, patients themselves are becoming better educated, not only about insurance options but also about medical treatments. Today, thanks to the Internet, trends in product advertising, and the massive proliferation of medical information, patients are better equipped to take part in their care than ever before. Rather than simplifying the physician's job, however, this increased patient knowledge base is creating new challenges."

We are transitioning toward a patient-directed health care system—if the federal and state governments don't intervene—in which all of the components cater to the patient, rather than the physician. It is impossible to overstate the magnitude of the change. We aren't there yet, but the system is moving—or being pulled—in that direction.

In the new system, insurers and employers, doctors and other health care providers, researchers and pharmaceutical companies will view the patient rather than the provider as the primary consumer. And in the new system:

- Insurers will have to create products that consumers rather than their employers want;
- Doctors will have to please their patients rather than insurers, reinvigorating the weakened doctor-patient relationship; and

- Pharmaceutical and medical device companies increasingly will market directly to the consumers who use their products.

Because health care consumers are becoming better informed, they will, on balance, make better decisions. And they will want even more information. But how do companies and providers reach individuals with the information the latter want and need? One way is through advertising.

Every Sunday newspaper is filled with advertising flyers for department stores, office products, computers, cars, food and clothing. Yet people don't complain they can't afford food because all the grocery stores advertise. And does anyone really think they would be able to get a computer for less money if none of the computer manufacturers and retail outlets advertised?

In virtually every sector of the economy, those with products or services to sell must get information to those who will buy. Advertising is the vehicle for getting information to the intended customers. It tells prospective customers about product availability, quality and cost—the information those prospects need in order to make comparisons. While some people may consider it annoying if they are not looking for a particular product, those in the market for the advertised item often will pay close attention to ads and other marketing techniques such as direct mail and communication from sales representatives.

The general assumption is that advertising raises the costs of products. This assumption recently has entered the debate over the impact of drug companies' advertisements aimed at consumers. But advertising can—and should—lower costs. For example, according to economist John Calfee of the American Enterprise Institute:

> A pioneering study compared the prices of eye-glasses in states that either permitted or restricted advertising for eyeglass services. Prices were about 25% higher where advertising was restricted or banned (and prices were highest for the least educated consumers). A later study by the Federal Trade Commission (FTC) staff showed that product quality in the states without advertising was not higher despite the higher prices. Studies also found higher prices in the absence of advertising for such diverse products as gasoline, prescription drugs and legal services.

How is it that advertising can actually lower prices? Most products have certain fixed costs, plus some variable costs. While variable costs are imputed to each item produced, fixed costs are divided by the number of products sold. The goal of advertising is to expand consumer awareness and increase sales. The more items sold, the greater the economies of scale and the lower the fixed costs per consumer.

Holman Jenkins of the Wall Street Journal explains the rationale: "The media also complain about advertising as if this were an extra cost borne by drug users. Drug companies spend on advertising because it's profitable—it pays for itself by generating additional sales, allowing development costs to be spread over a larger number of users. The average price to each user is lower."

In the absence of competition, advertising might raise prices. But in the absence of competition, vendors would likely raise prices whether they advertised or not. Competition keeps manufacturers from charging as much as they would like, except in cases where there is an unusually high demand for a particular product (as when everyone decides they want a Cabbage Patch doll, a Tickle Me Elmo or a Furby for Christmas). Thus, even when advertising doesn't increase sales, vendors cannot add the cost on top of the product if there are other competitively priced alternatives on the market.

DTC ads and the health care system   Putting information in the hands of consumers who didn't have that information before is a revolutionary business—and revolutions engender change. Critics know this and raise concerns that DTC advertising will increase health care spending, strain doctor-patient relationships and confuse consumers and patients. Worst of all, they believe going directly to the consumer is only a drug company technique to increase prices and therefore profits. Are any of these concerns valid?

Will DTC advertising increase health care spending?   Probably, but that is not necessarily bad. Increased health care spending is bad only when it is wasteful and inefficient. For example, if doctors were to prescribe medicines for patients who had no medical need, that would be wasteful—and unethical. However, very few doctors would prescribe medicines their patients do not need. In fact, a new *Prevention* magazine survey found that about half of those who talk to a doctor as a result of a DTC ad receive no drug therapy.

A greater concern is that patients, having seen an expensive brand-name drug advertised, will want it rather than a generic equivalent. When patients or their doctors choose brand names over generics, their choices may increase total health care spending. But, again, that may not be bad. The brand name may be higher in quality or slightly different in composition. And it may have fewer side effects. Thus it may offer additional benefits, in which case the additional cost may be justified.

If an expansion of DTC advertising means that we are treating more people who otherwise might have just suffered in pain or endured a debilitating condition, then increased medical spending is positive. Some have argued that increased drug spending may lower total health care costs if less expensive drug therapy replaces more expensive surgery or other procedures. This may be true for individual patients, but it cannot be aggregated to apply to the whole health care system. Total spending will continue to rise because the American health care system will continue to do more and more for patients.

Will DTC advertising strain the doctor-patient relationship?   Historically, doctors informed and patients performed. That is, doctors diagnosed and issued instructions that patients followed—or at least were supposed to. With more information at the patients' fingertips, that relationship is changing. Patients are asking questions, and doctors are beginning to see the questions as opportunities to enhance patients' understanding and sense of responsibility about their own health. (The author himself has asked a physician about an advertised prescription drug, and neither he nor the doctor saw anything unusual or unethical about the exchange.)

Doctors may have to take more time to discuss with their patients why Drug A, which the patient saw advertised on TV, would not in the doctor's opinion be as good a choice as Drug B. Cost, efficacy and suitability all may play a role in that discussion. Some irascible patients may refuse to accept the doctor's advice. But this occurs even without DTC advertising. Indeed, current DTC advertising is very subtle. No announcer tells the audience to demand Drug A from a doctor because it has been clinically proven to be better than Drug B. DTC ads tend to convey too little information rather than too much. This may change, but the medical community already is learning to deal with people who come to the doctor not just as patients but as consumers.

Will DTC ads confuse patients?   Economist John Calfee contends that three decades of research on advertising has led to two basic understandings:

> First, advertising has an unsuspected power to improve consumer welfare. As a market-perfecting mechanism, advertising arises spontaneously to attack serious defects in the marketplace. Advertising is an efficient and sometimes irreplaceable mechanism for bringing consumers information that would otherwise languish on the sidelines. Advertising's promise of more and better information also generates ripple effects in the market. These include enhanced incentives to create new information and develop better products. Theoretical and empirical research has demonstrated what generations of astute observers had known intuitively, that markets with advertising are far superior to markets without advertising.
>
> The second finding is that competitive advertising is fundamentally a self-correcting process. Some people may find this surprising. Well informed observers once thought that unregulated advertising would bring massive distortion of consumer information and decisions. Careful research, however, has shown these fears to be groundless. Self-correcting competitive forces in advertising generate markets in which information is richer and more fundamentally balanced than can be achieved through detailed controls over advertising and information.

Is DTC just a way to increase drug prices?   Drug companies advertise for the same reason every other company and industry advertises: to increase sales with a view to increasing profits. The consumer benefit is that, as competition grows, prices usually fall. By contrast, in the absence of marketing, prices would not go down, but up. Just consider under which scenario a manufacturer is more likely to charge high prices for low quality: where there is no advertising and consumers have no way to comparison-shop without taking their own time to go from store to store to compare price and quality, or where advertising takes that information directly to the consumer? It is not advertising that increases the price of products, it's the lack of it. High prices thrive in an atmosphere of ignorance. If critics want to see the price of prescription drugs fall, they should encourage even more advertising and competition.

The missing ingredient: value   As long as patients are insulated from the cost of medical care and doctors stand between patients and their prescriptions, the health care marketplace cannot work exactly like a normal market in which consumers demand from vendors quality, service and reasonable prices—that is, value.

But the U.S. health care system can take on some of the dynamics of a market, and in fact is already doing so. There is some competition; there is some DTC advertising; and prices at least for some health care products and services are relatively low.

As we continue to move into a patient-directed system, market forces may become more apparent. For example, if most people chose to combine a Medical Savings Account (MSA) for small expenses with a catastrophic health insurance policy for large expenses, patients would pay for their prescription drugs out of the MSA and thus be more cost-conscious.

In addition, the realization is growing in Washington that the current tax subsidy for health insurance causes problems. As a result, Congress may pass a tax credit that will help the uninsured purchase a policy. This in turn may lead to a fundamental shift in the type of health insurance policy people purchase—and facilitate the move to a patient-directed system.

NO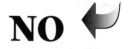

The Direct-to-Consumer Advertising Dilemma

How does DTC [direct-to-consumer] marketing affect the patient-physician relationship? Do the ads serve a valuable educational purpose? How has DTC advertising changed physicians' liability in suits brought by patients? Two experts answer these and other questions.

Direct-to-consumer (DTC) advertising of prescription medications has rapidly become one of the most contentious issues facing the medical profession in the United States. Changes in the political and regulatory climate, cultural shifts emphasizing the patient's role in making medical decisions, and expanding profits from drug sales have encouraged the pharmaceutical industry to pursue more direct marketing strategies. Currently, companies are spending close to $2 billion a year on DTC advertising in this country.

Proponents argue that DTC promotion provides a service by increasing public awareness of medical conditions and encouraging informed communication between patients and providers. Critics fear that drug companies will trade on the public's lack of medical knowledge to obscure products' risks and adverse effects. Some physicians report that they must devote increasing amounts of time to dissuading patients from taking drugs that DTC advertising has led them to believe are free of problems. [1]

Rise of DTC Advertisements

The increase in DTC advertising was motivated in part by the desire of manufacturers to more aggressively market their products and by the willingness of regulators to clarify broadcast advertising regulations in order to lessen the confusion surrounding vague reminder ads. Recent years have seen the erosion of physicians' authority to prescribe specific drugs as a result of the proliferation of drug formularies, utilization review systems, and pharmaceutical risk-sharing agreements.

A consumer empowerment movement led by an aging baby boomer population has also contributed to the growth of DTC advertising. Driven by the

From Anne B. Brown, "The Direct-to-Consumer Advertising Dilemma," *Patient Care,* vol. 35, no. 6 (March 30, 2001). Copyright © 2001 by Thomson Medical Economics. Reprinted by permission.

information explosion of the Internet, these consumers want to participate in decisions concerning their health care.

The Role of the FDA [U.S. Food and Drug Administration]

In the 1980s, pharmaceutical companies sponsored reminder advertisements— naming the product but not the illness—which avoided the FDA requirement of lengthy risk disclosure. Critics charged that these reminder commercials were often confusing and provided little information that consumers could use to improve their health. Public input and the FDA's own experience with DTC promotion prompted the agency to draft guidance designed to encourage more informative commercials.

In 1997, the FDA clarified its interpretations of broadcast advertisement regulations for television and radio, allowing manufacturers to mention both the drug's trade name and the disease or condition for which it had been approved (without requiring the disclosure of all risk information). Advertisers, however, are required to mention the important risks and to provide a statement explaining that additional information is available from other resources— such as a toll-free 800 number, a Web site, a magazine or newspaper ad, or a health care professional.

Although pharmaceutical companies are not required to submit the content of their DTC promotional materials to the FDA before using them, they often voluntarily seek FDA review during the broadcast production process. In the past 4 years, the FDA has sent more than 75 notices to sponsors, informing them that their DTC print and broadcast promotion advertisements violate regulations, usually by presenting insufficient or understated risk information and, in some cases, by overstating the product's effectiveness or the extent of its approved use.

FDA Evaluations

The FDA continues to examine the effects of DTC advertising on health care. The results of a recent FDA survey suggest that DTC prescription drug promotion offers public health benefits that may outweigh the potential negative effects. [2] For example, advertisements prompt patients to ask physicians about their medical conditions, with half of the consumers stating they looked for more information about a drug or a health condition after noticing an ad; 81% said they spoke to a doctor.

But while 62% of respondents said that DTC advertisements prompted them to discuss health concerns with their physicians, not all the responses were favorable. Fifty-eight percent said that the advertisements "make the drugs seem better than they are." About one fourth of the consumers agreed with the statement that "only the safest prescription drugs are allowed to be advertised to the public." The law does not allow the FDA to prohibit sponsors from advertising products that may be unsafe.

The survey results also suggested that DTC promotions may not always work to the advertiser's benefit. Requests for advertised products may result in prescriptions for competing products. Half of the consumers who had asked about an advertised product received a prescription for that product, but 32% received a different prescription. The FDA survey also highlighted concerns about whether the multiple-page lists of risks that are required for printed advertisements—and ignored by as many as 33% of patients—are optimal.

More research is needed on the clinical effects of DTC promotions, including the types of patients who are receiving prescriptions largely as a result of DTC ads and the cost-effectiveness of specific agents in these patients. By summer 2001, the FDA hopes to have enough data on the impact of DTC drug advertising to finalize its guidance to the pharmaceutical industry.

The Impact of DTC Advertisements

Studies have shown that increased consumer interest in advertised drugs and conditions leads to more office visits and tests. For example, IMS Health, a health care information company in Plymouth Meeting, Pa, reported that 1 year after a DTC campaign for alendronate (Fosamax), physician visits for osteoporosis evaluation nearly doubled. [3] Clearly increased consumer demand leads to more prescriptions. But are ad-induced prescriptions cost-effective? An inexpensive drug that is not needed or that treats a trivial condition adds to health spending, whereas a very expensive drug that prevents or cures a costly disease could be a bargain.

Several studies have examined the effect of DTC ads on prescription patterns. In a 1999 survey of 1200 people by *Prevention* magazine with technical assistance from the FDA, 31% of respondents said they had talked with their doctor about a prescription drug they had seen advertised. Of those 372 people, 8.7% asked their doctor for a drug they saw advertised, and 7.3% said their doctor wrote a prescription for it. [4]

In a recent AARP Public Policy Institute study, older consumers (particularly those aged 60 and older) appeared to obtain less information from DTC ads than younger persons. At the same time, older consumers also tended to report fewer discussions about medications with their physicians and pharmacists. This suggests that older consumers, along with other groups such as low-income and less educated persons, may be more vulnerable than others to the "medication information gap" in the prescription drug marketplace. This gap has important implications for older consumers because they tend to use more prescription drugs than younger ones. [5]

Studies of the full impact of DTC advertising have generally yielded more questions than answers because of the potentially diverse, widespread effects of these promotions. The likely impact of DTC advertisements is not limited to consumers but extends to the patient-physician relationship and affects drug spending and physician liability.

Educating Patients and Consumers

Proponents believe that advertising helps meet consumer demand for information about health conditions and possible treatments. Often, this information prompts people to seek medical attention, promotes informed discussions with medical professionals, and further enhances the dialogue between physicians and their patients. Pharmaceutical Research and Manufacturers of America (PhRMA) further argues that since prescription drugs are available only under a doctor's supervision, there is little danger that advertising will lead to inappropriate use. Also, DTC advertising fosters competition among products, which can lead to improved quality and lower prices for consumers. In summary, say its proponents, DTC advertising improves the public health and should be allowed its full voice in the marketplace.

Critics charge that few consumers have the clinical and pharmacologic background to properly understand and evaluate DTC advertisements, and this leads to confusion and inaccurate perceptions of a drug's efficacy and safety. Further, DTC advertising may cultivate the belief among the public that there is a pill for every ill and contribute to medication of trivial ailments.

Changing Patient-Physician Relationship

A majority of physicians believe that DTC advertising can have an inappropriate effect on prescribing. [6] They worry that people are beginning to ask their doctor for newer and costlier medicines when less expensive drugs may work just as well in many cases. When patients are told that there is an older, cheaper drug that is just as effective, they may be disappointed and may even change doctors.

In one study consumers were asked how they would respond if their physician turned down their request for an advertised drug:

- 46% of consumers said they would try to persuade the physician.
- 24% would attempt to obtain the prescription from a different physician.
- 15% said they might switch physicians. [7]

Others worry that DTC advertisements erode public trust in physicians. Patients may lose faith in their physicians when advertising messages conflict with professional advice. [8] Recent studies have shown beyond a doubt that DTC advertising motivates discussions between patients and their physicians about pharmaceutical products, which is beneficial if the discussions focus on the patient's presenting complaint, the diagnostic implications, the meaning of the diagnosis in the context of the patient's life, and the full range of available treatment options. . . . If discussions focus on specific brand-name drugs, trivial complaints, or procurement issues, however, they could detract from more meaningful interactions concerning the patient's health.

Another concern is that ads rarely mention behavior changes or other nonpharmacologic interventions, which are often as important as drug therapy in improving outcomes. A low-fat diet, stress management, or allergen avoidance may be more useful than a prescription.

Increasing Drug Spending

Concerns have been raised about whether mass media ads are inducing inappropriate demand for some new prescription medicines. The 25 drugs that contributed most to the increase in retail sales of pharmaceuticals in 1999 accounted for 40.7% of the overall $17.7 billion increase in spending. Most of these drugs were heavily advertised to the public and experienced a sharp growth in sales—an aggregate 43% in a single year.

In contrast, the growth in sales for all other prescription drugs from 1998 to 1999 was 13.3%. The strong growth in revenues and spending for heavily promoted drugs was driven largely by the rise in the volume of prescriptions. Pharmacies dispensed 34.2% more prescriptions in 1999 than in 1998 for the 25 drugs that contributed most to the rise in spending in 1999. In comparison, pharmacies dispensed just 5.1% more prescriptions for all other medications in 1999. [9]

In September 1999, the Health Insurance Association of America (HIAA) issued a white paper entitled "Prescription Drugs: Cost and Coverage Trends," predicting that increasing outlays for prescription drugs will drive up health insurance premiums and consumer out-of-pocket spending over the next decade. HIAA attributes soaring drug costs to several factors. Greater efficiency within the FDA is accelerating approvals of more effective but expensive treatments. The growth in third-party payment for prescription drugs has encouraged consumer demand for high-priced medications, as have the aging of Americans and implementation of disease management programs. But the most significant new development, according to HIAA, is the expansion of DTC advertising because of relaxed FDA regulations.

Similarly, a recent study from the National Institute for Health Care Management Foundation links the rise in pharmaceutical advertising to increased spending on prescription drugs. [9] Four pharmaceutical categories—oral antihistamines, antidepressants, cholesterol reducers, and antiulcer drugs—led the drug sales surge and included those medications most heavily advertised to consumers in 1998. In summary say its opponents, DTC advertising interferes with physician prescribing practices, has a deleterious impact on the public health, and should be more closely regulated.

Limiting Physician Liability

One potential benefit of DTC advertisements is that they may remove the physician as an intermediary between the sponsor and the patient in liability suits. In the past, drug companies were protected from adverse effects of their drugs experienced by patients because the doctor was "a learned intermediary" who informed patients of risks and benefits. Recently, the Supreme Court of New Jersey took a controversial stand challenging the foundation of pharmaceutical liability litigation. In *Perez v Wyeth Laboratories Inc.,* the court argued that the "learned intermediary doctrine," which has historically shielded pharmaceutical companies from any obligation to warn patients directly about their prescription products, does not apply when companies engage in DTC advertising. [10]

In the current era of time-limited medical visits, appealing new "lifestyle" prescription drugs, and widespread advertising opportunities, a physician's ability to influence the "preconceived expectations about treatment" was found to be significantly diminished. Arguing that these developments compromised the role of the learned intermediary, the court found that companies engaging in DTC marketing were legally responsible for providing adequate warning to consumers about the potential dangers of their products.

In addition to making pharmaceutical companies more accountable for the ways they market products directly to consumers, the court's ruling also provides a reminder of the growing limitations physicians may face in helping the patients make informed medical decision. Although physicians may be elated at the prospect of sharing some of the legal burdens placed on them, this landmark decision reflects the growing inability of physicians to serve as effective learned intermediaries in a health care system in which this function may be more necessary then ever.

References

1. Huang AJ. The rise of direct-to-consumer advertising of prescription drugs in the United States [editorial]. JAMA. 2000; 284:2240.
2. Attitudes and behaviors associated with direct-to-consumer (DTC); promotion of prescription drugs: preliminary survey results. Food and Drug Administration Web site. Available at: http://www.fda.gov/cder/ddmac/research.htm. Accessed October 5, 2000.
3. National Disease and Therapeutic Index [database online]. Plymouth Meeting, Pa: IMS Health: 1996.
4. Year Two: A national survey of consumer reactions to direct-to-consumer advertising. Prevention Magazine with technical assistance from the FDA. 1999.
5. AARP Executive Summary: Are consumers well informed about prescription drugs? The impact of printed direct-to-consumer advertising. Available at: http://www.research.aarp.org/health/2000_04_advertising_1.html.   Accessed October 5, 2000.
6. Spurgeon D. Doctors feel pressurised by direct to consumer advertising. BMJ. 1999; 319:1321.
7. Wilkes MS. Bell RA. Kravitz RL. Direct-to-consumer prescription drug advertising: Trends, impact and implications. Health Aff. 2000; 19:110–128.
8. Perri M, Shinde S, Banavali R. The past, present, and future of direct-to-consumer prescription drug advertising. Clin Ther. 1999; 21:1798–181.
9. National Institute for Health Care Management (NIHCM) Foundation research brief: Prescription drugs and mass media advertising. Available at: http://www.nihcm.org/index2.html. Accessed October 7, 2000.
10. Perez v Wyeth Laboratories Inc. Supreme Court of NJ, No. A-16-98 (August 9, 1999).
11. Gemperli MP. Rethinking the role of the learned intermediary: The effect of direct-to-consumer advertising on litigation. JAMA. 2000; 284:2241.

POSTSCRIPT

Do Consumers Benefit When Prescription Drugs Are Advertised?

O pponents of prescription drug advertising contend that drug companies' promotions are frequently inaccurate or deceptive. Furthermore, they maintain that drug companies are more interested in increasing their profits, not in truly providing additional medical benefits to the average consumer. Drug companies do not deny that they seek to make profits from their drugs, but they argue that they are offering an important public service by educating the public about new drugs through their advertisements.

An important issue is whether or not the average consumer is capable of discerning information distributed by pharmaceutical companies. Are people without a background in medicine, medical terminology, or research methods sufficiently knowledgeable to understand literature disseminated by drug companies? With the help of the Internet and other media, prescription drug advertising proponents maintain that the average consumer is indeed capable of understanding information about various drugs.

When drug manufacturers introduce a new drug, they get a patent on the drug to protect their investment. Drug companies, therefore, receive financial rewards for introducing new drugs. Of course, drug companies also take financial risks when developing new drugs. However, some critics maintain that many of these new drugs are merely "me too" drugs (similar to existing drugs) and that they do not provide any additional benefits. Are consumers being fooled into requesting more expensive drugs that are no better than drugs that are already on the market?

Two articles that explore the benefits of prescription drug advertising are "Promotion of Prescription Drugs to Consumers," by Meredith Rosenthal et al., *The New England Journal of Medicine* (February 14, 2002) and "What You Should Know About Direct-to-Consumer Advertising of Prescription Drugs," by David E. Dukes, James F. Rogers, and Eric A. Paine, *Defense Counsel Journal* (January 2001). Articles critical of direct-to-consumer prescription drug advertisements are "Pharmaceutical Advertisements: How They Deceive," by Ashish Chandra and Gary Holt, *Journal of Business Ethics* (February 15, 1999) and "Peddling Pills: The Rise of Direct-to-Consumer Prescription Drug Advertising and the Dangers to Consumers," by Larry Sasich, *Multinational Monitor* (January/February 1999). Finally, whether or not Great Britain will allow direct-to-consumer drug advertising is discussed in "Consumer Choice or Chaos?" *Chemist & Druggist* (June 10, 2000).

National Institute on Alcohol Abuse and Alcoholism (NIAAA)

This site provides research on the causes, consequences, treatment, and prevention of alcoholism and alcohol-related problems.

http://niaaa.nih.gov

National Clearinghouse for Alcohol and Drug Information (NCADI)

Information on a variety of drugs and research published by the federal government are available at this site. Up-to-date developments in drug use are also available through the NCADI.

http://www.health.org

The Weiner Nusim Foundation

This private foundation, which is located in Easton, Connecticut, publishes free information about drug education.

http://www.weinernusim.com

DrugHelp

This site, which is a service of the American Council for Drug Education (an affiliate of the Phoenix House Foundation), provides information, counsel, and referrals to treatment centers.

http://www.drughelp.org

Partnership for a Drug-Free America

The effects of drugs and the extent of drug use by young people are discussed at this Web site.

http://www.drugfreeamerica.org

National Council on Alcoholism and Drug Dependence

This site contains objective information and referrals for individuals, families, and others who seek intervention and treatment.

http://www.ncadd.org

PART 3

Drug Prevention and Treatment

*I*n spite of their legal consequences and the U.S. government's interdiction efforts, drugs are widely available and used. Two common ways of dealing with drug abuse is to incarcerate drug users and to intercept drugs before they enter the country. However, many drug experts believe that more energy should be put into preventing and treating drug abuse. An important step toward prevention and treatment is to find out what contributes to drug abuse and how to nullify these factors.

By educating young people about the potential hazards of drugs and by developing an awareness of social influences that contribute to drug use, many drug-related problems can be averted. The debates in this section focus on different prevention and treatment issues, the effects that alcohol advertisements have on young people's drinking behavior, and the effectiveness of needle exchange programs in reducing the transmission of the human immunodeficiency virus (HIV).

- Should Nonsmokers Be Concerned About the Effects of Secondhand Smoke?

- Is Total Abstinence the Only Choice for Alcoholics?

- Should Needle Exchange Programs Be Supported?

- Should Employees Be Required to Participate in Drug Testing?

- Does Drug Abuse Treatment Work?

- Do Alcohol Advertisements Influence Young People to Drink More?

ISSUE 14

Should Nonsmokers Be Concerned About the Effects of Secondhand Smoke?

YES: U.S. Department of Health and Human Services, from *Reducing Tobacco Use: A Report of the Surgeon General* (2000)

NO: J. B. Copas and J. Q. Shi, from "Reanalysis of Epidemiological Evidence on Lung Cancer and Passive Smoking," *British Medical Journal* (February 12, 2000)

ISSUE SUMMARY

YES: The U.S. Department of Health and Human Services identifies numerous health consequences associated with secondhand smoke. Secondhand smoke is a human carcinogen, accounting for 3,000 lung cancer deaths annually, and it also causes bronchitis, pneumonia, middle ear diseases, asthma, and heart disease.

NO: Statisticians J. B. Copas and J. Q. Shi argue that research demonstrating that secondhand smoke is harmful is biased. They contend that journals are more likely to publish articles if secondhand smoke is shown to be deleterious and that the findings of many studies exaggerate the adverse effects of secondhand smoke.

The movement to restrict secondhand smoke—the smoke that a person breathes in from another person's cigarette, cigar, or pipe—is growing. Smoking is banned on all commercial airplane flights within the continental United States. Canada, Australia, and many other countries have enacted similar bans. Smoking is prohibited or restricted in all federal public areas and workplaces. The right to smoke in public places is quickly being eliminated. Is this fair, considering tobacco's addictive hold over smokers? Former surgeon general C. Everett Koop and many researchers point out that smoking is an addiction that is as difficult to overcome as an addiction to cocaine or heroin. Should smokers be penalized—prevented from smoking or isolated from nonsmokers—for having a nicotine addiction?

Articles describing secondhand smoking, or passive smoking, can be confusing because several terms frequently are used to describe it. *Passive smoking* has been referred to as involuntary smoking, and the smoke itself has been identified as both *secondhand smoke* and *environmental tobacco smoke*, or *ETS*. Secondhand smoke can be further broken down into *mainstream smoke* and *sidestream smoke*. Mainstream smoke is the smoke that the smoker exhales. Sidestream smoke is the smoke that comes off the end of the tobacco product as it burns. Sidestream smoke has higher concentrations of carbon monoxide and other gases than mainstream smoke. Scientists also believe that sidestream smoke contains more carcinogens than mainstream smoke.

The issue of passive smoking is extremely divisive. On one side of the debate are the nonsmokers, who strongly believe that their rights to clean air are compromised by smokers. Their objections are based on more than aesthetics; it is not simply a matter of smoke being unsightly, noxious, or inconvenient. Nonsmokers are becoming more concerned about the toxic effects of secondhand smoke. Groups of nonsmokers and numerous health professionals have initiated a massive campaign to educate the public on the array of health-related problems that have been associated with inhaling the smoke generated by those who smoke tobacco products.

On the other side are smokers, who believe that they should have the right to smoke whenever and wherever they wish. This group is backed by the tobacco industry, which has allocated vast sums of money and resources to conduct research studies on the effects of secondhand smoke. Based on the results of these studies, smoking rights groups contend that the health concerns related to secondhand smoke are based on emotion, not scientific evidence. They argue that there are too many variables involved to determine the exact impact of secondhand smoke. For example, to what extent does a polluted environment or a poorly ventilated house contribute to the health problems attributed to secondhand smoke? Isolating the effects of secondhand smoke, these groups maintain, is difficult, and any studies concluding that secondhand smoke is harmful are questionable.

Many smokers who acknowledge that smoking may have adverse effects on health argue that their freedoms should not be limited. They feel that they should have the right to engage in behaviors that affect only themselves, even if those behaviors are unhealthy. Some smokers reason that if smoking behavior is regulated, perhaps other personal behaviors also will become regulated. They fight against the regulation of smoking because they believe that behavior regulation is a potentially harmful trend.

If smoking is restricted, many people employed in the tobacco industry may lose their livelihoods. What may be a health benefit for some people may be detrimental to the economic health of others. Are the people who want to restrict smoking willing to help those individuals who would be economically affected by such a restriction?

In the following selections, the U.S. Department of Health and Human Services stresses that the dangers associated with secondhand smoke are clear and that even exposure to low doses of secondhand smoke is toxic. J. B. Copas and J. Q. Shi maintain that much of the information about the health hazards of secondhand smoke has been distorted and accepted as fact without adequate critical questioning.

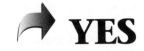 **YES**

Clean Indoor Air Regulation

Introduction

If the regulation of tobacco products themselves has been characterized by slow and incremental advances, the regulation of where and how tobacco products are used—that is, the regulation of exposure, particularly of nonsmokers, to ETS [environmental tobacco smoke]—has encountered comparatively little resistance. Public and private steps to regulate ETS have become both more common and more restrictive over the past several decades.

There are various reasons for this broad and rapid implementation. One reason is that the public health necessity of regulating ETS exposure is manifest: ETS is known to cause acute and chronic diseases in nonsmokers (National Academy of Sciences 1986; USDHHS 1986; National Institute for Occupational Safety and Health 1991; EPA 1992; California EPA 1997). Moreover, this demonstrated health threat is unentangled with legal or ethical issues of "informed choice" or "informed consent" . . . —hence a popular name for this exposure, *passive* smoking. Regulating ETS exposure also has important implications for reducing smoking: studies have shown that restricting smoking in public settings increases the likelihood that smokers in these settings smoke fewer cigarettes or quit smoking entirely (Petersen et al. 1988; Borland et al. 1990a; Stillman et al. 1990; Sorensen et al. 1991a; Woodruff et al. 1993). It has been estimated that the combined effect of general smoking cessation and smoking reduction in public settings could decrease total cigarette consumption by as much as 40 percent (Woodruff et al. 1993), although this conclusion may be questioned based on assessment of worksite interventions. . . . A second reason for the expansion of ETS regulations is that their public support, a key marker for successful implementation, is implicit: national studies suggest that most of the U.S. public experiences discomfort and annoyance from ETS exposure (CDC 1988, 1992b), and smaller-scale surveys have found that the great majority of both nonsmokers and smokers favors smoking restrictions in various public locations, including the workplace, restaurants, and bars (CDC 1991). A third reason is that employers might be expected to support ETS regulations, because prohibiting smoking in the workplace can help employers realize lower maintenance and repair costs of buildings and property, lower insurance costs, and

From U.S. Department of Health and Human Services, *Reducing Tobacco Use: A Report of the Surgeon General* (2000). Atlanta, Georgia: U.S. Department of Health and Human Services, Centers for Disease Control and Prevention, National Center for Chronic Disease Prevention and Health Promotion, Office on Smoking and Health, 2000. References omitted.

higher productivity among nonsmokers (Mudarri 1994). Employer support, however, may be influenced by other factors. . . .

Not surprisingly, during the 1980s the tobacco industry identified ETS regulation as the single most important issue confronting the industry's economic future (Chapman et al. 1990). The industry is concerned that the increasing focus on ETS may cause the public and policymakers to view smoking as an environmental issue with broad social consequences instead of as a personal behavior involving individual choice. The tobacco industry is also concerned about legal backlash from possible ETS-related litigation against employers and about revenue losses from possible decreased cigarette consumption due to smoking restrictions (Chapman et al. 1990). An example of the latter concern may be found in California, where workplace restrictions extant in 1990 have reduced consumption by an estimated 148 million packs per year, at a value of $203 million in pretax sales (Woodruff et al. 1993).

Health Consequences of Exposure to ETS

The detrimental health effects of exposure to ETS are well established (National Research Council 1986; USDHHS 1986, 2000b; EPA 1992; California EPA 1997). The most comprehensive review of the respiratory effects of ETS to date is the 1992 report of the EPA, which states that ETS is a human lung carcinogen that annually accounts for approximately 3,000 lung cancer deaths among adult nonsmokers in the United States. Autopsy reviews (Trichopoulos et al. 1992) and studies of ETS metabolites in body fluids (Hecht et al. 1993) provide biologic support for epidemiologic studies linking ETS and lung cancer. ETS also has subtle but significant effects on the respiratory health (including cough, phlegm production, and reduced lung function) of adult nonsmokers.

Among children, ETS has far-reaching health effects. ETS causes bronchitis and pneumonia, accounting for an estimated 150,000–300,000 annual cases in infants and young children, and causes middle ear diseases (infections and effusions). ETS causes additional episodes of asthma and increases its severity, worsening an estimated 400,000–1,000,000 cases annually. As a risk factor for new cases of asthma, ETS may account for 8,000–26,000 annual cases (EPA 1992; California EPA 1997).

In an important ruling, Judge Osteen of the U.S. District Court annulled Chapters 1–6 and the Appendices to the EPA's 1992 report (EPA 1992; *Flue-Cured Tobacco Cooperative Stabilization Corp. v. United States Environmental Protection Agency*, 4 F. Supp. 2d 435 [M.D.N.C. 1998]). The decision was a mix of procedural and scientific concerns. Judge Osteen found that the EPA had not complied with the procedural requirements of the Radon Gas and Indoor Air Quality Research Act of 1986, had acted beyond congressional intent, and had violated administrative law procedure by drawing conclusions about ETS prior to concluding a scientifically sound risk-assessment study. The judge was also concerned with the amount of evidence in the record supporting EPA's final basis for its plausibility hypothesis, with some of the animal laboratory tests that he felt were inconclusive but were cited as compelling evidence of the dangers of ETS, and with the EPA's choice of epidemiologic studies to support its findings.

Considerable information appeared after the EPA's 1992 report that supported its general conclusions (Brownson et al. 1992a; Stockwell et al. 1992; Fontham et al. 1994; Cardenas et al. 1997). A recent meta-analysis of workplace ETS exposure and increased risk of lung cancer also provided needed epidemiologic support (Wells 1998). The ninth EPA report on carcinogens was released in the year 2000 and lists ETS as a known carcinogen for the first time (USDHHS 2000).

Since the 1992 EPA report, further evidence linking ETS and heart disease has been assembled as well. (Glantz and Parmley 1995; Steenland et al. 1996; California EPA 1997; Kawachi et al. 1997; Law et al. 1997; Howard et al. 1998; Valkonen and Kuusi 1998; Wells 1998). If ETS is a causal risk factor for coronary heart disease, it likely accounts for many more deaths from heart disease than from lung cancer (EPA 1992; Wells 1994). A review of 12 epidemiologic studies has estimated that ETS accounts for as many as 62,000 annual deaths from coronary heart disease in the United States (Wells 1994). However, because smoking is but one of the many risk factors in the etiology of heart disease, quantifying the precise relationship between ETS and this disease is difficult.

Strong evidence is also accumulating that ETS is a risk factor for sudden infant death syndrome (Jinot and Bayard 1994; DiFranza and Lew 1995; Klonoff-Cohen et al. 1995; Anderson and Cook 1997; California EPA 1997; Alm et al. 1998; Dybing and Sanner 1999). In a large U.S. study, maternal exposure during pregnancy and postnatal exposure of the newborn to ETS increased the risk of this syndrome (Schoendorf and Kiely 1992).

Other Consequences of ETS

Separate from their concerns about direct health effects, most nonsmokers are annoyed by ETS exposure (CDC 1988; Brownson et al. 1992b). U.S. survey data have suggested that 71 percent of all respondents, including 43 percent of current smokers, are annoyed by ETS (CDC 1988). Similarly, data from urban St. Louis and Kansas City, Missouri, have shown that 66 percent of all respondents and nearly 40 percent of current smokers were annoyed by ETS exposure (Brownson et al. 1992b). The term "annoyance," a seemingly minor attribute, has some nontrivial ramifications. Public attitudes toward smoking, an amalgam of concerns about health and social interactions, have changed in the past decade, as is discussed in greater detail in the section "Effectiveness of Clean Indoor Air Restrictions," later in this [selection]. The findings from one survey suggested that the proportion of Americans who favored a total ban on smoking in restaurants and workplaces increased from less than one-fifth in 1983 to almost one-third in 1992 (Gallup Organization, Inc. 1992). The proportion favoring no restrictions fell from as high as 15 percent in 1983 to 5 percent in 1992. Similarly, by 1992, more than 90 percent of respondents favored restrictions or a total ban on smoking in trains and buses as well as in hotels and motels. More than 90 percent "agreed" or "strongly agreed" that ETS is injurious to children, pregnant women, and older adults. Thus, an important consequence of information on ETS has been a changing social norm regarding smoking and an evolving foundation for clean indoor air regulations.

Because of the consequences of ETS, employers are likely to save costs by implementing policies for smoke-free workplaces. Savings include those associated with fire risk, damage to property and furnishings, cleaning costs, workers compensation, disability, retirement, injuries, life insurance, absenteeism, productivity losses, and synergistic occupational risks such as asbestos exposure (Kristein 1989). Such costs were estimated at $1,000 per smoking employee in 1988 dollars. In a recent report on the savings associated with a nationwide, comprehensive policy on clean indoor air, the EPA estimated that such a law would save $4 billion to $8 billion per year in operational and maintenance costs of buildings (Mudarri 1994).

Prevalence of Exposure to ETS

Exposure to ambient tobacco smoke is widespread. The 1988 National Health Interview Survey reported that an estimated 37 percent of the 79.2 million U.S. nonsmoking workers worked in places that permitted smoking in designated and other areas and that 59 percent of these experienced moderate or great discomfort from ETS exposure in the workplace (National Center for Health Statistics 1989). Since the advent of urinary cotinine screening, firmer documentation of ETS has become available. In a study of 663 nonsmokers attending a cancer screening, Cummings and colleagues (1990) found that 76 percent of participants were exposed to ETS in the four days preceding the interview. The authors concluded that the workplace and the home were the primary sources of ETS exposure among these nonsmokers. The best single predictor of urinary cotinine was the number of smokers among friends and family members seen regularly by the study participant. In a study of 881 nonsmoking volunteers, Marcus and colleagues (1992) found that employees in workplaces that were "least restrictive" (i.e., allowed smoking in numerous locations) were more than four times more likely to have detectable saliva cotinine concentrations than employees from smoke-free workplaces were (p. 45).

The largest study of population exposure to ETS with biochemical markers is the CDC's Third National Health and Nutrition Examination Survey, conducted from 1988 to 1991 on a nationally representative sample of 16,818 persons aged 2 months and older (Pirkle 1996). Serum cotinine was measured in 10,642 participants aged 4 years and older. The data indicate high concordance between reported ETS exposure and serum cotinine level. Among nontobacco users, 87.9 percent had detectable levels of serum cotinine, and the level was significantly and independently associated with both the number of smokers in the household and the number of hours of work exposure. The authors concluded that both the work and the household environments make important contributions to the widespread exposure to ETS experienced by children and adults.

Some improvement in ETS exposure has been noted. A study from California found that nonsmokers' self-reported exposure to ETS at work declined from 29 percent in 1990 to 22 percent in 1993 (Patten et al. 1995b). This decline was not as pronounced, however, among some sociodemographic subgroups, such as African Americans, Asian Americans, and persons with less than a high school education. During the same period, the percentage of employees reporting that they worked in smoke-free workplaces greatly increased (from 35 to 65 percent). Survey data from Missouri in 1993 indicated that 41 percent of the population were exposed to ETS in the workplace and 18 percent in the home environment (Brownson et al. 1995a). Among subgroups, younger persons, men, Hispanics, and persons with less than a high school education had more workplace exposure to ETS. Similarly, data from rural Missouri showed higher prevalence of workplace ETS exposure among younger persons, men, African Americans, and persons with less than a high school education (Brownson et al. 1995a). Emmons and colleagues (1992) analyzed entries in diaries recording ETS exposure among 186 persons who were former smokers or had never smoked. Approximately 50 percent of the daily ETS exposure was attributed to the workplace, and 10 percent was attributed to the home environment. However, for persons who lived with a smoker, more exposure occurred in the home than in the workplace.

Relatively few population-based data that specifically examine the levels of ETS exposure in the workplace have been collected. Such data may be important, because exposure levels likely vary greatly by workplace, and recent studies have indicated that higher levels of ETS (measured by intensity or duration of ETS exposure) increase the risk of lung cancer in nonsmokers (Brownson et al. 1992a; Stockwell et al. 1992; Fontham et al. 1994). In a review of existing studies, Siegel (1993) found that ETS concentrations varied widely by location; mean levels of nicotine measured in the ambient air were 4.1 $\mu g/m^3$ for offices overall, 4.3 $\mu g/m^3$ for residences with at least one smoker, 6.5 $\mu g/m^3$ for restaurants, and 19.7 $\mu g/m^3$ for bars. In a survey of 25 Massachusetts worksites, Hammond and colleagues (1995) found that the type of worksite smoking policy had a great effect on nicotine concentrations. Levels of nicotine ranged from 8.6 $\mu g/m^3$ in open offices that allowed smoking to 0.3 $\mu g/m^3$ in worksites that banned smoking.

Legal Foundation for Regulation of Public Smoking

The legal foundation for regulating public smoking is based on case law pertaining mainly to the protection of the health of workers. Under common law (the body of law based on court decisions rather than government laws or regulations), employers must provide a work environment that is reasonably free of recognized hazards. Courts have ruled that common-law duty requires employers to provide nonsmoking employees protection from the proven health hazards of ETS exposure (Sweda 1994).

Three pioneering cases have demonstrated the basis for this protection. In *Shimp v. New Jersey Bell Telephone Co.* (368 A.2d 408, 145 N.J. Super. 516 [1976]), a secretary who was allergic to cigarette smoke sought an injunction requiring a smoking ban. The court ordered the employer to provide a safe working environment by restricting smoking to a nonwork area. Similarly, in the case of *Smith v. Western Electric Co.* (643 S.W.2d 10 [Mo. App. 1982]), the Missouri Court of Appeals overturned a lower court and forced the employer to "assume its responsibility to eliminate the hazardous conditions caused by tobacco smoke" (p. 13). Finally, in *Lee v. Department of Public Welfare* (No. 15385 [Mass. Mar. 31, 1983], *cited in* 1.2 TPLR 2.82 [1986]), a social worker sued her employer, seeking relief from ETS exposure at work. The Massachusetts Superior Court ruled in favor of the plaintiff and required a smoke-free workplace. Additional protections to employees are extended by federal statute, such as the Americans with Disabilities Act of 1990 (ADA) (Public Law 101-336), and by rulings in workers compensation claims.

Status of Restrictions to Limit Smoking in Public Places

Although the health risks of ETS exposure began to be publicized in the early 1970s (NCI 1991), momentum to regulate public smoking increased only in 1986, when reports by the Surgeon General (USDHHS 1986) and the National Academy of Sciences (1986) concluded that ETS is a cause of lung cancer in non-smokers. Since then, government and private business policies that limit smoking in public places have become increasingly common and restrictive (Rigotti and Pashos 1991). The designation of ETS as a class A (known human) carcinogen by the EPA (1992) stimulated further restrictions on smoking in public places (Brownson et al. 1995a), but a recent court ruling set aside that report (see "Health Consequences of Exposure to ETS," earlier in [this selection]).

Although many of the regulatory efforts discussed herein focus on government's passage of a law or an ordinance, other regulations can be implemented by agencies with special authority. An example of a non-government regulatory action is the recent adoption of an accrediting standard that prohibits smoking in hospital buildings (Joint Commission on Accreditation of Healthcare Organizations 1992; Longo et al. 1995). . . .

Federal Laws and Regulations

The most notable federal regulation of ETS is the requirement that domestic airline flights be smoke free. The regulation was first enacted in 1988 for domestic flights lasting two hours or less and was renewed in 1989 for domestic flights lasting six hours or less. Since the early 1970s, the Interstate Commerce Commission (ICC) has required that smoking on interstate buses be confined to the rear of the bus and that smoking sections constitute no more than 10 percent of total seating capacity. Similar ICC regulation for trains was repealed in 1979. In 1987, congressional legislation that threatened to withhold federal funds influenced the State of New York's Metropolitan Transportation Authority to ban smoking on the MTA Long Island Rail Road (USDHHS 1989). Currently, the Occupational Safety and Health Administration is considering regulations that would either prohibit smoking in all workplaces or limit it to separately ventilated areas (*Federal Register* 1994). Furthermore, the federal government has instituted increasingly stringent regulations on smoking in its own facilities, and the Pro-Children's Act of 1994 (Public Law 103-227, secs. 1041–1044) prohibits smoking in facilities in which federally funded children's services are provided on a regular or routine basis.

State Laws and Regulations

As of December 31, 1999, smoke-free indoor air to some degree or in some public places was required by 45 states and the District of Columbia. These restrictions vary widely, from limited restrictions on public transportation to comprehensive restrictions in worksites and public places (CDC, Office on Smoking and Health, State Tobacco Activities Tracking and Evaluation System, unpublished data). In 1973, Arizona became the first state in which public smoking was regulated in recognition of ETS as a public health hazard. Five states (Alabama, Kentucky, New Mexico, North Carolina, and Wyoming) have either no legislation or legislation that preempts localities from enacting any law to restrict smoking in public places.

As of December 31, 1999, laws restricting smoking in government worksites were present in 43 states and the District of Columbia: 29 limit smoking to designated areas, 2 require either no smoking or designated smoking areas with separate ventilation, and 11 prohibit smoking entirely. Twenty-one states have laws restricting smoking in private worksites: 20 limit smoking to designated areas, and 1 (California) requires either no smoking or separate ventilation for smoking areas. Thirty-one states have laws that regulate smoking in restaurants; of these, only Utah and Vermont completely prohibit smoking in restaurants, and California requires either no smoking or separate ventilation for smoking areas (CDC, Office on Smoking and Health, State Tobacco Activities Evaluation System, unpublished data).

In 1994, Maryland proposed a regulation that would prohibit smoking in most workplaces in the state, including restaurants and bars (*Maryland Register* 1994). Despite strong support among both nonsmokers and smokers for restrictions on public smoking in the state (Shopland et al. 1995), this proposal was aggressively challenged by the tobacco industry (Spayd 1994), which questioned the state's legal authority to regulate smoking through administrative rule rather than law. In early 1995, the original regulation was modified by legislative action to permit some exceptions for the hospitality industry, and the rules went into effect. In October 1994, the state of Washington also enacted an extensive indoor workplace ban. In this instance, a temporary injunction was dismissed by the state court, and the ban went into effect without litigation (CSH 1994b).

In North Carolina, legislation was enacted on July 15, 1993 (HB 957), that required that smoking be permitted in at least 20 percent of space in state-controlled buildings but also formally required nonsmoking areas. An important preemption clause prohibited local regulatory boards from enacting more restrictive regulations for public or private buildings after October 15, 1993. During that three-month "window of opportunity," 89 local agencies passed new measures providing some increased protection from ETS. Despite the rush to new restrictions, researchers estimated that by the year 2000, the preemption would prevent 59 percent of private employees in North Carolina from being protected from ETS (Conlisk et al. 1995).

Local Ordinances

The modern era of local ordinances for clean indoor air began in the early 1970s (Pertschuk 1993). In 1977, Berkeley, California, became the first community to limit smoking in restaurants and other public places. After the release of the 1986 Surgeon General's report on the health consequences of ETS, the rate of passage of local ordinances accelerated. By 1988, nearly 400 local ordinances to restrict smoking had been enacted throughout the United States (Pertschuk and Shopland 1989). The trend toward smoke-free local ordinances has accelerated since 1989 (Rigotti and Pashos 1991; Pertschuk 1993). As of June 30, 1998, public smoking was restricted or banned in 820 local ordinances. Of those that specified which agency was responsible for enforcement, 44 percent cited health departments or boards of health, 19 percent named city managers, 5 percent said police departments, and 6 percent identified other agencies (Americans for Non-smokers' Rights, unpublished data, June 30, 1998). The effectiveness of various enforcement mechanisms and the level of compliance achieved are not known. Data from Wisconsin suggest that implementation may be just as important as legislation in achieving policy goals (Nordstrom and DeStefano 1995).

One study examined the impact a local ordinance had on restaurant receipts (CDC 1995a). Contrary to some prior claims, an analysis of restaurant sales after a ban on smoking in this community (a small suburb of Austin, Texas) showed no adverse economic effect. In a series of ecologic analyses, Glantz and Smith (1994, 1997) analyzed the effect of smoke-free restaurant and bar ordinances on sales tax receipts. Over time, such ordinances had no effect on the fraction of total retail sales that went to eating and drinking places. The authors asserted that claims of economic hardship for restaurants and bars that establish smoke-free policies have not been substantiated.

Private Sector Restrictions on Smoking in Workplaces

Two national data sets are available to ascertain the level of workplace smoking restrictions among private firms in the United States. A survey conducted by the Bureau of National Affairs, Inc. (1991), estimated that 85 percent of large workplaces had policies restricting smoking. The percentage of smoke-free workplaces has increased dramatically, from 2 percent in 1986 to 7 percent in 1987 and to 34 percent in 1991. Similarly, data from the 1992 National Survey of Worksite Health Promotion Activities indicated that 87 percent of workplaces with 50 or more employees regulated smoking in some manner and that 34 percent were smoke free (USDHHS 1993). The 1995 Update of the Business Responds to AIDS Benchmark Survey conducted by CDC also found that 87 percent of worksites with 50 or more employees had a smoking policy of some kind (National Center for Health Statistics 1997).

The prevalence of smoking policies in small workplaces, where the majority of Americans work, is less well studied. A comprehensive examination of workplace smoking policies from the NCI's tobacco use supplement to the Current Population Survey (n = 100,561) indicated that most indoor workers surveyed (81.6 percent) reported that an official policy governed smoking at their workplaces, and nearly half reported that the policy could be classified as "smoke-free"—that is, that smoking was not permitted either in workplace areas or in common public-use areas (Gerlach 1997). This proportion varied by sex, age, ethnicity, and occupation: blue-collar and service occupations had significantly less access to smoke-free environments. Though data were not specifically reported by workplace size, the range of occupations suggests that the survey included a substantial proportion of persons who work in smaller workplace environments. But for all workplace sizes, the data suggest that access to smoke-free environments could be substantially improved.

Effectiveness of Clean Indoor Air Restrictions

Although it is generally accepted that regulatory changes influence nonsmokers' exposure to ETS and smokers' behavior, relatively few evaluation studies quantify these effects over time. Evaluating such changes is hampered by the complex interaction of social forces that shape behavior, by the decline in smoking and smoke exposure in the overall population, and by the overlapping effects of concomitant regulatory policies (e.g., a new law for clean indoor air passed at or around the time of an increase in the cigarette excise tax). Controlling for such potential confounding factors in studies is difficult.

Population-Based Studies

Effects on Nonsmokers' Exposure to ETS

Despite the widespread implementation of restrictions against public smoking, few population-based studies have examined whether these restrictions have reduced nonsmokers' exposure to ETS. One such study from California used data collected in 1990 and 1991 to examine the association between the strength of local ordinances for clean indoor air and cross-sectional data on nonsmokers' exposure to ETS in the workplace (Pierce et al. 1994b). Exposure to ETS in the workplace ranged from 25 percent of workplaces in areas with a strong local ordinance to 35 percent in areas with no local ordinance.

In measuring the impact of a statewide law for clean indoor air, researchers in Missouri examined self-reported data on ETS exposure from 1990 through 1993 (Brownson et al. 1995a). Nonsmokers' exposure to ETS in the workplace declined slightly the year the law was passed and substantially more after the law went into effect. Exposure to ETS in the home remained constant over the study period; this finding suggests that the declining workplace exposure was more likely linked to the smoking regulations than to the overall declining smoking prevalence observed during the study period. Despite improvements over time, ETS exposure in the workplace remained at 35 percent in the final year of the study (1993). Other data from California indicate that nonsmokers employed in workplaces with no policy or a policy not covering their part of the workplace were eight times more likely to be exposed to ETS (at work) than those employed in smoke-free workplaces (Borland et al. 1992).

NO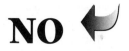

J. B. Copas and J. Q. Shi

Reanalysis of Epidemiological Evidence on Lung Cancer and Passive Smoking

Objective   To assess the epidemiological evidence for an increase in the risk of lung cancer resulting from exposure to environmental tobacco smoke.

Design   Reanalysis of 37 published epidemiological studies previously included in a meta-analysis allowing for the possibility of publication bias.

Main outcome measure   Relative risk of lung cancer among female lifelong non-smokers, according to whether her partner was a current smoker or a lifelong non-smoker.

Results   If it is assumed that all studies that have ever been carried out are included, or that those selected for review are truly representative of all such studies, then the estimated excess risk of lung cancer is 24%, as previously reported (95% confidence interval 13% to 36%, P < 0.001). However, a significant correlation between study outcome and study size suggests the presence of publication bias. Adjustment for such bias implies that the risk has been overestimated. For example, if only 60% of studies have been included, the estimate of excess risk falls from 24% to 15%.

Conclusion   A modest degree of publication bias leads to a substantial reduction in the relative risk and to a weaker level of significance, suggesting that the published estimate of the increased risk of lung cancer associated with environmental tobacco smoke needs to be interpreted with caution.

Introduction

Exposure to environmental tobacco smoke (passive smoking) is widely accepted to increase the risk of lung cancer, but different epidemiological studies have produced varying estimates of the size of the relative risk. Hackshaw et al reviewed the results of 37 such studies that estimated the relative risk of lung cancer among female lifelong non-smokers, comparing those whose spouses (or partners) were current smokers with those whose spouses had never smoked.[1]

From J. B. Copas and J. Q. Shi, "Reanalysis of Epidemiological Evidence on Lung Cancer and Passive Smoking," *British Medical Journal,* vol. 320 (February 12, 2000). Copyright © 2000 by The BMJ Publishing Group. Reprinted by permission. Notes omitted.

Of the 37 studies, 31 reported an increase in risk, and the increase was significant in seven studies. The remaining six studies reported negative results, but none of these was significant. Pooling these results using a method which allows for statistical heterogeneity between studies, Hackshaw et al concluded that there is an overall excess risk of 24% (95% confidence interval 13% to 36%).[1] This is strong epidemiological evidence for an association between lung cancer and passive smoking (P < 0.001).

The approach used by Hackshaw et al does not allow for the possibility of publication bias—that is, the possibility that published studies, particularly smaller ones, will be biased in favour of more positive results. We reanalysed the results and looked for evidence of publication bias.

Methods and Results

. . . [T]he relative risks from the 37 epidemiological studies analysed by Hackshaw et al[1] [were] plotted against a measure of the uncertainty in that relative risk. This uncertainty (s) decreases as the size of the study increases so that large studies are on the left of the plot and small studies on the right. The plot shows a trend for smaller studies to give more positive results than the larger studies (correlation = 0.35, P < 0.05, or P = 0.012 by Egger's test[2]). This graph is similar to the funnel plot used in the meta-analysis of clinical trials, when a trend such as this is interpreted as a sign of publication bias.[3] This bias arises when a study is more likely to be written up and submitted to a journal and more likely to be accepted for publication if it reports positive results than if its results are inconclusive or negative. Since it is reasonable to assume that publication is more likely for larger (small s) than smaller (large s) studies, the problem of publication bias will be most evident among the smaller studies, as suggested by the figure. By "publication" we mean the whole process of selecting a study for review.

We reanalysed the results of the 37 epidemiological studies to allow for the trend evident in the figure. Our method describes the apparent relation between relative risk and study size by a curve. This gives a good fit to the observed points. The basic idea of the method is that there is no real relation between study outcome and study size, the relation that we observe is simply an artefact of the process of selecting these studies.

Our method has been published,[4] and further details are available from us on request. The estimated average relative risk depends on a statistical parameter that can be interpreted as the probability that a paper with a certain value of s is published (publication probability). If the publication probability is 1, all papers are published and so there is no possibility of publication bias; the relative risk is then estimated as 1.24 (24% risk excess), agreeing as expected with Hackshaw et al's result.[1] But smaller values of publication probability give smaller estimates of relative risk. We do not know how many unpublished studies have been carried out. Therefore there is no way of estimating the publication probability from any data: all we know is that there is a significant correlation in the funnel plot, so that some degree of publication bias is needed to explain this trend.

Table 1 gives the estimated relative risk for values of publication probability between 0.6 and 1, together with 95% confidence intervals and P values. The P value is less than 5% only when the publication probability is more than about 0.7. The indirect estimate of 19% excess risk derived from studies on biochemical markers (table 5 of Hackshaw et al's paper[1]) agrees with the epidemiological analysis when the publication probability is about 0.9.

Table 1

Estimated Relative Risk and Number of Unpublished Smaller and Larger Studies for Various Values of Publication Probability

Publication probability	Relative risk (95% CI)	P value	No of unpublished studies (*)	
			Small	Large
0.6	1.11 (0.97 to 1.27)	0.110	36	24
0.7	1.13 (1.00 to 1.27)	0.052	23	15
0.8	1.15 (1.03 to 1.28)	0.014	14	9
0.9	1.18 (1.07 to 1.31)	0.002	7	4
n	1.24 (1.13 to 1.36)	<0.001	0	0

(*) Smaller studies $s > 0.4$; larger studies s [is less than or equal to] 0.4.

For any given value of publication probability it is possible to estimate the number of studies which have been undertaken but not published. This is shown in the final two columns of Table 1. If the publication probability is 0.8 then there are a total of 23 unpublished studies so that the 37 selected ones represent a sample of 37/60 = 62% of all such studies that have been undertaken. If this is the case, then the excess risk is likely to be closer to 15% than 24%. . . .

Conclusions

Although the trend . . . seems clear, Bero et al suggest that the number of unpublished studies is unlikely to be large,[5] and so the problem of publication bias may be less severe here than in systematic reviews of other aspects of medicine. However, the possibility of publication bias cannot be ruled out altogether, and at least some publication bias is needed to explain the trend we found. Our results show that the publication probability does not have to fall much below 1.0 before there is quite a substantial reduction in the estimated risk.

References

1. Hackshaw AK, Law MR, Wald NJ. The accumulated evidence on lung cancer and environmental tobacco smoke. BMJ 1997;315:980–988.
2. Egger M, Smith GD, Schneider M, Minder C. Bias in meta-analysis detected by a simple graphical test. BMJ 1997;315:629–634.

3. Egger M, Smith GD. Misleading meta-analysis. BMJ 1995;310:752–754.
4. Copas JB. What works; selectivity models and meta analysis. J R Stat Soc Am 1999; 162:95–109.
5. Bero LA, Glantz SA, Rennie D. Publication bias and public health policy on environmental tobacco smoke. JAMA 1994;272:133–136.

POSTSCRIPT

Should Nonsmokers Be Concerned About the Effects of Secondhand Smoke?

In today's health-conscious society, many people seem to be more aware of what they eat, whether or not they get enough exercise, if they get an adequate amount of sleep, and how much stress they experience. Thus, it is only logical that people are also concerned about possible environmental threats to their health, such as secondhand smoking.

Whether or not secondhand smoke is injurious to nonsmokers is relevant because many businesses have adopted policies and many states have passed laws based on the premise that secondhand smoke is a health risk. A number of states restrict smoking in the workplace; most shopping malls prohibit smoking; the military has banned or restricted smoking in many of its facilities; some cities have even banned smoking in bars; many colleges prohibit smoking in residence halls; and numerous restaurants forbid smoking in their establishments.

The issue of smoking has also become a point of contention in child custody cases. It has been argued that parents who smoke around their children are unfit parents. Is smoking around children a form of child abuse? Should parental smoking be a consideration in child custody cases?

Increasingly, smokers are being isolated in society; they are pictured almost as social outcasts. There appears to be a growing contempt and disdain shown toward smokers. The emotionality of this issue often puts smokers on the defensive. This confrontational stance is not conducive to addressing the issue of smokers' rights in a constructive way.

In "Second Hand Smoke and Risk Assessment: What Was in It for the Tobacco Industry?" *Tobacco Control* (December 2001), Norbert Hirschhorn and Stella A. Bialous discuss how the tobacco industry tries to refute the claims regarding the harms related to secondhand smoke. An overview of the government's position and that of the tobacco industry on the issue of passive smoking is discussed in Elisa Ong and Stanton Glantz, "Tobacco Industry Efforts Subverting International Agency for Research on Cancer's Second-Hand Smoke Study," *The Lancet* (April 8, 2000). Scott Gottlieb, in "Study Confirms Passive Smoking Increases Coronary Heart Disease," *British Medical Journal* (1999), reviews numerous studies demonstrating that heart disease among nonsmokers is caused by passive smoking. A thorough examination of secondhand smoke can be found in a report by the California Environmental Protection Agency entitled *Health Effects of Exposure to Environmental Tobacco Smoke* (September 1997).

ISSUE 15

Is Total Abstinence the Only Choice for Alcoholics?

YES: Thomas Byrd, from *Lives Written in Sand: Addiction Awareness and Recovery Strategies* (Hallum, 1997)

NO: Heather Ogilvie, from "A Different Approach to Treating Alcoholism," *Consumers' Research Magazine* (June 2002)

ISSUE SUMMARY

YES: Professor of health Thomas Byrd maintains that Alcoholics Anonymous (AA) provides more effective treatment for alcoholics than psychiatrists, members of the clergy, or hospital treatment centers. Byrd contends that AA is the most powerful and scientific program, in contrast to all other therapies.

NO: Journalist Heather Ogilvie states that a number of studies support the concept that alcoholics can learn to drink moderately. Abstinence is not the only option for alcoholics, she argues, although it is important for alcoholics to identify the treatment that is best for them.

According to government figures, there are an estimated 10 to 20 million alcoholics in the United States. Cocaine addicts number between 250,000 and 1 million. Eating disorders, sexual addictions, compulsive gambling, excessive spending, and compulsive working affect millions more people. Knowing the best way to help people who engage in these compulsive or addictive behaviors is difficult. One way to control addictive behavior is to abstain from it. However, is total abstention, which is promoted by Alcoholics Anonymous (AA), the best or only viable treatment goal?

The concept of helping people with addictions can be approached from opposing perspectives. Some critics take the view that addiction occurs when people lose control over their addictive behavior. Moreover, there is always some kind of reward or payoff that fuels one's addictive behavior. The benefit may be security, sensation, or power, but as long as one or more of these benefits are experienced, people will not stop their behavior. Not everybody needs to abstain from unhealthy behaviors—only those people whose behaviors have reached the addiction stage. With some potentially addictive behaviors, such as eating or working, it is impossible to abstain. However, with behaviors that are not necessary for survival, such as alcohol consumption, abstention is, according to some viewpoints, the only path to follow.

If addiction leaves people powerless, as some professionals maintain, then the only way to gain personal power and control is through abstention. If alcoholics are powerless against alcohol, then they cannot drink simply for the enjoyment of alcohol; they will invariably drink to excess.

The abstinence model is currently the most popular approach for treating addiction. Abstinence is included in the 12-step model promoted by Alcoholics Anonymous and other self-help groups. Elements of this model include admitting to being powerless over one's addiction, accepting a higher power, and restructuring one's life. Opponents of the 12-step approach argue that it is not suitable for everyone and that it has not been proven effective. The idea of placing faith in a higher power, for example, is inconsistent with the values of many people, especially those who do not believe in the concept of a higher power. Another problem is that programs such as AA claim to be effective based on the testimonies of the program participants. However, because of the anonymity of people who attend or have attended AA meetings, follow-up studies are negligible.

A number of studies show that most people who stop addictive behavior do so on their own. Heroin addicts who quit using heroin generally do not go through any type of formal treatment. Likewise, the majority of individuals who quit smoking also stop without an organized program. Factors contributing to spontaneous remission are not well understood. It is believed that people stop self-destructive behaviors once they "hit bottom."

One criticism of the abstinence approach is that it stigmatizes people. The label "alcoholic" may deter people from receiving help because it connotes social deviance. Also, individuals who admit that they cannot control their own behavior are implying that they lack the strength to do so. That is, they are too weak to take care of their problems themselves. This stigma may prevent some people from seeking help.

In recent years alternative self-help groups to Alcoholics Anonymous have appeared. The Secular Organization for Sobriety (SOS), which does not emphasize belief in a higher power, is one such group for alcoholics. There is also Women for Sobriety/Men for Sobriety, which does not accept AA's disease model of addiction. Abstinence is a prominent aspect of this group, but overcoming alcoholism is based on self-acceptance and the role of love in relationships. Other programs are Rational Recovery (RR) and Moderation Management (MM). Unlike other models, RR and MM incorporate the belief that moderate alcohol use is possible.

In the selections that follow, Thomas Byrd makes the case that the abstinence-only, 12-step AA model is the only viable approach for overcoming alcoholism. Due to the findings of a number of studies, Heather Ogilvie supports moderate drinking. She maintains that treatment programs need to be matched to each person.

Thomas Byrd

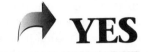 **YES**

Lives Written in Sand: Addiction Awareness and Recovery Strategies

Alcoholics Anonymous, What Works Best for Most

Finding the words to describe an organization which has saved millions of lives and countless relationships is difficult. Fundamentally, Alcoholics Anonymous provides hope to those in despair. The contents of the "program" focus on feelings, and how to cope with them throughout life. It is not an intellectual program, rather focusing on problem resolution and the subsequent spiritual rewards. The fellowship teaches a philosophy whose rewards are immediate and practical. AA is not a religion where prime benefits may be promised in the afterlife. It is a group of people who share a common problem and experience. Members are committed to living in the solution, not in the problem. Only a distinct minority of alcoholics are able to put their disease in remission and enter recovery. Most alcoholics do not recover. AA is a simple program for complicated people. New members frequently ask "how" does the program work. If you dissect the word, the first letter stands for an honest appraisal of the problem; the second letter refers to being openminded to new concepts from those in recovery; and the third letter stands for a willingness to devote the energy it takes to enter recovery. Members have committed two fundamental crimes. One is against the growth and development of another person. The second transgression is the indifference to the growth and development of self. Members are encouraged to make amends when possible and to carry the message to those still suffering. It is a program of attraction, not of promotion. The only requirement for membership is a desire to quit drinking.

Stopping drinking seems simple. You just don't drink. The problem is that there is a lot of failure. However, many of those who drink again will eventually stop drinking. Family members seem more likely to get their hopes up, only to suffer further discouragement if the alcoholic resumes drinking. The problem drinker seems to be less upset with relapse, probably because drinking has played such a major role in his or her life.

The physician may help identify the problem but is best at tending to physical problems. The alcoholic is generally not a desirable patient in most medical offices. Rejection of prescribed treatment, dishonesty, evasiveness, and rationalization of drinking are typical. Alcoholism is best treated by the specialist, a fellow recovering alcoholic, where there is no barrier of misunderstanding. Fears, guilt and self-condemnation and other psychiatric problems are minimized in this relationship.

Most rehabilitation programs encourage their patients to participate in Alcoholics Anonymous as part of an aftercare program. This organization exists because alcoholics need help and AA is more successful than psychiatry, the clergy, hospitals or jails in providing that needed aid. The organization works one day at a time for anyone who thinks help is needed. Membership is anonymous unless the member desires to drop the anonymity.

Alcoholics Anonymous was founded by two prominent men whose lives had been seriously affected by excessive drinking. They set out simply to survive. What they did was to try anything and everything, keeping what works and rejecting the rest.

John D. Rockefeller made a $5,000 contribution to the co-founders Bill Wilson and Dr. Bob Smith to help the fledging organization. Bill Wilson had grandiose ideas of establishing a network of recovery centers throughout the United States. These plans were stilled by Rockefeller's son. At a dinner presided over by Nelson Rockefeller he declined to make any further family donations to the organization, stating "this is too good to be destroyed by money." This decision ultimately led to the establishment of a non-profit organization, which became self-supporting through their own membership's contributions. Wilson acquiesced to the condition of the one time gift, and the wealthy and visionary New York politician salvaged the organization by replacing profit with humanity.

AA is at the basis of all good treatment simply because it is the most powerful, and because it is the most scientific of all therapies. The first months of membership in Alcoholics Anonymous are most critical. Getting to the first meeting is difficult. Continuing to participate in your own recovery is also difficult. There are erroneously preconceived attitudes that can form barriers to recovery. The alcoholic needs to keep attending until he or she wants to attend. In other words, they need to give it a chance.

Help from another alcoholic is something that can be depended on. Service to others is one of the components of recovery. The drinker is accepted without question into the AA group. The 12 steps of Alcoholics Anonymous constitute a recovery program that begins with the admission that the member is powerless over alcohol and that strength is needed from another source to overcome the problem. A searching, fearless moral self-inventory is also part of the program. Restitution to those who have been harmed gives the alcoholic emotional strength. Knowing there is help if a person wants to stop drinking can be vital.

There are no rules, no dues, and participation is voluntary. It is a fellowship based upon a common problem. Sponsors in the organization are available to give support to the newcomer. Suggestions on how to stay sober are exchanged between members. "Tomorrow may never come, yesterday is a canceled check." The alcoholic can't be cured, but is only an arrested case. If the alcoholic takes a drink again, the problem will surface and the member will be right back in the depths of active alcoholism. The objective is to stay sober today. Alcoholics understand this, simple as it is. Personality reorientation can come later. *The Big Book of Alcoholics Anonymous* is an excellent source of information. The author also recommends another book, authored by Nan Robertson. It's titled, *Getting Better: Inside AA,* published by Fawcett Crest, New York, New York, 1988.

Actions Among Equals

There are many approaches to the treatment of alcoholism, successful programs involve abstinence by whatever method it is achieved. Yet if one method of approaching a problem yields noticeably better and more striking results than others, then this method must contain some unique factor or factors that set it apart and form the basis of its supremacy.

"Alcoholics Anonymous is a fellowship of men and women who share their experience, strength and hope with each other that they may solve their common problem and help others to recover from alcoholism." The experiences of alcoholics are essentially the same, the theme is always the same: a progressive deterioration of the human personality. What then is the constant factor? What is AA's unique difference? I feel there are four distinctive characteristics that set apart this successful recovery program.

One of the answers lies in the manner in which this experience, strength and hope are shared and who is doing the sharing. Long before the average alcoholic walks through the doors of an AA meeting, help has been offered, in some instances even forced upon them. But these helpers are always superior beings. The moral responsibility of the alcoholic and the moral superiority of the helper, even though unstated, are always clearly understood. The overtone of parental disapproval and discipline in these authority figures is always present. Instead of the menacing, "This is what you should do," there is an instantly recognizable voice saying, "This is what I did." Therefore, one of the constant factors of a premium recovery program is where one alcoholic consciously and deliberately turned to another alcoholic, not to drink with, but to stay sober. I am personally convinced that the basic search of every human being is to find another human being, before whom one can stand completely without pretense or defense, and trust that person not to hurt them, because that person is exposed too. It is self-evident that the newcomer has been invited to share in the experience of recovery.

If the alcoholic responds to this invitation, the member then encounters a second unique factor: AA treats the symptoms first. The conviction that alcoholism is the symptom of deeper troubles. Even the cleverest diagnosis of these troubles is of little benefit if the patient dies. Autopsies do not benefit the persons upon whom they are performed. Total abstinence is the name of the game.

Recovery can only begin with a decision to stay away from the first drink. No one can or will make that decision for the ill. In fact, one soon further learns that if he makes the decision, no one can or will force fulfillment of the goal. There are reports of action taken, rather than rules not to be broken. Action is the magic word. There are steps to be taken which are suggested as a program for recovery. Quoting from Chapter Five of the book, *Alcoholics Anonymous: Step One,* "We admitted we were powerless over alcohol, that our lives had become unmanageable." The newcomer finally sees that they must take these Steps before being entitled to report on them. It is important to "utilize, not to analyze."

The desire to make this decision often results from what appears to be a third unique quality: The intuitive understanding the alcoholic receives, while compassionate, is not indulgent. The new member is not asked what they are thinking, rather they are told what they are thinking. The companion "therapists" already have their doctorates in the four fields where the alcoholic reigns supreme: phoniness, self-deception, evasion, and self-pity. There's not much point in trying to fool people who may have invented the game that's being played. In the end, the member begins to achieve honesty by default.

There is a fourth factor which I feel is significant, and that is the recovering alcoholic's infinite willingness to talk about alcoholism. Without the newcomer's ever becoming fully aware of it, the fascination with alcohol is literally talked to death. There is a reversal of form which the educational process takes. The participant is asked, not so much to learn new values, as to unlearn those that brought the seeker to the doors of recovery; not so much to adopt new goals, as to abandon old ones. The real answer is that this unique therapy occurs wherever two alcoholics meet: at home, at lunch, in the street, at work or school, and on the telephone. Members may faithfully attend meetings waiting for "something" to rub off, namely the "miracle of AA." The sad part about it is that "something" is rubbing off on them. Death. The real miracle is simply the willingness to act.

The formless flexibility of AA's principles as interpreted by their different adherents finally pushes the alcoholic into a stance where he must use only himself as a frame of reference for personal actions, and this in turn means there must be a willingness to accept the consequences of those actions. In my viewpoint, that is the definition of emotional maturity. True freedom lies in the realization and calm acceptance of the fact that there may very well be no perfect answer. The search for perfection is the hallmark of the neurotic. In the final analysis, we are all striving to be a better human beings. The future is that time when you will wish that you had used the time that you have now. Live in the present.

Other programs such as Rational Recovery and S.T.A.R.T. emphasize self-management and recovery training. Both programs do not incorporate the "higher power" aspect of the AA program, neither use a 12 Step format, reject the recovering concept, sponsorship, nor a "one at a time" philosophy.

Growth, a Day at a Time

Recovering people can become overwhelmed by new responsibilities. Sometimes too, members wonder why we can't ever be finished and just stop for awhile.

Feeling this way can mean it is time to stop and rest. The process of recovery has plateaus and detours along the way, and it's okay at times to take a break. But the "it's too much trouble" feeling also can be a signal that we need to pay more, not less, attention to ourselves and our recovery program.

Just as the chemically dependent person chooses not to drink or use drugs on a daily basis, so must a codependent person choose to continue recovery one day at a time. It is easy to see progress or lack of it in the big choices—to abstain from chemicals, to dissolve destructive relationships, to change careers. Less visible, but at least as important, are the little choices we all make every day.

Recovery means choosing to confront small instances of abusive behavior instead of letting them go. It means choosing to set boundaries to protect your time for recreation and rejuvenation. It means saying "no" to demands you can't meet. It means deciding every day to take care of yourself by paying attention to your needs for sleep, exercise, and healthy diet.

We can let all these choices overwhelm us if we focus on the "every single day for the whole rest of my life" aspect of them. Or we can take them one day at a time, recognizing that some days are easier than others. And we can remember that, as choosing growth becomes a pattern, it gets easier. Each seemingly insignificant daily choice is a separate affirmation that recovery is worth the trouble.

NO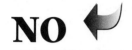

Heather Ogilvie

A Different Approach to Treating Alcoholism

Most Americans think of problem drinking as the disease of alcoholism. They believe the problem drinker is a sick person who requires treatment. The public is also under the impression that the primary evidence corroborating that a heavy drinker has the disease is his unwillingness to admit it—his denial. Treatments based on the classic disease concept of alcoholism, with its notions of irreversibility and loss of control, prescribe one goal: total abstinence.

Furthermore, when most Americans think of treatment for drinking problems, two things come to mind: 28-day inpatient recovery programs (such as the Betty Ford Center) and the "12 Step" program of Alcoholics Anonymous (AA). There are, however, at least a dozen alternative approaches to treatment that have been proven at least as effective as AA and inpatient programs (most of which are also based on the "12 Steps").

There is also another, strikingly different, concept of treatment that goes sharply counter to the now-traditional disease concept and its total abstinence prescription. This competing view, which has gained adherents in recent years, holds that what is called alcoholism is often a result of modifiable behavior patterns that are within the power of the individual to change, and that in such cases the optimum solution may well be, not total abstinence, but sensible moderation in drinking.

At issue in debates about these matters—and of urgent interest to anyone who must deal with them as they relate to family or friends—is which of these two different approaches is more effective in managing the problem. In some cases it may be one, in some cases it may be the other.

Since its founding in the mid-1930s, the fellowship of AA has undoubtedly saved countless lives. The people who are able to maintain sobriety through AA should certainly continue to attend meetings. But AA does not work for everyone. Various estimates suggest that more than half of the people who attend AA meetings drop out within the first year. Of the people who regularly attend meetings, only about 25% succeed in a goal of long-term abstinence. Most professionals performing alcohol-related research today aim to make available treatment options that can help the problem drinkers for whom AA does not work or does not appeal, as well as for those who never even try AA.

Unfortunately, few treatment options have better outcomes than AA: 25% is about the best any one program can boast. This is not great news, as it is estimated that a third of all problem drinkers cut down or quit drinking on their own. To even suggest that some problem drinkers recover on their own is heresy to the advocates of the disease model, as alcoholism is, by their definition, irreversible. They argue that those drinkers who appear to have reduced their drinking to moderate, nonproblematic amounts were never true alcoholics to begin with. This thinking is not particularly helpful, as it makes it impossible to tell a "true" alcoholic from a mere heavy drinker until serious damage has been done.

Are alcoholics diseased?   The idea of the irreversibility of alcoholism has been propagated by Alcoholics Anonymous with such phrases as "Once an alcoholic, always an alcoholic," "always recovering, never recovered," and "one drink, one drunk." Dr. D.L. Davies challenged that notion in his 1962 report that followed up on diagnosed "alcohol addicts" who had been treated in a London hospital seven to 10 years earlier. Dr. Davies noted in his report that seven out of the 93 male patients seemed to be drinking normally.

Nearly 80 studies had been published in the scientific literature prior to 1980, remonstrating that non-problem drinking is a stable treatment outcome. These studies reported rates of observed normal drinking among previously diagnosed alcoholics varying between 2% and 32%. The Rand Corporation assessed data collected from alcoholism treatment centers nationwide between 1970 and 1974, and found that the data suggested "the possibility that for some alcoholics, moderate drinking is not necessarily a prelude to a full relapse and that some alcoholics can return to moderate drinking with no greater chance of relapse than if they had abstained."

Dr. George Vaillant, analyzing data from Harvard Medical School's Study of Adult Development—which followed 660 men from 1940 to 1980, from their adolescence into late middle age—found that alcohol abuse among college-age men was a very poor predictor of heavy drinking at middle age. This finding supports other studies that have found that most college-age binge drinkers outgrow their heavy drinking behavior once they leave college and begin jobs or start families. K.M. Fillmore's follow-up of college students with drinking problems found that only 20% still had problems 20 years later. Dr. Vaillant wrote: "The course of alcohol abusers in the college sample contradicted my previous assertions that sustained alcohol abuse without abstinence is a progressive disorder."

The notion of loss of control also figures prominently in the classic disease model of alcoholism. Researchers have devised many experiments to assess whether a drinker has indeed experienced a physical loss of control following a "priming dose" of alcohol. An experiment conducted at Johns Hopkins University in 1971 tried to determine the incentives it would take to get an alcoholic not to drink. Researchers found that abstinence could be bought for as little as $7 and no more than $20 a day.

Other studies have replicated this finding. In a five-week experiment, inpatient subjects were given the option to drink up to 10 ounces of alcohol every weekday. Every other week, the subjects were given access to an improved environment—including telephone, television, pool table, games, and reading materials—provided they drank fewer than 5 ounces of alcohol for the day. If the subject exceeded that amount, he was put in a more Spartan environment and was not allowed to drink the following day. On the alternate weeks, the subjects remained in ascetic environments no matter how much they drank. All five subjects drank less during the weeks when privileges were available than during the weeks when no privileges were available.

A 1977 review of scientific literature cited 58 studies that have corroborated the finding that alcoholic drinking is a function of "environmental contingencies."

Can alcoholics control their drinking?   As the classic disease concept of addiction was eroded by reports of "normal" drinking among previously diagnosed alcoholics, researchers began to wonder whether "normal" or moderate drinking was a viable treatment goal for some alcoholics. The first widely cited report of successful training for controlled drinking appeared in 1970. Researchers applied behavioral therapy techniques in treating 31 alcoholics, after which 24 managed to drink in a "controlled" manner for periods ranging from four months to a little over one year (the length of follow-up). These results sparked an interest among other researchers who were eager to duplicate the study's outcome.

One study compared a controlled-drinking treatment program with one whose goal was abstinence. Roughly one-third of each treatment group was abstinent for a year following treatment. Immediately following treatment, the members of both groups who were not abstinent had cut down to approximately half their pre-treatment alcohol consumption. Three months later, the drinkers in the group trained for abstinence were drinking 70% as much as they had before treatment, while the drinkers in the controlled-drinking group had further reduced their consumption to about 20% of their pre-treatment levels. Over six months' time, the drinkers in the controlled-drinking group continued to reduce their consumption by a greater amount than did those in the abstinence-oriented group.

The most controversial controlled-drinking study was reported in 1972, by researchers Mark and Linda Sobell. Their 40 volunteer subjects were male inpatients at Patton State Hospital in California. The Sobells treated their controlled-drinking subjects with their own "Individualized Behavior Therapy" (IBT). The Sobells concluded: "Subjects who received the program of . . . IBT with a treatment goal of controlled drinking . . . functioned significantly better throughout the two-year follow-up period than did their respective control subjects . . . who received conventional abstinence-oriented treatment." They also noted: "Only subjects treated by IBT with a goal of controlled drinking successfully engaged in a substantial amount of limited, non-problem drinking during the two years of follow-up, and those subjects also had more abstinent days than subjects in any other group."[1]

Another controlled-drinking study involved randomly dividing 70 problem drinkers, who were each drinking roughly 70 ounces of alcohol per week, into an abstinence group and a controlled-drinking group (whose members were asked to abstain for the first four sessions of treatment). During the first three weeks, the members of the abstinence group drank much more than the controlled-drinking group and significantly more of the controlled-drinking group actually abstained. A year later, no significant difference existed between the groups, but the abstinence group had sought help more frequently than had the controlled drinkers.

Another study of male veterans divided participants into two groups: one receiving abstinence-oriented treatment and the other receiving controlled-drinking treatment. After six months, the severely dependent members of the controlled-drinking group experienced more days of heavy drinking than did those in the abstinence group; however, after one year, the differences disappeared, and at six years there were no significant differences between the two groups.

One might think that controlled-drinking treatment would appeal to every alcoholic, but this is not the case. In one study of 63 alcohol-dependent men given the choice in treatment goals between abstinence and controlled drinking, roughly 70% chose abstinence. Indeed, controlled-drinking studies have shown that most people who moderate their drinking eventually abstain. According to one researcher: "Our long-term follow-up research with clients treated with a moderation goal found that more wound up abstaining than moderating their drinking without problems."

Other researchers have reached similar conclusions. In one study, 75% of participants who reported previous drinking problems recovered without formal treatment (i.e., eliminated all problems resulting from overdrinking), and 50% achieved stable, moderate drinking. University of Washington Professor G. Alan Marlatt concludes: "Contrary to the progressive disease model, these findings indicate that a majority of individuals with drinking problems recover on their own . . . Even when they are trained in controlled drinking, many alcohol-dependent individuals choose abstinence. Over time, rates of abstinence (as compared to controlled drinking) tend to increase."

Who responds best to controlled-drinking therapy? In general, people under 40 who have suffered less severe dependence-related problems, people with stable marital or family relationships, people with stable employment, and women.

Younger people and those whose problems are not that severe are notoriously difficult to attract into conventional treatment and to persuade to adopt a goal of abstinence. One study found that young, unmarried men with a low level of dependence were 10 times more likely to relapse if they had adopted abstinence as a goal than if they had become moderate, nonproblem drinkers 18 months after treatment. Offering young drinkers the option of controlled-drinking counseling may therefore draw them into treatment sooner and thus prevent them from developing worse drinking problems down the line.

Even in cases in which abstinence is clearly the most pragmatic treatment goal (for example, for a 55-year-old male who has been in and out of detox wards for 35 years), offering the option of moderation may at least bring the person into treatment he might otherwise shun. Once the person is in treatment, a failed attempt at controlled drinking may prove the case for abstinence more persuasively than would a confrontational therapist citing disease-theory dogma for hours on end. As Dr. Marlatt puts it: "From a public health perspective, it makes sense to offer moderation-oriented programs to alcohol abusers and mildly dependent individuals as a means of increasing client recruitment and retention. Individuals who do not benefit from these programs can be "stepped up" to more intensive abstinence-oriented services."

How patient control can help recovery   In "12 Step" recovery programs, the client is told (a) his drinking is beyond his control—in fact, he is powerless against it, (b) his condition is irreversible and incurable, and (c) the success of the treatment depends solely on a Higher Power. While that Higher Power may be the god of any religion, the group, or another person, it must be a power other than the individual. A person who prefers to see himself as the effective power, therefore, would not find AA helpful in improving his sense of self-efficacy, his (supposedly absent) self-control, or his will power not to take another drink.

Disease theory proponents argue that attributing the drinker's problems to a disease outside her control frees her from the guilt and stigma of moral weakness. It clears her conscience enough to admit the problem and not be ashamed to seek help.

But doesn't the disease perspective merely swap one stigma—that of moral failing—for another—that of being diseased? By assigning responsibility for the problem to something outside the person, the disease perspective tells him, in effect, that he is powerless and therefore helpless. The person learns to think of himself as a victim.

Stanton Peele, one of the most outspoken critics of conventional addiction treatment, has observed that recovering alcoholics are able to "use their addicted identity to explain all their previous problems without actually doing anything concrete to improve their performance." He accuses traditional treatment of ignoring "the rest of the person's problems in favor of blaming them all on the addiction" and limiting clients' "human contacts primarily to other recovering alcoholics who only reinforce their preoccupation with drinking;" in effect, trapping them "in a world inhabited by fellow disease sufferers" until they "feel comfortable only with others in exactly the same plight."

Wouldn't it be more productive for the drinker to think he has a personality weakness he can overcome, rather than a lifelong disease he can never shake? Might not the shame of a moral failure be put to good use? Some people have wondered: Why shouldn't alcoholics feel ashamed of their behavior? Wouldn't a greater sense of shame have prevented the behavior in the first place?

What good is it to tell someone he is sick and powerless, but then send him to a self-help group, rather than to a doctor, for treatment? In his book, *Heavy Drinking,* Herbert Fingarette asks: "If the alcoholic's ailment is a disease that causes an inability to abstain from drinking, how can a program insist on voluntary abstention as a condition for treatment? (And if alcoholics who enter these programs do voluntarily abstain—as in fact they generally do—then of what value is the disease notion of loss of control?)"

The danger of constantly telling people that they have no control is that eventually they may come to believe it. Falling off the wagon thus only proves to the drinker what he has been told: that he has no control. Henceforth, what is his motivation to keep attending AA or to seek further treatment? Treatment professionals who advocate "12 Step" programs typically regard relapse not as a failure of treatment, but as a failure of the patient to comply with treatment. Given these conditions, it is no wonder so few people are able to maintain long-term sobriety through "12 Step" recovery programs.

On the other hand, when you tell someone that, with time and effort, he can change his habits, make improvements to troublesome aspects of his life, and reverse the course of his drinking problems, he will probably be more willing to give treatment a try and recognize the signs of his progress. By showing him he has choices for treatment, you provide more hope and give him back a sense of control simply by allowing him to choose.

Note

1. Mary Pendery, the director of an alcohol-treatment center in Southern California, did an extensive follow-up investigation of the Sobells' study. Ten years after the Sobell study, her findings were published in the respected journal *Science*. She and her co-authors all but accused the Sobells of fraud. Soon after, in March 1953, *60 Minutes* aired a segment on the Sobell study, interviewing Mary Pendery but not the Sobells. In response to media attacks, the Sobells asked the Addiction Research Foundation in Toronto to set up an independent committee to investigate the charges against them. The committee's findings became known as the Dickens Report.

   Among its many criticisms, the Dickens Report faulted Pendery's study for citing data out of context. Pendery reported, for instance, that four of the 20 subjects who received controlled-drinking training had died as the result of alcohol-related problems. The Dickens Report revealed, however, that Pendery had failed to point out that the deaths occurred between six and 11 years after treatment, and that more—in fact, six—of the 20 subjects in the abstinence-oriented control group had died during the same period. The Dickens Report found accusations that the Sobells had suppressed certain findings to be completely without merit and found no reasonable cause to doubt the scientific or personal integrity of the Sobells. A congressional investigation into the matter supported this conclusion.

POSTSCRIPT

Is Total Abstinence the Only Choice for Alcoholics?

The fundamental question here is, Must alcoholics totally abstain from alcohol use or can they benefit from other types of treatment? This issue was initially raised in the 1970s, when Linda and Mark Sobell presented research showing that alcoholics who were taught to drink socially were less likely to relapse than people who were told to abstain from alcohol. (This study was subsequently criticized for its methodology.) In another study supported by the RAND Corporation in the 1970s, it was found that the majority of alcoholics who went through formal treatment were drinking moderately or occasionally up to 18 months after treatment. Most did not resume their abusive use of alcohol. A criticism of this study was that it did not follow those in treatment long enough—a four-year follow-up revealed that many had relapsed.

Many people who attempt to completely stop addictive behaviors fail. If a person tries several times to abstain from drinking alcohol (or other self-destructive behaviors) and cannot stop, perhaps other forms of treatment may be worth pursuing. However, moderation as a treatment goal may not prove to be productive because alcohol—the central element to the addiction—is still present in the alcoholic's life.

Rather than trying to identify the one best type of treatment for alcoholics, it may be better to match people with the type of treatment that is best for them. Kimberly Walitzer and Gerard Connors review various forms of alcohol treatment in "Treating Problem Drinking," *Alcohol Research and Health* (vol. 23, no. 2, 1999). Keith Humphrey, in "Professional Interventions That Facilitate 12-Step Self-Help Group Involvement," *Alcohol Research and Health* (vol. 23, no. 2, 1999), discusses the benefit of Alcoholics Anonymous when used in conjunction with other types of therapy. Two articles that are critical of Alcoholics Anonymous are Stanton Peele's "All Wet: The Gospel of Abstinence and Twelve-Step, Studies Show, Is Leading American Alcoholics Astray," *The Sciences* (March/April 1998) and Michael Lemanski's "The Tenacity of Error in the Treatment of Addiction," *The Humanist* (May/June 1997).

A number of drugs, such as Antabuse, Buspar, and Naltrexone, have been used to treat alcoholism. The effectiveness of the drug Naltrexone is discussed in the article "Naltrexone Treatment for Alcohol Dependence," by R. K. Fuller and E. Gordis, *New England Journal of Medicine* (December 13, 2001).

ISSUE 16

Should Needle Exchange Programs Be Supported?

YES: David Vlahov and Benjamin Junge, from "The Role of Needle Exchange Programs in HIV Prevention," *Public Health Reports* (June 1998)

NO: Office of National Drug Control Policy, from "Needle Exchange Programs: Are They Effective?" *ONDCP Bulletin No. 7* (July 1992)

ISSUE SUMMARY

YES: In their review of various studies, David Vlahov, professor of epidemiology and medicine, and Benjamin Junge, evaluation director for the Baltimore Needle Exchange Program, found that needle exchange programs successfully reduced the transmission of the virus that causes acquired immunodeficiency syndrome (AIDS). In addition, many people who participated in needle exchange programs reduced their drug use and sought drug abuse treatment.

NO: The Office of National Drug Control Policy, an executive agency that determines policies and objectives for the U.S. drug control program, sees needle exchange programs as an admission of defeat and a retreat from the ongoing battle against drug use, and it argues that compassion and treatment are needed, not needles.

Both selections presented here refer to intravenous drug use as a factor in the escalating incidence of acquired immunodeficiency syndrome (AIDS). One point needs to be clarified: Any type of drug injection, whether it is intravenous (mainlining), intramuscular, or just below the surface of the skin (skin popping), can result in the transmission of AIDS. Technically, what is transmitted is not AIDS but the human immunodeficiency virus (HIV), which ultimately leads to the development of AIDS.

Until a cure for AIDS is found or a vaccine against HIV has proven to be effective, the relationship between AIDS and injecting drugs will remain a cause of great concern. According to the Centers for Disease Control and Prevention (CDC), approximately one-third of AIDS cases in the United States are directly or indirectly associated with drug injection, and half of all new HIV infections occur among users of injected drugs.

No one disagrees that the spread of AIDS is a problem and that the number of people who inject drugs is also a problem. The issue that needs to be addressed is, What is the best course of action to take to reduce drug injection and the transmission of AIDS? Is it better to set up more drug treatment facilities, as the Office of National Drug Control Policy (ONDCP) suggests, or to allow people who inject drugs access to clean needles?

One concern of needle exchange opponents is that endorsement of these programs conveys the wrong message concerning drug use. Instead of discouraging drug use, they feel that such programs merely teach people how to use drugs or encourage drug use. Needle exchange advocates point to studies showing that these programs have not resulted in an increase in intravenous drug users. Other studies indicate that many drug users involved in needle exchange programs drop out and that drug users who remain in the programs are not as likely to share needles in the first place.

Proponents of needle exchange programs argue that HIV is easily transmitted when needles are shared and that something needs to be done to stem the practice. Opponents argue that whether or not needle exchange programs are available, needles will be shared. Three reasons cited by drug users for sharing needles are (1) they do not have access to clean needles, (2) they do not own their own needles, and (3) they cannot afford to buy needles. If clean needles were readily available, would drug addicts necessarily use them? Some studies show that people who inject drugs are concerned about contracting AIDS and will alter their drug-taking behavior if presented with a viable alternative.

Although needle exchange programs may result in the use of clean needles and encourage people to obtain treatment, they do not get at the root cause of drug addiction. Drug abuse and many of its concomitant problems stem from inadequate or nonexistent employment opportunities, unsafe neighborhoods, underfunded schools, and insufficient health care. Some argue that until these underlying causes of drug abuse are addressed, stopgap measures like needle exchange programs should be implemented. Needle exchange programs, however, may forestall the implementation of other programs that could prove to be more helpful.

Needle exchange programs generate a number of legal and social questions. Because heroin and cocaine are illegal, giving needles to people for the purpose of injecting these drugs contributes to illegal behavior. Should people who are addicted to drugs be seen as criminals or as victims who need compassion? Should drug users, especially drug addicts, be incarcerated or treated? The majority of drug users involved with needle exchange programs are members of minority groups. Could needle exchange programs promote the continuation of drug use and, hence, the enslavement of minorities?

In the following selections, David Vlahov and Benjamin Junge address the benefits of needle exchange programs and respond to criticisms of these programs. The ONDCP reports on the inadequacies of previous research regarding needle exchange programs and argues that these programs exacerbate drug abuse problems by facilitating drug use.

David Vlahov and Benjamin Junge 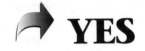 **YES**

The Role of Needle Exchange Programs in HIV Prevention

Synopsis

Injecting drug users (IDUs) are at high risk for infection by human immunodeficiency virus (HIV) and other blood-borne pathogens. In the United States, IDUs account for nearly one-third of the cases of acquired immunodeficiency syndrome (AIDS), either directly or indirectly (heterosexual and perinatal cases of AIDS where the source of infection was an IDU). IDUs also account for a substantial proportion of cases of hepatitis B (HBV) and hepatitis C (HCV) virus infections. The primary mode of transmission for HIV among IDUs is parenteral, through direct needle sharing or multiperson use of syringes. Despite high levels of knowledge about risk, multiperson use of needles and syringes is due primarily to fear of arrest and incarceration for violation of drug paraphernalia laws and ordinances that prohibit manufacture, sale, distribution, or possession of equipment and materials intended to be used with narcotics. It is estimated that in 1997 there were approximately 110 needle exchange programs (NEPs) in North America. In part, because of the ban on the use of Federal funds for the operation of needle exchange, it has been difficult to evaluate the efficacy of these programs. This [selection] presents data from the studies that have evaluated the role of NEPs in HIV prevention.

Evidence for the efficacy of NEPs comes from three sources: (1) studies originally focused on the effectiveness of NEPs in non-HIV blood-borne infections, (2) mathematical modeling of data on needle exchange on HIV seroincidence, and (3) studies that examine the positive and negative impact of NEPs on HIV and AIDS. Case-control studies have provided powerful data on the positive effect of NEPs on reduction of two blood-borne viral infections (HBV and HCV). For example, a case-control study in Tacoma, Washington, showed that a six-fold increase in HBV and a seven-fold increase in HCV infections in IDUs were associated with nonuse of the NEP.

The first federally funded study of needle exchange was an evaluation of the New Haven NEP, which is legally operated by the New Haven Health Department. Rather than relying on self-report of reduced risky injection drug use,

From David Vlahov and Benjamin Junge, "The Role of Needle Exchange Programs in HIV Prevention," *Public Health Reports* (June 1998). Washington, D.C.: U.S. Government Printing Office, 1998. References omitted.

this study utilized mathematical and statistical modeling, using data from a syringe tracking and testing system. Incidence of HIV infection among needle exchange participants was estimated to have decreased by 33% as a result of the NEP.

A series of Government-commissioned reports have reviewed the data on positive and negative outcomes of NEPs. The major reports are from the National Commission on AIDS; the U.S. General Accounting Office; the Centers for Disease Control/University of California; and the National Academy of Sciences. The latter two reports are used in this [selection].

The aggregated results support the positive benefit of NEPs and do not support negative outcomes from NEPs. When legal restrictions on both purchase and possession of syringes are removed, IDUs will change their syringe-sharing behaviors in ways that can reduce HIV transmission. NEPs do not result in increased drug use among participants or the recruitment of first-time drug users.

⚜

Injecting drug users (IDUs) are at risk for human immunodeficiency virus (HIV) and other blood-borne infections. The principal mode of transmission is parenteral through multiperson use of needles and syringes. The mechanism of contamination is through a behavior called registering, whereby drug users draw back on the plunger of a syringe after venous insertion to ensure venous placement before injecting drug solutions. Strategies to prevent or reduce parenteral transmission of HIV infection need to focus on reducing, if not eliminating altogether, the multiperson use of syringes that have been contaminated. The principle underlying these strategies has been stated clearly in the recommendations of the 1995 National Academy of Sciences Report on preventing HIV infection as follows: "For injection drugs the once only use of sterile needles and syringes remains the safest, most effective approach for limiting HIV transmission." This principle was echoed in the 1996 American Medical Association's booklet *A Physician's Guide to HIV Prevention* and in 1995 in the booklet of the U.S. Preventive Services Task Force *Guide to Clinical Preventive Services*. More recently, this principle has been codified in a multiagency *HIV Prevention Bulletin*.

The first line of prevention is to encourage IDUs to stop using drugs altogether. However, for drug users who cannot or will not stop drug use, owing to their addiction, other approaches are needed. Two major approaches have been developed to provide sufficient sterile needles and syringes to drug users to reduce transmission of HIV and other blood-borne infections. The first is needle exchange programs (NEPs), and the second is modification of syringe prescription and paraphernalia possession laws or ordinances. Hereafter, we will refer to the latter as deregulation of prescription and paraphernalia laws.

NEPs   There are now more than 110 NEPs in the United States. By comparison, there are 2000 or more outlets in Australia and hundreds in Great Britain. The exchange programs are varied in terms of organizational characteristics. Some operate out of fixed sites; others are mobile. Some are legally authorized; others are not. Funding, staffing patterns, policies, and hours of operation vary considerably among the different programs.

Despite different organizational characteristics, the basic description and goals of NEPs are the same. They provide sterile needles in exchange for contaminated or used needles to increase access to sterile needles and to remove contaminated syringes from circulation in the community. Equally important, needle exchanges are there to establish contact with otherwise hard-to-reach populations to deliver health services, such as HIV testing and counseling, as well as referrals to treatment for drug abuse.

Over time, numerous questions have arisen about NEPs, such as whether these programs encourage drug use and whether they result in lower HIV incidence. These questions have been summarized and examined in a series of published reviews and Government-sponsored reports. The Government-sponsored reports include those from the National Commission on AIDS in 1991, the U.S. General Accounting Office in 1993, the University of California and Centers for Disease Control (CDC) Report in 1993, and the National Academy of Sciences in 1995.

As to whether NEPs increase drug use among participants, the 1993 California report examined published reports that involved comparison groups (Table 1). Because the sampling and data collection methods varied considerably among studies, the summary has been reduced here to show whether needle exchange was associated with a beneficial, neutral, or adverse effect. Of the eight reports that examined the issue of injection frequency, three showed a reduction in injection frequency, four showed a mixed or neutral effect (no change), and one initially recorded an increase in injection frequency.

Table 1

Summary of Studies of Behavioral Change Within NEPs

Outcome measures	Beneficial NEP effect	Mixed or neutral NEP effect	Adverse NEP effect
Drug risk:			
Sharing frequency	10	4	–
Give away syringes	3	1	1
Needle cleaning	3	1	–
Injection frequency	3	4	1
Sex risk:			
Number of partners	2	1	–
Partner choice	1	1	–
Condom use	1	1	1

In terms of attracting youth or new individuals into NEPs in the United States, programs that have no minimum age restriction have reported that recruitment of participants who are younger than 18 years old was consistently less than 1%; this low rate of use was noted in studies that were conducted in San Francisco and New Haven and in our recent studies in Baltimore. However, recent studies also have shown that new injectors who are adolescent or young adults also are at extremely high risk for HIV infection. In response to this problem, Los Angeles has recently developed an NEP specifically directed at new initiates into injection drug use (P. Kerndt, personal communication, February 10, 1996).

Another question is whether the presence of NEPs in a community conveys a message to youth that condones and encourages drug use. This issue is particularly difficult to study. In 1993, the authors of the University of California-CDC report examined longitudinal national drug use indicator data (data from the DAWN Project), which monitors emergency-room mentions of drug-abuse-related admissions. Comparisons of data before and after the opening of needle exchanges and between cities with and without NEPs showed no significant trends.

The only systematic study to date of trends in drug use within a community following the opening of a needle exchange comes from Amsterdam. Using data on admissions to treatment for drug abuse, Buning and colleagues noted that the proportion of drug users younger than 22 declined from 14% in 1981 to 5% in 1986; the NEP opened in 1984. The opening of the needle exchange increased neither the proportion of drug users overall nor the proportion of those younger than 22 years. Thus, the currently available data argue against the belief that needle exchange encourages drug use.

Another issue is whether needle exchanges will result in more contaminated syringes found on the street. If a needle exchange is designed as a one-for-one exchange, the answer is no. In Baltimore, a carefully designed systematic street survey showed no increase in discarded needles following the opening of an NEP. An update following two years of surveys has shown a similar trend of no increase.

Findings of behavioral change associated with needle exchange are varied. A number of published studies have compared levels of risky behavior among IDUs participating and those not participating in needle exchange. As the University of California-CDC report noted, methods varied considerably among these published reports, so that the summary here (Table 1) sorts the studies into whether and how the needle exchange has shown an effect—risk reduction, no effect, or adverse effect.

In terms of drug risks, Table 1 shows that there were 14 studies that looked at the frequency of needle sharing, the most dangerous behavior in terms of drug-related risk of HIV transmission. In those studies, 10 showed a reduction in needle sharing frequency, four had no effect, and none showed any increase in needle sharing.

Similar trends were noted for the practice of giving away syringes: three showed a reduction in this practice, one no effect, and one an increase. Three out of four studies reporting on this needle cleaning showed a positive effect.

Finally, in terms of sexual risk behavior, few studies overall have examined the impact of needle exchange on sexual risks. Sexual transmission among IDUs is an important area that merits further investigation.

The next question about NEPs is whether such programs actually reduce the incidence of HIV infection in IDUs. While the idea of using only sterile needles makes the question of efficacy seem obvious, the real question centers on how effective the programs are in practice and how subject such programs are to the ubiquitous "law of unintended consequences."

Studies of the impact of needle exchange on the incidence of HIV infection in the United States are few, primarily because funding for such evaluations is relatively recent and sample size requirements are large. The first study (shown in Table 2) was conducted by Hagan and colleagues in Tacoma, Washington. In that city, the prevalence and, therefore, the incidence of HIV were extremely low. A needle exchange was initiated with the goal of maintaining HIV incidence at a low level. Two case-controlled analyses used hepatitis B and hepatitis C virus infection as outcome variables because the epidemiology of these two viruses is similar to HIV, although transmission of hepatitis is more efficient than HIV. In these studies, needle exchange participation was associated with more than an 80% reduction in the incidence of hepatitis infection. Over time, HIV prevalence has not risen.

Table 2

Impact of NEPs on Incidence of Blood-Borne Infections in the United States

Author	City	Design	Outcome	Percent reduction
Hagen et al.	Tacoma	Case-control	HBV HCV	83 86
Kaplan et al.	New Haven	Mathematical modeling based on testing of syringes returned to NEP	HIV	33
Des Jarlais et al.	New York	Prospective study of seroconversion; NEP is external cohort and IDUs in neighboring regions	HIV	70

In terms of HIV studies, Kaplan and Heimer at Yale utilized information about HIV test results of washes from syringes returned to the New Haven Needle Exchange Program by constructing an elegant statistical model to estimate that needle exchange reduced HIV incidence by 33%. This model has been reviewed by three independent statistical reviewers who have judged the model sound in estimates as reasonable or even conservative.

More recently, Des Jarlais and colleagues from New York City published a prospective study of seroconversion between attendees and nonattendees of needle exchange. In this study, they estimated a 70% reduction in HIV incidence. Several other studies are ongoing in San Francisco, Chicago, and Baltimore, but their findings are too preliminary to present at this time.

In terms of HIV seroconversion studies from needle exchanges with comparison groups from outside the United States, data are available from Amsterdam and Montreal. In Amsterdam, data from a case-control study nested within an ongoing cohort study identified a slightly increased risk of HIV seroconversion with needle exchange use. However, when the analyses were examined by calendar time, the needle exchange was initially protective, but the association reversed over time. The authors attributed their results to the needle exchange losing lower risk users to pharmacy access over time, leaving a core of highest risk users within the exchange.

More recently a study was published using a case-control analysis nested within a cohort study in Montreal. Of 974 HIV-seronegative subjects followed an average of 22 months, 89 subjects seroconverted. Consistent use of needle exchange compared with nonuse was associated with an odds ratio for HIV seroconversion of 10.5, which remained elevated even during multivariate adjustment. The authors concluded that NEPs were associated with higher HIV rates and speculated that the exchange may have facilitated formation of new social networks that might have permitted broader HIV transmission. In an accompanying commentary, Lurie criticized the Montreal study saying that the more likely explanation for the findings was that powerful selection forces attracted the most risky IDUs as evidenced by substantial differences in the baseline data for the exchangers *vs.* nonexchangers: exchangers had higher injection frequencies, were less likely to have a history of drug abuse treatment, were more likely to share needles and use shooting galleries, and had a high HIV prevalence. Lurie attributed the differences to the hours and locations of the exchange (late night in the red-light district) attracting only a select subset of users.

In Vancouver, Strathdee reported on HIV incidence in a cohort of IDUs of whom 92% were enrolled in needle exchange. The incidence of 18.6 (100 person-years) was associated with low education, unstable housing, commercial sex, borrowing needles, injecting with others, and frequent use of needle exchange. The related study by Archibald and colleagues demonstrates a selection of higher risk individuals into needle exchange in Vancouver.

The point to consider is what accounts for the discrepancy between the U.S. and non-U.S. studies. From a methodological perspective, selection factors could be operating. For example, in Vancouver, a study compared characteristics of exchangers with those of nonexchangers, or high frequency *vs.* low frequency exchangers; this study showed that the high frequency exchangers were more likely to engage in high risk activities. While the Vancouver study showed that self-selection into needle exchange results in leaving a comparison group that is not similar in other respects, the data do suggest that needle exchange has been successful in recruiting high risk users.

At another level, the U.S. studies involve evaluation of a needle exchange in comparison with people who do not have access to an NEP or to sterile needles through other sources. In contrast, the Canadian and Dutch studies have involved comparisons that do have an alternative source for sterile needles, principally through pharmacies; their studies may have selected into the needle exchange the people who cannot get needles from pharmacies. The effectiveness of NEPs depends on understanding who constitutes the comparison group.

More recently, an ecological analysis was published with serial HIV seroprevalence data for 29 cities with NEPs and 52 cities without such programs. The results, although subject to a possible ecological fallacy, indicated a 5.8% decline in HIV prevalence per year in cities with NEPs and a 5.9% increase in cities without exchange.

Deregulating syringe prescription and paraphernalia laws   In 1992, Connecticut changed the state laws to permit sale and possession of up to 10 syringes at a time. The CDC, in conjunction with the state of Connecticut, conducted initial studies that examined whether IDUs utilized pharmacies and discovered that they did. The CDC and the state of Connecticut then examined how pharmacy utilization affected needle-sharing behaviors in the two samples of IDUs that were interviewed: 52% reported sharing needles before the law changed, and 31% did so after the law changed. While these data are encouraging, data on needle disposal and HIV incidence are not yet available.

Summary

Access to sterile needles and syringes is an important, even vital, component of a comprehensive HIV prevention program for IDUs. The data on needle exchange in the United States are consistent with the conclusion that these programs do not encourage during use and that needle exchanges can be effective in reducing HIV incidence. Other data show that NEPs help people stop drug use through referral to drug treatment programs. The studies outside of the United States are important for reminding us that unintended consequences can occur. While changes in needle prescription and possession laws and regulations have shown promise, the identification of organizational components that improve or hinder effectiveness of needle exchange and pharmacy-based access are needed.

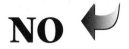

Office of National Drug Control Policy

Needle Exchange Programs: Are They Effective?

When President Bush took office, most Americans regarded the use of illegal drugs as the most serious problem confronting the Nation. Since that time, the Nation has made substantial progress in reducing drug use. But now, in response to the AIDS epidemic, there are those who are ready to sound a retreat in the war against drugs by distributing clean needles to intravenous drug users in the hope that this will slow the spread of AIDS. I believe this would be a serious mistake. We must not lose sight of the fact that illegal drugs still pose a serious threat to our Nation. Nor can we allow our concern for AIDS to undermine our determination to win the war on drugs.

In 1988, 14.5 million Americans and nearly two million young people, aged 12–17, were using drugs. In response to the devastation caused by drug use, the President boldly announced the first National Drug Control Strategy in a televised address to the Nation in 1989. That Strategy was a landmark document. Not only did it establish a coherent, coordinated policy for the national effort against drugs, but it committed unprecedented new resources for fighting drug use.

The Strategy is working; the use of illegal drugs by Americans is declining. Between 1988 and 1991, almost two million fewer Americans were using drugs, a drop of almost 13 percent. And by 1991, about half a million fewer young people were current users of drugs, a drop of 27 percent. Since 1985, the number of Americans using drugs has fallen by over 10 million.

Key to the success of the Strategy has been increasing Americans' intolerance of illicit drugs. But, for those already caught in the deadly web of addiction, we must act with compassion. The Administration therefore vigorously supports efforts to provide effective drug treatment to those who want it and can benefit from it, and has increased funding for drug treatment from $1.1 billion in 1989 to a proposed $2.1 billion for 1993.

Our gains against drug use have been hard-won, and this is no time to jeopardize them by instituting needle exchange programs. Despite all the arguments made by proponents of needle exchange, there is no getting around the fact that distributing needles facilitates drug use and undercuts the credibility

From Office of National Drug Control Policy, Executive Office of the President, "Needle Exchange Programs: Are They Effective?" *ONDCP Bulletin No. 7* (July 1992). Washington, D.C.: U.S. Government Printing Office, 1992. Some notes omitted.

320 ISSUE 16 / Should Needle Exchange Programs Be Supported?

of society's message that using drugs is illegal and morally wrong. And just as important, there is no conclusive evidence that exchange programs reduce the spread of AIDS.

The Administration's concerns about needle exchange are widely shared. Recently, for example, the Congress extended a prohibition on the use of most Federal drug treatment funds to support needle exchange programs. And in June 1992, the National Association of State Alcohol and Drug Abuse Directors informed every member of Congress of its support for continuing this prohibition. Also, in February 1992, the National District Attorneys Association passed an official policy position condemning needle exchange.

The Administration will continue to work with the Congress, and with State and local officials to support alternatives to needle exchange, including expanded and improved drug treatment and aggressive outreach programs. These efforts will provide addicts with something that needle exchange programs cannot: hope and a chance for real recovery from drug addiction.

Needle Exchange Programs in the United States

Intravenous drug use and HIV/AIDS[1]   Intravenous drug users in the United States are one of the groups most at risk for contracting AIDS. AIDS prevention and education programs, which have had a measurable effect on the behavior of other high-risk groups, have not been so successful with intravenous drug users. In fact, the Centers for Disease Control estimates that about 32 percent of the diagnosed AIDS cases in this country, involving nearly 70,000 individuals, resulted from intravenous drug use or sexual contact with intravenous drug users. In addition, intravenous drug use is responsible for half of the AIDS cases among women.

AIDS is spread among intravenous drug users primarily through the sharing of hypodermic syringes, or "needles," and other drug-using paraphernalia (e.g., cotton and water) that have been contaminated with the AIDS virus, and secondarily by high-risk sexual behavior. Thus, intravenous drug users pose a threat not only to themselves, but to their sexual partners and offspring as well. In fact, 58 percent of all reported pediatric AIDS cases are associated with intravenous drug use.

Faced with the growing link between intravenous drug use and AIDS, some cities and communities have instituted or are contemplating programs to provide clean needles to addicts in the hope that this will help reduce the sharing of needles, and hence, the spread of the HIV virus.

Needle exchange programs   Needle exchange programs provide free, clean needles to intravenous drug users in an attempt to reduce the likelihood that they will share needles with other users. Some programs operate from fixed locations such as city government offices or pharmacies. Others are mobile, using outreach workers in vans, on foot, and at temporary sites. Some programs provide a new needle only in exchange for an old one, while others provide at least one "starter" needle. Most programs limit the number of needles that can be exchanged at any one time. Some programs provide needles to persons only if they have a verifiable history of drug injection, and most have age limits. Most programs are privately funded; others are supported with State or municipal government funds.[2]

Needle exchange programs also differ in scope. Some only exchange needles, while others are more comprehensive and provide counseling, referral to testing and drug treatment, bleach to clean needles, and safer sex information.

Needle exchange and the law In 39 States and the District of Columbia, sterile needles can be purchased inexpensively without a prescription in many pharmacies.[3] In most of the remaining 11 States, a prescription is required. However, four of the 11 are considering legislation that would broaden access to needles. Only one State, Alabama, is considering legislation that would restrict accessibility by making it a criminal offense for those other than licensed pharmacists or practitioners to sell needles.

Forty-nine States, the District of Columbia, and numerous local jurisdictions have laws to prohibit the sale and distribution of drug paraphernalia. The majority of these laws conform with the Model Drug Paraphernalia Act, which was released by the Drug Enforcement Administration in August 1979. The Model Drug Paraphernalia Act would make it a crime to possess, deliver, or manufacture needles with the intent to violate anti-drug laws. Therefore, operating needle exchange programs may be a violation of the law in many States and local jurisdictions. Furthermore, operating such programs may subject municipalities to civil liability in some jurisdictions.

What the research shows Several studies on the efficacy of needle exchange programs have been conducted in the United States and abroad. Some of these studies have been cited by proponents of needle exchange as evidence that such programs work. However, all of the needle exchange programs studied have yielded either ambiguous or discouraging results. Moreover, the methodology used to conduct these studies has been flawed. For example:

- Many studies make long-term projections of addict behavior based on short-term results;
- Many use a small or insufficient sample size and then project results to larger populations;
- Despite claims that needle sharing was reduced, none of the studies conducted objective tests (e.g., analysis of blood types on returned needles) to determine whether needles were shared;
- Most do not use valid comparison or control groups; and
- Most have program staff, rather than independent evaluators, conduct client interviews on which the findings of the studies are based.

There are four other significant problems with the research. First, needle exchange programs are plagued by high levels of attrition. Programs may have initial contact with intravenous drug users who are at the highest risk of sharing needles and contracting AIDS, but only as few as 20 percent may return for a second or third visit.

Second, needle exchange programs tend to attract and retain a self-selecting group of older, long-term intravenous drug users who are less likely to share needles than less experienced, more promiscuous users. Therefore, positive reports on the effectiveness of exchange programs may be due *more* to the behavior of this less risky subset of the intravenous drug using population and *less* to the availability of clean needles.

Third, programs offering needle exchange often provide bleach for cleaning needles, referrals to testing and treatment, and other services. However, the research conducted to date has not isolated the specific impact that exchanging needles has had on reducing the transmission of AIDS compared with these other factors. Most researchers have simply attributed positive results to needle exchange.

The fourth weakness with the research relates to the dynamics of addiction. No matter what addicts promise when they are not on drugs, they may still share needles when they shoot up heroin or cocaine. In many cases it is simply part of the ritual of taking drugs. More often, a drug-induced state overwhelms rational thinking. Many addicts know that they can get AIDS from dirty needles. Yet hazards to their health—even deadly ones—do not weigh heavily on their minds. Rather, they are primarily concerned with the instant gratification of drugs.

To expect an individual locked in the grip of drug addiction to act responsibly by not sharing needles is unrealistic. Such a change in behavior requires self-discipline and a willingness to postpone gratification and plan for the future—all of which are contrary to the drug-using lifestyle. The fact that addicts can purchase clean needles cheaply, without prescription, in many pharmacies in most States, but often fail to do so, is evidence of their irresponsible behavior.[4] In fact, the only proven way to change an addict's behavior is through structured interventions, such as drug treatment.

The New Haven study   A 1991 interim study of a needle exchange program in New Haven, Connecticut, is cited by many needle exchange advocates as evidence of the benefits of needle exchange.[5] The study asserts numerous positive findings, most of which are not supported by the data.

The study states that retention rates stabilized after a high attrition rate early in the program. But, of the 720 addicts who initially contacted the New Haven program over an eight-month period, only 288 (40 percent) returned at least once to exchange a used needle (Figure 1). The New Haven study defines the 288 returning intravenous drug users as "program participants," but does not distinguish between those who exchanged needles once and those who exchanged needles more frequently.[6] The loose definition of "program participation" exaggerates the program's reported retention rate and calls into question the claim that participation in the program stabilized. In addition, the study does not provide information on the 288 individuals who remained in the program and whether they shared needles before the program started. In fact, the

Figure 1

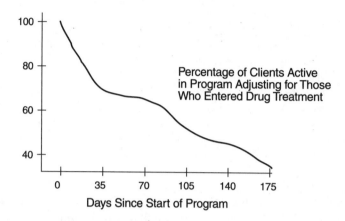

Percentage of Clients Active
in Program Adjusting for Those
Who Entered Drug Treatment

Days Since Start of Program

Source: The New Haven Study, July 1991.

study reports that of the 720 addicts who contacted the program, 436 (61 percent) reported never sharing needles before the program began (Table 1).

The study also states that about half of the 10,180 needles distributed by the program between November 1990 and June 1991 were returned, and that an additional 4,236 "street" or nonprogram needles were brought in for exchange. However, the study fails to account for the 4,917 needles—50 percent of those given out—that were not returned. Based on this information, the study claims that the circulation time for needles was reduced and that fewer contaminated needles were appearing in public places. However, no data are presented to directly support such conclusions.

The authors also report that 107 intravenous drug users (about 15 percent of those who contacted the program) entered treatment over an eight-month period through contact with the New Haven program, but there are no data on how many of these individuals were "program participants" (e.g., had exchanged needles more than once). Therefore, the study does not present any basis for correlating the *exchange* of needles to entry into drug treatment. Also, no data on treatment retention or completion are presented.

The study also claims that intravenous drug use in the community did not increase. Although this may be true, it is not supported by convincing data. The study indicates that 92 percent of those who initially contacted the program were experienced users who had been injecting drugs for one year or more. The study uses this statistic to demonstrate that the availability of free needles did not entice individuals to begin using intravenous drugs. However, there is no evidence to verify that experienced users did not use needles distributed by the program to initiate new users. The study also cites an unchanged rate in drug

Table 1

Extent of Needle Sharing Reported at Initial Contact With Program

How Often Shared Works		
Always (100%)	16	(2%)
Almost Always (67–99%)	16	(2%)
Half the Time (34–66%)	43	(6%)
Sometimes (1–33%)	196	(27%)
Never (0%)	436	(61%)
(Missing)	13	(2%)

Sources: The New Haven Study, July 1991.

arrests as evidence that no increase in intravenous drug use occurred due to the program. However, the New Haven program had only been in operation for two months and had been contacted by fewer than 200 addicts at the time statistics on drug arrests were recorded. Therefore, it is unlikely that the program could have had any impact on the rate of drug arrests.

The most striking finding of the New Haven study—that the incidence of new HIV infections was reduced by one-third among those participating in the program—is based on tenuous data. The study indicates that 789 needles—581 from the program, 160 from the street, and 48 from a local "shooting gallery"[7]—were tested for the presence of HIV.[8] The tests found that program needles were much less likely to be HIV positive than street or gallery needles. The tests also indicated that "dedicated" program needles (e.g., those returned by the original recipient) were much less likely to be HIV positive than other program needles. Based on this information, the study concludes that "dedicated" needles were not shared, *although no tests were conducted to determine if different blood types appeared on the needles or the blood type on the needle matched that of the program participant.* Without conducting such tests, accurate conclusions as to whether needles were shared cannot be drawn, and a reduction in the spread of HIV cannot be attributed to needle exchange.

Finally, the study projects that expanding the availability of clean needles to New Haven's entire intravenous drug using population would also reduce the incidence of new HIV infections by one-third. The projection is based on a highly complex mathematical model involving eight different factors that are supported by numerous assumptions, estimates, probabilities, and rates. While the model may be valid, its projections are based on the tenuous assumption that the 288 intravenous drug users "participating" in the New Haven program are representative of the general intravenous drug using population. However, the high attrition rate of the New Haven program demonstrates that such an assumption cannot be made.

Foreign Needle Exchange Programs

In recent years, other countries—most notably the Netherlands and the United Kingdom—have established needle exchange programs. Studies of these programs have also produced mixed results. Most reflect the problems noted in existing research on needle exchange. Many report anecdotal or other unquantified information. Furthermore, some base "success" on the number of needles distributed.

In Amsterdam, a program started in 1984 reported that the number of participants grew more than tenfold in four years. The program also reported that during the first four years participants shared fewer needles, the HIV prevalence rate among intravenous drug users stabilized, and instances of Hepatitis B decreased.

In England, about 120 exchange programs distribute approximately four million needles annually. These programs reportedly reach users who have not been in contact with drug treatment services, decrease needle sharing, and increase contact with other social services by participants.

Sweden's three needle exchange sites reported after three years that no project participant had become infected with HIV, that needle sharing had declined, and that many users not previously in contact with drug treatment had been attracted to the program.

Although generally positive, the reports on these programs are scientifically weak and present very few objective indicators of success. All claim that needle exchange reduced the number of needles shared, but none of the programs conducted the tests (e.g., blood-type tests) necessary to make that determination.

In addition, the attrition rates in foreign programs are extremely high. A 1989 study of 15 needle exchange programs in England and Scotland reported that only 33 percent of intravenous drug users who initially contacted the programs returned up to five times. As in the United States, needle exchange programs in other countries are more likely to attract and retain intravenous drug users who are already predisposed not to share needles, and who therefore are at lower risk of contracting AIDS than other, less cautious, users.

Alternatives to Needle Exchange

The challenges to society presented by drug use and HIV/AIDS require the steady development of scientific understanding and the promotion of effective interventions. Requested Federal funding for AIDS prevention, treatment, research, and income maintenance in 1993 is $4.9 billion—a 69 percent increase since 1990 (Figure 2). The President's National Drug Control Strategy supports using a portion of these funds for research, experiments, and demonstrations to seek out high-risk drug users; to encourage and support their entry into drug treatment; and to provide them with information on the destructiveness of their behavior and ways to change it. The Strategy also supports efforts to expand the capacity and effectiveness of drug treatment for intravenous drug users.

Figure 2

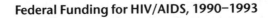

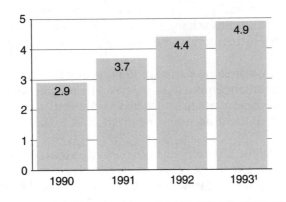

Federal Funding for HIV/AIDS, 1990–1993

[1]Requested

Source: Office of Management and Budget, 1992

Outreach programs   The most effective method of reducing the spread of AIDS among intravenous drug users is to treat successfully their drug addiction. However, Federal studies estimate that more than 40 percent of intravenous drug users have never been in treatment, even though many have used drugs intravenously for more than 10 years. Therefore, it is essential to continue efforts to aggressively recruit intravenous drug users into treatment.

Since 1987, the Department of Health and Human Service's National Institute on Drug Abuse has funded projects in more than 40 cities to help identify intravenous drug users and persuade them to enter treatment. In these cities, squads of outreach workers contact addicts and encourage them to avoid sharing needles and other risky behaviors and to enter treatment. Outreach workers also provide addicts with information on the threat of AIDS and dispense materials (e.g., bleach and condoms) to reduce the risk of HIV infection.

Between 1987 and 1992, outreach workers contacted approximately 150,000 intravenous drug users. Of these, 45,000 addicts (54 percent of whom reported regularly sharing needles) and 9,500 sexual partners were provided with information on treatment, counseling and methods for reducing the risk of infection. Program participants were assigned to standard and enhanced interventions. Follow-up surveys were conducted six months after the assignments were made, and the results of those surveys indicated that:

- 31 percent of the intravenous drug users had enrolled in formal drug treatment programs;
- 38 percent were sharing needles less frequently;

- 44 percent had begun to always clean their needles, always use a new needle, or had stopped injecting completely; and
- 47 percent had stopped injecting or reduced their frequency of injection.

The success of this effort demonstrates that outreach programs are highly effective in persuading intravenous drug users to avoid sharing needles and to seek treatment. By comparison, only 15 percent of those who contacted the New Haven program entered treatment. The Federal government will continue to support outreach programs by awarding approximately 60 grants in 1992 and 1993.

The Centers for Disease Control also administers an extensive outreach program for preventing the spread of the HIV virus among intravenous drug users. This program, which is operated through State departments of health and community-based organizations, offers intravenous drug users counseling, testing, and referral to treatment. An evaluation of the program will be completed in about two years.

Expanding treatment capacity   The Federal government continues to support expanded treatment capacity for intravenous drug users, primarily through the Alcohol, Drug Abuse and Mental Health Services Block Grant program, which requires States to use at least 50 percent of their drug allotment for outreach and treatment of these drug users. Also, the Capacity Expansion Program, which was created by the Bush Administration in Fiscal Year 1992, will increase the number of drug treatment slots for areas and populations in the greatest need of treatment, including intravenous drug users. If Congress fully funds this program in Fiscal Year 1993 (the Administration has requested $86 million), an additional 38,000 addicts—many of whom will be intravenous drug users—will be provided with drug treatment.

Medications development   The Federal government is continuing its efforts to develop medications to treat heroin addiction. New pharmacological therapies, such as LAAM (a longer-acting alternative to methadone), depot naltrexone, and buprenorphine, are showing considerable promise in treating heroin addiction and should be available within the next few years.[9] In addition, performance standards and clinical protocols are being developed for methadone treatment programs to enhance their safety and effectiveness in treating heroin addiction.[10]

Conclusion

The rapid spread of AIDS has prompted officials of some of America's cities to institute programs that distribute clean needles to intravenous drug users. Such programs are questionable public policy, however, because they facilitate addicts' continued use of drugs and undercut the credibility of society's message that drug use is illegal and morally wrong. Further, there is no compelling research that needle exchange programs are effective in preventing intravenous drug users from sharing needles, reducing the spread of AIDS, or encouraging addicts to seek drug treatment.

Research does show, however, that aggressive outreach efforts are an effective way to get intravenous drug users to end their high-risk behavior and seek treatment. Therefore, the National Drug Control Strategy will continue to support such outreach programs. It also will continue to support expanded treatment capacity for high-risk populations, including intravenous drug users; the development of medications for treating heroin addiction; and the exploration of other options that may offer intravenous drug users a real chance for recovery.

Notes

1. Human Immunodeficiency Virus/Acquired Immunodeficiency Syndrome.

2. Federal law prohibits the use of Alcohol, Drug Abuse, and Mental Health Services Block Grant funds—the major source of Federal support for drug treatment—to pay for needle exchange programs.

3. In some States, such as California, needles may be sold without prescription for the administration of insulin or adrenaline if the pharmacist can identify the purchaser and records the purchase.

4. Syringes cost about $.30 each. For example, in a recent study of pharmacies in St. Louis, Compton et al. found the cost of a package of 10, 28-gauge, 100-unit insulin syringes to range from $1.92 to $4.28.

    See Compton, W., et al. "Legal Needle Buying in St. Louis," *American Journal of Public Health,* April 1992, Vol. 82, No. 4.

5. In Fiscal Year 1992, the National Institute on Drug Abuse awarded a grant to Yale University to conduct a rigorous evaluation of the New Haven program over a three-year period. Results of the evaluation will be available in 1995.

6. Researchers estimate that intravenous heroin users on average inject two or more times a day, heavy users four to six times a day. Intravenous cocaine users invariably inject more frequently. There is very little data yet available on the number of injections an average user gets from a needle before it is discarded, although a 1989 California survey of 257 users found a mean of 22.5 uses (with 27 reporting one use and 15 reporting over 100).

7. A "shooting gallery" is a communal injection site notorious for inadequate sterilization of injection equipment.

8. The study does not specify the method used to select program and street needles or whether they are considered random or representative samples.

9. LAAM is a longer-acting alternative to methadone, depot naltrexone is a long-acting heroin blocker, and buprenorphine is being investigated for treating individuals addicted to both heroin and cocaine.

10. Methadone is a synthetic medication used to treat heroin addicts by relieving withdrawal symptoms and craving for heroin for 24 hours. Methadone is only administered as part of a supervised treatment program.

POSTSCRIPT

Should Needle Exchange Programs Be Supported?

The implementation of needle exchange programs arouses several ethical and practical concerns. Opponents challenge the wisdom of giving drug addicts needles to inject themselves with illegal drugs. They ask, What might impressionable adolescents think if the government funds programs in which drug addicts are given needles? Some people reason that those who inject drugs into their bodies know the risks and should live with the consequences of their actions. Others wonder whether the distribution of needles will lead to an increase or a decrease in drug use.

One potential advantage of needle exchange programs is that needles may be safely discarded after they have been used. Unsafely discarded needles may accidentally prick someone (including nonusers) and lead to HIV transmission. A second potential benefit is that when people come to needle exchange sites, they can be encouraged to enter drug treatment programs.

Despite the difficulties of studying people who inject drugs, long-term studies are needed to determine the impact of needle exchange programs on (1) the incidence of AIDS, (2) the continuation or reduction of drug use, (3) whether or not these programs attract new users to the drug culture, (4) the likelihood of program participants entering drug treatment programs, and (5) the impact on other high-risk behaviors. Preliminary studies on the effectiveness of needle exchange programs are contradictory. One such program was introduced in Tacoma, Washington, and needle sharing declined 30 percent. Programs in New York City and New Haven, Connecticut, resulted in fewer reports of HIV infection without an increase in drug use. Conversely, in a program in Louisville, Kentucky, nearly two-thirds of people who inject drugs continued to share needles. In Louisville, however, needles are obtained through a prescription, which may have a different effect in the long run than receiving needles through an exchange program. If needle exchange programs are implemented, who should organize and finance them? Is this the responsibility of government? Should public funds be used? Would these programs save taxpayers money over time?

Two articles that address the benefits of needle exchange programs are "Harm Reduction and Injection Drug Use: Pragmatic Lessons From a Public Health Model," by Robert Reid, *Health and Social Work* (August 2002) and "On Pins and Needles," by Will Van Sant, *National Journal* (May 15, 1999). Articles that oppose needle exchange programs include "Killing Them Softly," by Joe Loconte, *Policy Review* (July/August 1998) and "Clean Needles May Be Bad Medicine," by David Murray, *The Wall Street Journal* (April 22, 1998).

ISSUE 17

Should Employees Be Required to Participate in Drug Testing?

YES: Todd Nighswonger, from "Just Say Yes to Preventing Substance Abuse," *Occupational Hazards* (April 2000)

NO: Leslie Kean and Dennis Bernstein, from "More Than a Hair Off," *The Progressive* (May 1999)

ISSUE SUMMARY

YES: Writer Todd Nighswonger supports workplace drug testing because most people between ages 18 and 49 who use illicit drugs work full time. Also, drug-using employees are more than three times more likely to be involved in a workplace accident and five times more likely to submit a claim for worker's compensation.

NO: Authors Leslie Kean and Dennis Bernstein oppose drug testing because many employees, especially African Americans, falsely test positive for drugs. As a result, too many employees with false positive findings are unfairly discharged.

In 1986 President Ronald Reagan first called for a drug-free federal workplace, ordering all federal employees in "sensitive" jobs to submit to random drug testing. The goals were to begin attacking the drug problem by reducing the demand for drugs and by involving all employees, both public and private, in the fight against drugs. Today, an overwhelming percentage of major corporations in the United States require drug testing as a condition of employment. In addition, government agencies, including the military, have adopted the practice of random urine testing to screen its personnel for illicit drugs.

One event that served as a springboard for random drug testing was a 1987 collision between an Amtrak train and a Conrail train near Baltimore, Maryland, which killed 16 people. Because the Conrail engineer and brakeman had used marijuana just prior to the wreck, the cause of the crash was immediately tied to drug use, even though the warning indicators on the Conrail train were malfunctioning at the time. This accident was a strong indication to many people that drug testing was necessary—if not for the sake of deterring employees from using illicit drugs for their own well-being, then to ensure the safety of others.

The Fourth Amendment of the U.S. Constitution guarantees citizens the right to be protected from unreasonable searches and seizures. With regard to drug testing, the Fourth Amendment protects citizens from being tested unless probable cause, or a reason to suppose that an individual is engaged in criminal behavior, is shown. Many people feel that random drug testing is unreasonable because it involves testing even those employees who are not drug users and who have shown no cause to be tested. On the other hand, if one is not using drugs, then one should not have to worry about drug testing.

One problem with a positive drug test result is that it may not clearly differentiate between on-the-job drug use and off-the-job drug use. Many people contend that an infringement of personal liberties and an unwarranted invasion of privacy for the sake of the government's drug battle agenda are at stake. However, should companies be required to keep employees if those employees use drugs while off the job?

One could argue that all people are affected by individuals' use of illicit drugs. For example, the public pays higher prices due to lost productivity from work-related accidents and job absenteeism caused by drug use. Also, innocent people are often directly victimized by individuals on drugs who inadvertently make dangerous mistakes. From this perspective, random drug tests are not unreasonable searches. Proponents for drug testing contend that the inherent dangers of drug use, particularly while on the job, necessitate drug testing. Accidents and deaths can and do occur because of drug-induced losses of awareness and judgment. The fact that a majority of Americans who use illicit drugs are employed has convinced many that random drug testing at the workplace should be mandatory.

In the following selections, Todd Nighswonger argues that the benefits of drug testing outweigh its drawbacks. He maintains that workplace safety should take precedence over the concern of whether or not someone's right to privacy might be violated. Leslie Kean and Dennis Bernstein argue that drug testing is subject to too many errors and that people are unfairly dismissed because of these errors. They also say that drug testing is prejudicial in that it may be biased against African Americans. Thus, although drug use is a problem in society, drug testing is not the fairest and most efficient way of dealing with the problem.

Todd Nighswonger

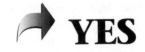 **YES**

Just Say Yes to Preventing Substance Abuse

Safety remains a key reason to keep up the fight against workplace drug and alcohol abuse.

A booming economy, resulting in low unemployment, and a six-year decline in injury and illness rates have resulted in prosperous and safe workplaces across the country.

Despite this optimistic scenario, substance abuse experts say this is not the time for U.S. businesses to let down their guard against the use of dangerous drugs and alcohol by employees. Drug and alcohol abuse is a societal problem that never will go away completely in the workplace, no matter how comprehensive a company's substance abuse program.

Even though these programs have existed for years, government studies reveal that 70 percent of illicit drug users age 18 to 49 work full time, more than 60 percent of adults know people who have gone to work under the influence of drugs or alcohol, and drug-using employees are 3.6 times more likely to be involved in a workplace accident and five times more likely to file a workers' compensation claim.

Yet, because it has become more difficult to fill job openings in many industries, there have been rumblings that some companies are considering eliminating drug testing as part of their substance abuse program. The reason: They fear they will not be able to keep or find enough workers otherwise.

Moreover, attempts to use adulterants, designed to alter drug test results, have increased in the last few years. For example, clean urine samples can be purchased through Web sites. As a result, drug testing companies have had to develop new ways of detecting adulterated samples.

Put Safety First

While the vast majority of workers are not substance abusers, it still is a significant enough problem—nearly 14 million Americans are illicit drug users—that employers should have a substance abuse program, said Garen Dodge, assistant director of the Institute for a Drug-Free Workplace. More employers are not only establishing these programs, he added, but are doing so for safety reasons.

"One of the trends I'm seeing is companies being proactive, realizing that the abuse of drugs and alcohol is a safety concern and, on that basis, establishing comprehensive substance abuse programs," said Dodge, who regularly assists companies in developing such programs. "Co-workers are recognizing that working next to somebody who's high on drugs or under the influence of alcohol is unsafe for that person and, potentially, for themselves."

The symptom that concerns Elena Carr the most is reports that some employers may abandon drug testing. Carr, substance abuse coordinator for the Department of Labor's Working Partners for an Alcohol- and Drug-Free Workplace, worries that employers will take this route instead of increasing treatment efforts.

"It is an employer's choice that probably is affected by the state of the economy," said Carr, formerly director of AFL-CIO's Substance Abuse Institute. "In the early 1990s, when there were lots of workers to choose from, testing and firing people was definitely the route of choice for many employers."

Now, the testing pendulum may begin swinging the other way. Dodge, who is a partner with the Washington, D.C., law firm of Littler Mendelson, also has heard the argument that testing should be relaxed if companies cannot fill their job openings.

"The counterargument is that a company will spend more money on a bad employee than if a position is not filled," Dodge said. "Is it cost-effective to relax drug testing and take on the chronic drug abuser who is more likely to be sick, late, unproductive, use drugs on the job and introduce drugs to co-workers?"

Numerous studies, reports and surveys suggest that substance abuse is having a profoundly negative effect on the workplace in terms of decreased productivity and increased accidents, absenteeism, turnover and medical costs. One accident costs a business an average of $12,000 to $16,000, according to the National Safety Council. Accidents caused by substance abuse also represent an area of high liability. In 80 percent of serious accidents caused by substance abuse, the injured party is not the abuser.

Yet, it is up to companies to decide whether to do drug testing because there are few federal workplace substance abuse rules. Apart from industries regulated by the Department of Transportation and federal contractors subject to the Drug-Free Workplace Act of 1988, employers mostly are left on their own to determine what type of substance abuse program to have or whether to have one at all.

While OSHA [Occupational Safety and Health Administration] embraces the idea that having a drug-free workplace contributes to the safety of workers, Carr said, the agency has issued no standards for substance abuse programs and only provides information and assistance to employers and employees. "The impact of drugs in the workplace affects a small population of workers," she said. "It pales in comparison to other issues that OSHA traditionally deals with."

Despite a lack of regulations, most employers address substance abuse in some fashion. In a study released [in 1999] by the Substance Abuse and Mental Health Services Administration (SAMHSA), 70 percent of full-time workers age 18 to 49 reported that their workplaces had a written policy concerning drug or alcohol use. The study indicated that smaller companies were much less likely to provide information or have a written policy.

The percentage of full-time workers age 18 to 49 who indicated that their employer conducted any type of drug testing programs, whether at hiring, randomly, upon suspicion or post-accident, was 48.5 percent in 1997, according to the SAMHSA study. Drug tests, typically of urine, detect stimulants (such as amphetamines, cocaine), hallucinogens (marijuana, LSD), opiates and morphine derivatives, and depressants (alcohol, barbiturates).

No-Nonsense Approach

Many companies not only have substance abuse programs for safety reasons but are avoiding the urge to soften their stance on drug testing in a low-unemployment job market.

Two companies—United States Gypsum (USG) of Chicago and BE&K Construction of Birmingham, Ala.—have a no-tolerance policy toward substance abuse in the workplace. Employees who test positive for drug or alcohol use are fired, while job applicants who test positive are not hired.

Both companies, members of the Institute for a Drug-Free Workplace, established substance abuse programs in the mid-1980s.

"We didn't start this program because we necessarily had a big drug problem," said Jeffrey Rodewald, director of employer relations for 13,000-employee USG. "We just felt it was necessary to do for safety reasons. Our drug and substance abuse policy is not based on a moral issue. That's not the concern. The concern is that we don't want people hurt on the job."

In the past three years at USG, a maker of wallboard and ceiling products, management has seen an increase in employees requesting assistance for substance abuse. "Part of the reason might be who's left to hire," Rodewald said.

Rodewald has seen job applicants stay off drugs long enough to pass a mandatory pre-employment drug test, then use drugs once they have been hired. That may be one reason why USG's positive rate for post-incident test results (almost 10 percent) is about double that of its pre-employment positive rate (5 percent), said Donald Schaefer, USG's director of occupational safety.

"With a full-employment economy, even though we're being selective and not seeing a real big change in our (pre-employment) rates, once they're in the work force, that may be part of what's driving up that post-incident number," Schaefer said.

The best way to combat the increase in post-incident positive test results, Rodewald contends, is through random drug testing, which is not allowed in some states. USG's employees have asked for, and received, increased random testing. "We had to find a way to deal with this problem from a safety standpoint and not wait for an accident to occur," he said.

USG employs drug testing at several stages as one element of a workplace substance abuse program (see "Five Steps to a Substance Abuse Program"). The company's multistage testing is representative of workplaces across the country. The SAMHSA study revealed that 38.6 percent of respondents reported drug testing was part of their hiring process, 25.4 percent were subject to random testing, and 28.7 percent worked at companies that tested after accidents.

As with a positive test result at any stage, someone with an adulterated sample is subject to dismissal. "We're not giving the person another opportunity to be re-tested," Rodewald said. The same goes for anyone who refuses to take a test. Any positive results are rechecked and confirmed before action is taken against an employee.

At BE&K Construction, the goal of its substance abuse policy is to provide and maintain a work environment free from the effects of substance abuse for all employees. That can be easier said than done, especially in an industry that has one of the U.S. work force's highest rates of illicit drug use at 14.1 percent and heavy alcohol use at 12.4 percent, according to the SAMHSA study. The core age group of substance users, 18 to 34, constitutes the bulk of construction workers.

Even so, BE&K does not back down from its goal of being 100 percent drug-free at its sites in more than 15 states, said Bill Harris, personnel manager for the company's 3,000 construction workers. "We have a very strict program," Harris said. "There are no exceptions. From our chairman of the board down to the newest laborer, we're all subject to drug testing."

Like USG, BE&K does pre-employment, random, post-accident and for-cause testing to the tune of 1,200 to 1,500 samples per year. Each month, random sampling involves 10 percent of a project's work force.

A worker cannot be rehired for 90 days after the first confirmed, positive test result and for a year after the second offense. During that time, and before, the company's employee assistance program offers counseling. A worker will not be rehired if tested positive a third time.

Because marijuana is the most prevalent illicit drug, BE&K sets its cutoff level at 20 nanograms per milliliter. Most companies' policies set a threshold of 50 or 100 nanograms.

"I think we're the trendsetter and go above and beyond what's normal," Harris said, adding that BE&K's overall positive test results have dropped from 14 percent in the program's beginning to less than 5 percent today. "Other companies have modeled their policy after ours."

Alcohol Abuse

Not to be forgotten in any substance abuse policy is alcohol consumption. More than 11 million employed Americans are self-admitted heavy drinkers, the SAMHSA study revealed. Heavy drinking was defined as five or more drinks on five or more days in the past 30 days. In fact, 59 percent of U.S. workers believe that alcohol abuse is a major problem in the workplace.

Up to 40 percent of industrial fatalities and 47 percent of industrial injuries can be linked to alcohol consumption and alcoholism, according to the 1989 Occupational Medicine article "Management Perspectives on Alcoholism: The Employer's Stake in Alcoholism Treatment."

USG's policy allows for temporary suspension and testing of a worker who has a "detectable presence" of alcohol, Rodewald said. If a test is positive, the worker's job status depends on the blood alcohol content from a test. If the test result is at or above 0.08 percent, the employee is dismissed. If below 0.08 or there is no detectable presence, the worker is returned to work with back pay.

If a presence is repeatedly detectable, but always measures less than 0.08, it becomes a performance issue. "Just because you're under the legal limit doesn't mean you can keep coming in to work in that condition," Rodewald said, adding an employee is subject to discipline for repeated measurable presences of alcohol below the legal limit.

Employers who do not have a substance abuse program or may be thinking of doing away with drug testing should reconsider, Working Partners' Carr said. "Drug and alcohol use and abuse is something you can't afford to ignore," she said. "Even though it may not be required, having a drug-free workplace program is the right and the smart thing to do."

Five Steps to a Substance Abuse Program

A comprehensive substance abuse program typically includes five components: a written policy, supervisor training, employee education and awareness, an employee assistance program, and drug and alcohol testing.

Step 1: Write a Substance Abuse Policy

Before writing the policy, Working Partners for an Alcohol- and Drug-Free Workplace suggests conducting a needs assessment to better understand your company's situation and determine what you want the program to accomplish. Remember, workers should be your allies in this process.

A written policy has three basic parts: an explanation of why you are implementing a program, a description of substance abuse-related behaviors that are prohibited and an explanation of consequences for policy violators. The policy should identify all elements of the substance abuse program.

Step 2: Train Supervisors

Supervisors are responsible for identifying and addressing performance problems that may be the result of substance abuse. While not expected to diagnose conditions, supervisors should be able to identify the signs of poor job performance.

Train supervisors to understand the company's substance abuse policy and procedures, to identify and help resolve employee performance problems, and to know how to refer employees to available assistance.

Step 3: Educate Employees

Educating workers is considered a critical step in achieving the program's objectives. A basic program should achieve several objectives:

- Provide information about the dangers of alcohol and illicit drugs.

- Describe the impact that substance abuse can have on workplace safety, accident rates, health care costs, absenteeism, productivity, product quality and the bottom line.
- Explain, in detail, how the policy applies to every employee and consequences for policy violations.
- Describe how the basic components of the program work. Components might include an employee assistance program (EAP) and drug and alcohol testing.
- Explain how employees and their dependents, if included, can get help for their substance abuse problems.

Step 4: Provide Employee Assistance

Many companies use EAPs to assist workers whose job performance is negatively affected by personal problems, including substance abuse. Employers have found that EAPs are cost-effective because they help reduce accidents, workers compensation claims, absenteeism and employee theft.

EAPs, if they are to be successful, should be viewed as a confidential source of help. Workers, though, should understand that it will not shield them from disciplinary action for continued poor performance or policy violations.

Step 5: Drug and Alcohol Testing

By itself, testing is not a substance abuse program, but it can be an effective deterrent to drug use and an important tool to help employers identify workers who need help. Consider who will be tested, when testing will take place, what substances will be tested, what consequences workers will face who test positive and who will administer the testing.

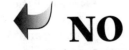 **NO**

More Than a Hair Off

Althea Jones, an African-American mother of two, always wanted to go to police school. "It was my lifelong dream to be a police officer, ever since I was a little girl," she says. When she applied for admission to the Chicago Police Academy, it requested a sample of her hair, which it sent to Psychemedics, the largest hair-testing company in the country. The results came back positive for drug use.

"I was shocked. I couldn't believe it," says Jones. "I don't even smoke or drink. I was heartbroken by this." She was denied admission to the academy and is now a criminal justice major at Chicago State University.

Adrian McClure, an African-American woman, was also keen on a career with the Chicago police department. When she was a senior in college in 1997, she submitted a hair sample to the academy, which sent it to the Psychemedics Corporation. Her test came back positive, too. She says she tried to explain that it was an error and requested a new test, but was rebuffed. "Everybody knows I don't use drugs," McClure says. "This thing has a hold of me. They have shattered me."

Last August, Althea Jones and Adrian McClure, along with six other Chicago African-Americans who say they received erroneous hair test results when applying for the Police Academy, filed complaints of racial discrimination with the Equal Employment Opportunity Commission. The complaints are currently under investigation, and the group is considering suing both the city of Chicago and Psychemedics.

Jones and McClure are just two of many who have lost out as a result of hair testing. Numerous scientific studies have shown hair testing to be inaccurate and unreliable. And the procedure appears to give false positives disproportionately to African-Americans. Nevertheless, use of hair tests is expanding nationwide. Psychemedics reports that business is booming. The Cambridge, Massachusetts, firm more than doubled sales of its hair test between 1993 and 1997, and in 1997 *The Boston Globe* named Psychemedics one of the "Top Fifty Growth Companies" of Massachusetts. "The total annual market for drug testing in the United States has been estimated at between $500 and $600 million, and is growing fast," says Psychemedics CEO Raymond C. Kubacki Jr.

Psychemedics services 1,400 businesses that use hair testing on their employees and job applicants. These include General Motors, Anheuser Busch, BMW, Rubbermaid, and Steelcase Corporation. The company is also conducting hair tests for forty to fifty schools, five Federal Reserve banks, and the police departments of New York City, Chicago, Boston, and San Francisco.

Whites and blacks have complained about the tests.

Three Police Academy members were given hair tests in New York City as part of their application to the police department. The three Caucasian men claim that they did not take drugs and that the test was flawed. Two of the men had clean urine tests within months prior to the New York police department test. To bolster their assertions, these two men sent hair samples off for a second test to Laboratory Corporation of America and Metropolitan Drug Screening. According to Peter Coddington, an attorney retained by the Patrolmen's Benevolent Association to represent the men, the tests from the other labs produced opposite results. "They were clean," he said.

"It is quite clear that the police got the wrong results, either through the mishandling of the samples or through the laboratory techniques," says Coddington. "My clients should be reinstated, based on the contradictory tests." Coddington says that the men's lives have been devastated. "There is no question that they don't use drugs. They are three clean-cut, all-American boys. It was their lifetime goal to become police officers, and two of them are from police families. Now their whole lives are on hold."

New York attorney Regina Felton is representing a group of nine police officers, all African-American, dismissed in 1996 due to a positive Psychemedics hair test. All nine had random urinalysis tests throughout their two-year probationary period, which were negative. According to court transcripts, one of Felton's clients sent her hair to National Medical Services within three weeks after the New York Police Department sent her hair sample to Psychemedics. As in the Patrolmen's Benevolent Association cases, the test came back positive from Psychemedics and negative from National Medical Services.

Felton's clients appeared at hearings to seek unemployment compensation from the New York Department of Labor.

Ann Marie Gordon, the Director of Quality Assurance from Psychemedics, testified in each case as the expert on the accuracy of hair testing. As a result, the dismissed officers are not receiving any unemployment compensation. "The person who testified as the expert actually has a proprietary interest in Psychemedics," says Felton. "This person works for Psychemedics, and if she doesn't testify appropriately, she may not have a job."

◦◦◦

The Food and Drug Administration (FDA), the Department of Transportation, the National Institute of Drug Abuse, and the Society of Forensic Toxicologists (the preeminent professional association in the field of drug testing) all raise serious questions about the accuracy of hair testing. "The consensus of scientific opinion is that there are still too many unanswered questions for [hair analysis] to be used in employment situations," said Edward Cone, the National Institute of Drug Abuse's leading researcher on the test, in June 1998. In a recent interview, Cone said that hair testing "is not ready for use yet, where people's lives are at stake."

The Society of Forensic Toxicologists stands by its 1990 report, which said: "The use of hair analysis for employees and pre-employment drug testing is premature and cannot be supported by the current information on hair analysis for drugs of abuse."

According to a 1996 letter from Secretary of Health and Human Services Donna Shalala to the U.S. Senate, her agency "has not approved the use of hair testing for drugs of abuse." Shalala stated that "the available research suggests there are significant scientific and procedural concerns that must be addressed," and that these problems "make it impossible for us to recommend at this time its use in the federal program."

D. Bruce Burlington, a medical doctor who is director of the FDA's Center for Devices and Radiological Health, spoke before the House Committee on Commerce on July 23, 1998. "Many scientific questions remain . . . about the effectiveness of hair testing for detecting drug use," he said. "The agency [FDA] has not been presented with adequate independent data on the effectiveness of such tests."

Some of the tests appear to give false positives to people who don't consume drugs. More disturbing yet, test results appear to vary according to ethnicity. "Dark hair, blond hair, and dyed hair react differently [from each other], thus creating questions of equity among ethnic groups and genders," Burlington testified.

A U.S. Navy study released by the National Institute of Drug Abuse in 1995 shows that the dark, coarse hair of many African-Americans, Hispanics, and Asians is more likely to retain external contamination, such as drug residues absorbed from the environment. Since these residues can be absorbed into hair even when they are not ingested, these groups could face a greater chance of error when subjected to the test. The issue of external contamination is particularly serious for police officers, who may be exposed to drugs during day-to-day law-enforcement operations.

A 1997 study by the National Institute of Drug Abuse supports the Navy's study, stating that "significantly greater nonspecific and specific radioligand binding occurred in dark colored hair compared to light hair." It concludes: "There may be significant ethnic bias in hair testing for cocaine." National Institute of Drug Abuse scientists showed in May 1998 that melanin is the most likely binding site for cocaine in human hair. The study found that cocaine binding was greater "in male Africoid hair than in female Africoid hair and in all Caucasoid hair types."

More recently, Douglas Rollins, director of the Center for Human Toxicology at the University of Utah, gave equal amounts of drugs to rats with black hair and white hair. He found that the black hair retained the drugs at a rate up to fifty times higher than the white hair. He is beginning comparable studies on humans.

William Minot, director of marketing communications at Psychemedics Corporation, says his company is "very conscious" about concerns that a person's race may affect the outcome of the test. The current test, he says, is "fail-proof" because Psychemedics extracts all the melanin from the hair before testing it. Minot says that hair samples are washed thoroughly to remove the hair surface, a procedure that also totally removes any external environmental contaminants before testing.

But the March/April 1998 issue of the *Journal of Analytical Toxicology* reported that scientists studied the effect on the hair of cocaine users when the melanin was removed. By measuring the cocaine content of the hair both with and without the melanin, the scientists observed that "removal of melanin from hair digests by centrifugation does not eliminate hair color bias when interpreting cocaine concentrations."

Psychemedics's corporate profile claims that its "no-nonsense" hair test is "five to ten times more effective at detecting drug abusers than urinalysis." But Psychemedics, like other hair-testing companies, provides little in the way of hard evidence to support such assertions.

Psychemedics has refused to disclose its testing and analysis procedures to the scientific community, says Leo Cangianelli, who headed the U.S. Navy drug testing division from 1980 to 1990 and is currently vice president of the Walsh Group, a research firm that studies drug and alcohol testing. This makes the hair test difficult for scientists to replicate and makes it almost impossible to establish a system of quality assurance for hair testing, Cangianelli says. And no hair testing labs have been federally certified, according to Burlington.

⋅⟨⊙⟩⋅

Sergeant Duane Adens, an African-American father of five, was a fourteen-year employee of the Pentagon. Adens was less than six years away from retirement and had received the highest possible rating for overall performance in his last job evaluation when his life was turned upside down by a drug test.

In October 1996, two agents from the Army's Criminal Investigation Division called Adens to a meeting and asked him to testify against an associate of his, who the agents said was stealing and selling computers. Adens says he told them he could not do this, since he had no knowledge of the crimes. "The agent told me that I was obstructing justice and they would play hardball with me," recalls Adens. He says one of the agents then accused him of using drugs and threatened him with the loss of his Pentagon job. At that point, the agent asked Adens to provide him with a sample of his body hair, which he intended to have tested for drugs. Adens refused to provide the hair, and following the suggestion of his commander, the Army conducted a urine test on him the next day. That test came back negative.

In January 1997, two new agents came to Adens's home. "They told me they had a warrant," says Adens. This time, Adens's attorney advised him to provide the hair. They took Adens to a hospital and laid him on a table. One of the agents asked him if he would prefer the hair to be taken from his head or his pubic area. When Adens requested that it be taken from his head, the agent "said he would take it from my pubic area anyway so as not to mess up my haircut," says Adens, who believes the agent intended to humiliate him. A medical doctor removed the pubic hair, which the agent put in a small box in his pocket. After a delay of twenty days and without Adens signing off on the hair to identify it as his own—in violation of custody regulations—the hair was sent to National Medical Services in Willowborough, Pennsylvania. The results came back positive.

Adens was stunned. He says he does not use drugs and had not been exposed to environmental contaminants. Seven urinalysis tests he had taken over the course of a year and a half—most of them random tests required by the military—all came back negative. Adens took these tests between October 1996 and May 1998. He also did more tests once he knew the Army's Criminal Investigation Division was after him and can document the negative results.

Adens was brought before an Army court martial. He and his new attorney, Charles Gittins, requested a DNA test to verify the identity of the hair, which Adens believes was not even his. The U.S. Army denied his request. Because of the hair-test results, Sergeant Adens received a bad conduct discharge in July 1998.

◦◉◦

Representative Cynthia McKinney, Democrat of Georgia, has taken up the issue. In a July 22, 1998, letter to Secretary of Defense William Cohen, McKinney told the Secretary that the case of Sergeant Adens "has the potential to trigger hearings before the House National Security Committee" and that she is "exploring a possible legislative remedy to prohibit human hair testing for drugs in the military" until guidelines are established. "Hair testing has been proven by forensic toxicologists to be racially biased," she wrote.

McKinney received a response to her inquiry from Under Secretary of Defense Rudy de Leon on October 1. He reported that the Army had "contracted for hair analysis in six cases in the last two years involving five African-American subjects." In response to McKinney's letter, de Leon responded, "I understand your concern that hair color and other factors may affect hair absorption and extraction rates, and the ability of the test to detect the presence of illegal drugs. While this does not invalidate test results, DOD does not plan to use these tests in administrative drug testing programs until this matter is thoroughly studied and adequately addressed."

Representative Charles Rangel, Democrat of New York, wrote to the Army in behalf of Adens in September. Rangel's personal assistant Albert Becker wrote to Lieutenant Colonel Aaron B. Hayes: "Something is wrong with our military system of equal justice when an individual can pass all the required blood tests on Monday and fail the same procedure on Tuesday using a method that has not been approved by a branch of the federal government (the FDA). For a soldier to lose his self-esteem, family and military respect is a bit too much based on the strength of a body hair." Deputy Under Secretary of Defense Jeanne Fites declined to comment on the specifics of the Adens case.

The issue of hair testing has recently been brought to the House Judiciary Committee through the office of ranking committee member John Conyers, Democrat of Michigan. Conyers is concerned about the ethnic bias of the hair test, and Judiciary Committee staff members are looking into it.

Adens was removed from his position at the Pentagon at the beginning of his ordeal. He says he has been demoted to "doing odds and ends jobs like driving for people, filing, office work. . . . I've tried through my contacts to get some other jobs in the military, but they don't want to touch me at this point." Since his removal, Adens has missed out on two promotions that would have increased his income substantially. As soon as the Army approves the transcript of his case, he will be put on involuntary leave, which means he will lose his job and his government-subsidized home.

"One of the things that really, really bothers me is that this is a federal conviction," says Adens. "I will never be able to get a good job. I lose my voting rights. Something I worked hard at for fourteen years is all going to be taken away from me—for no reason at all."

POSTSCRIPT

Should Employees Be Required to Participate in Drug Testing?

As a follow-up to the discussion of whether or not employees should be required to submit to drug testing, one needs to ask what should be done with people who test positive for drugs. Should they be dismissed or treated? Do companies have the right to punish workers for activities they engage in away from work?

Many questions surround the legalities of drug testing. Over the past two decades the courts have been divided over whether or not drug testing is reasonable and whether or not it constitutes a search under the Fourth Amendment. Most courts have concluded that a mandatory urine, blood, breath, and hair test can be considered a search under the Fourth Amendment; the focus now is on the extent to which drug searches may be reasonable.

Advocates of random drug testing argue that testing at the workplace will prevent illicit drug use and problems associated with drug use. Proponents believe that it is not a violation of civil rights when the government acts to protect all citizens from the problems of illicit drug use. However, drug tests are not always accurate. To avoid a positive result, some drug users may submit another person's urine or put salt and detergent in their own samples, which affect the accuracy of the test. People on both sides of the argument contend that more reliable tests and better handling by laboratory workers are needed if drug testing is to be allowed.

Drug testing raises other questions: How should the confidentiality of drug test results be maintained? Should drug testing be implemented at the worksite or at a neutral location? Who should be allowed access to employees' files regarding drug test results? How could employees be assured of their privacy? In addition, will job discrimination or employee stigmatization come about from positive test results?

Articles that examine the advantages and disadvantages of drug testing are "Drug Testing Laws and Employment Injuries," by Randall Kesselring and Jeffrey Pittman, *Journal of Labor Research* (Spring 2002); "An Assessment of Drug Testing Within the Construction Industry," by Jonathon Gerber and George Yacoubian, *Journal of Drug Education* (vol. 32, no. 1, 2002); and "Testy, Testy," by Chris Pentilla, *Entrepreneur* (June 2000). Criticisms of employee drug testing can be found in Jacob Sullum's "Pissing Contest," *Reason* (January 2000) and in Lee Fletcher's "Employer Drug Testing Has Pitfalls," *Business Insurance* (October 23, 2000).

ISSUE 18

Does Drug Abuse Treatment Work?

YES: Bernadette Pelissier et al., from "Triad Drug Treatment Evaluation Project," *Federal Probation* (December 2001)

NO: Robert Apsler, from "Is Drug Abuse Treatment Effective?" *The American Enterprise* (March/April 1994)

ISSUE SUMMARY

YES: Social science research analyst Bernadette Pelissier and her colleagues found that males and females in federal prisons who were provided with drug treatment, as well as some type of follow-up treatment, were less likely to be rearrested or to test positive for drugs than others who were not provided with drug treatment.

NO: Psychology professor Robert Apsler questions the effectiveness of drug abuse treatment. He also questions whether or not drug addicts would go for treatment if services were expanded.

Numerous drug experts feel that more funding should go toward preventing drug use from starting or escalating and toward treating individuals who are dependent on drugs. Today, when budget battles loom and taxpayers dispute how their tax monies are spent, the question of whether or not government funds should be used to treat people who abuse drugs is especially relevant. Questions surrounding this debate include: Does drug abuse treatment reduce criminal activity associated with drugs? Will drug addicts stop their abusive behavior if they enter treatment? Will more drug addicts receive treatment than currently do if services are expanded? Will the availability and demand for illegal drugs decline?

The research on the effectiveness of drug treatment is mixed. In *The Effectiveness of Treatment for Drug Abusers Under Criminal Justice Supervision* (National Institute of Justice, 1995), Douglas S. Lipton states that drug abuse treatment not only reduces the rate of arrests but also reduces crime and lowers the cost to taxpayers over the long run. Also, it has been shown that illicit drug use is curtailed by drug abuse treatment and that treated drug addicts are better able to function in society and to maintain employment. Perhaps most important, drug treatment may prove beneficial in curbing the escalation of the human immunodeficiency virus (HIV), the virus that causes AIDS. The logic here is that when drug users (a high-risk population for HIV) enter treatment, they can be advised about the behaviors that lead to HIV transmission. Drug treatment is less costly than hospitalization and incarceration.

Some experts contend that reports regarding the effectiveness of drug treatment are not always accurate and that research on drug abuse has not been subjected to rigorous standards. Some question how effectiveness should be determined. If a person relapses after one year, should the treatment be considered ineffective? Would a reduction in an individual's illegal drug use indicate that the treatment was effective, or would an addict have to maintain complete abstinence? Also, if illegal drug use and criminal activity decline after treatment, it is possible that these results would have occurred anyway, regardless of whether or not the individual had been treated.

There are a variety of drug treatment programs. One type of treatment program developed in the 1960s is *therapeutic communities.* Therapeutic communities are usually residential facilities staffed by former drug addicts. Although there is no standard definition of what constitutes a therapeutic community, the program generally involves task assignments for residents (the addicts undergoing treatment), group intervention techniques, vocational and educational counseling, and personal skill development. Inpatient treatment facilities, such as the Betty Ford Center, are the most expensive type of treatment and are often based on a hospital model. These programs are very structured and include highly regimented schedules, demanding rules of conduct, and individual and group counseling.

Outpatient treatment, the most common type of drug treatment, is less expensive, less stigmatizing, and less disruptive to the abuser's family than other forms of treatment. Vocational, educational, and social counseling is provided. Outpatient treatment is often used after an addict leaves an inpatient program. One type of treatment that has proliferated in recent years is the self-help group. Members of self-help groups are bound by a common denominator, whether it is alcohol, cocaine, or narcotics. Due to the anonymous and confidential nature of self-help groups, however, it is difficult to conduct follow-up research to determine their effectiveness.

Individuals who are addicted to narcotics are often referred to methadone maintenance programs. Methadone is a synthetic narcotic that prevents narcotic addicts from getting high and eliminates withdrawal symptoms. Because methadone's effects last about 24 hours, addicts need to receive treatment frequently. Unfortunately, the relapse rate is high once addicts stop treatment. Because there is much demand for methadone maintenance in some areas, there are lengthy waiting lists.

In the following selections, Bernadette Pelissier et al. report that drug treatment provided in prisons reduced drug use and rates of rearrest. Robert Apsler contends that the benefits of drug treatment are not as significant as proponents of drug treatment profess.

Bernadette Pelissier et al.

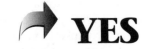 **YES**

Triad Drug Treatment Evaluation Project[1]

The Federal Bureau of Prisons (BOP) has provided drug abuse treatment in various forms for almost two decades. The current residential drug abuse treatment programs (DAP) were developed following passage of the Anti-Drug Abuse Acts of 1986 and 1988,[2] both of which reflected an increased emphasis on and resources for alcohol and drug abuse treatment. Participation in DAP compels inmates to identify, confront, and alter the attitudes, values, and thinking patterns that lead to criminal and drug-using behavior. The current residential treatment program also includes a transitional component that keeps inmates engaged in treatment as they return to their home communities.

The Bureau of Prisons undertook an evaluation of its residential drug abuse treatment program by assessing the post-release outcomes of inmates who had been released from BOP custody. The evaluation, conducted with funding and assistance from the National Institute on Drug Abuse, reveals that offenders who completed the residential drug abuse treatment program and had been released to the community for three years were less likely to be re-arrested or to be detected for drug use than were similar inmates who did not participate in the drug abuse treatment program. Specifically, 44.3 percent of male inmates who completed the residential drug abuse treatment program were likely to be re-arrested or revoked within three years after release to supervision in the community, compared to 52.5 percent of those inmates who did not receive such treatment. For women, 24.5 percent of those who completed the residential drug abuse treatment program were arrested or revoked within three years after release, compared to 29.7 percent of the untreated women.[3] With respect to drug use, 49.4 percent of men who completed residential drug abuse treatment were likely to use drugs within three years following release, compared to 58.5 percent of those who did not receive treatment. Among female inmates who completed the residential drug abuse treatment, 35.2 percent were likely to use drugs within the three-year post-release period in the community, compared to 42.6 percent of those who did not receive such treatment.[4] Overall, females are less likely to relapse or recidivate regardless of treatment.

We also found that women who completed residential drug treatment were employed for 70.5 percent of their post-release period, whereas untreated

From Bernadette Pelissier, William Rhodes, William Saylor, Gerry Gaes, Scott D. Camp, Suzy D. Vanyur, and Sue Wallace, "Triad Drug Treatment Evaluation Project," *Federal Probation*, vol. 65, no. 3 (December 2001). Copyright © 2001 by *Federal Probation*. Reprinted by permission.

women were employed for 59.1 percent of the time. No statistically significant effect was found among the men.

The findings for recidivism and drug use three years after release are consistent with the positive results reported in our preliminary report based on six months following release. Drug treatment provided to incarcerated offenders reduces the likelihood of future criminal conduct and drug use as well as increasing the employment rate among women. This study is consistent with the results of other evaluations of prison drug treatment; however, these findings are bolstered by the use of multiple treatment sites, a rigorous research design, a large sample size (2,315), and the opportunity to examine the effects of drug treatment on men and women separately. We note that the effects of treatment in reducing recidivism and drug use were less clear for women than for men. There are several plausible explanations, including methodological reasons (i.e., smaller sample size, lower overall rates) and substantive differences between the causes of drug abuse in men and women and their respective responses to existing treatment programs. Our treatment curriculum is currently being modified to better address these differing treatment needs.

Residential Drug Abuse Treatment

This report analyzes the results of the Bureau of Prisons' residential drug abuse treatment programs, which are designed for inmates with moderate to severe substance abuse problems. The Bureau also provides a variety of other substance abuse programs, including drug education and non-residential individual and group treatment. Treatment often continues when an inmate is released from Bureau custody to the supervision of U.S. Probation Service.

The residential drug abuse treatment program includes three stages:

- Stage 1: Drug abuse treatment is provided within the confines of a designated drug abuse treatment unit for 9 or 12 months, depending on the particular program. The treatment strategies employed are based on the premises that the inmate is responsible for and can effectively change his or her behavior.
- Stage 2: Upon successful completion of the unit-based drug abuse treatment program, inmates are required to continue drug abuse treatment for up to 12 months when returned to general population. During this stage of institution drug abuse programming, known as institutional transition, inmates meet with drug abuse program staff at least once a month for a group activity consisting of relapse prevention planning and a review of treatment techniques learned during the intensive phase of the residential drug abuse program.
- Stage 3: All inmates who participate in the residential drug abuse program are required to participate in community transitional services when they are transferred from the institution to a Community Corrections Center (halfway house sometimes followed by home confinement) prior to release from custody. The Bureau contracts with community

drug abuse treatment providers for group, individual, and/or family counseling as appropriate for individual inmates. Generally, these contractors offer the same type/philosophy of treatment offered in the institution.[5]

The current evaluation focuses on two types of residential treatment programs for alcohol and other drug problems. The first type offers 1,000 hours of treatment over a 12-month period with a staff-to-inmate ratio of 1:12. The second offers 500 hours of treatment over a 9-month period with a staff-to-inmate ratio of 1:24. Most of the subjects in this study participated in the 9-month program.[6]

All residential DAPs are unit-based; that is, all program participants live together—separate from the general population—for the purpose of building a treatment community. Each unit has a capacity of approximately 100 inmates. Ordinarily, treatment is conducted on the unit for a half day in two, two-hour sessions. The other half of the day, inmates participate in typical institution activities (e.g., work, school). During these times, as well as during meals, treatment participants interact with general population inmates.

The goal of the DAP programs is to attempt to identify, confront, and alter the attitudes, values, and thinking patterns that led to criminal behavior and drug or alcohol use. Most program content is standardized and the following modules comprise 450 hours of programming: Screening and Assessment; Treatment Orientation; Criminal Lifestyle Confrontation; Cognitive Skill Building; Relapse Prevention; Interpersonal Skill Building; Wellness; and Transitional Programming. The remaining program hours are structured at the discretion of each program.

Inmates with a recent history of alcohol or substance abuse or dependence are strongly encouraged to participate in treatment. At the outset of program implementation, there were few additional incentives for residential drug treatment program participation beyond the recovery from dependence or addiction. However, over time various incentives were implemented. These included nominal financial achievement awards, consideration for a six-month halfway house placement for successful DAP program completion, and tangible benefits such as shirts, caps, and pens with program logos to program participants in good standing.

The incentives for drug treatment significantly changed with the passage of the Violent Crime Control and Law Enforcement Act of 1994, which allows eligible inmates who successfully complete the BOP's residential drug treatment program to earn up to a one-year reduction from their statutory release dates.[7]

Sample

The three-year outcome results contained in this report relate to inmate subjects who were released between August 1992 and December 1997. More than half of these inmates were within one year of release from BOP custody when they completed the program.[8] The sample contained in this report includes 2,315 individuals—1,842 men and 473 women—for whom comprehensive data were available and who were released to supervision.[9]

Treatment Subjects

Treatment subjects were sampled from 20 different institutions with a residential drug treatment program. This represents approximately 40 percent of the institutions that currently operate residential treatment programs. These institutions represent all security levels, except maximum security, and serve both male and female populations.

The four types of residential DAP participants are as follows: 1) inmates who completed the treatment, 2) inmates who dropped out of their own volition, 3) inmates who were discharged from treatment for disciplinary reasons, and 4) inmates who, for a variety of other reasons, did not complete the program. This last category, in general, comprises inmates unable to complete the residential program because they were transferred to another institution or to a halfway house (CCC), had their sentences shortened toward the end of their incarceration, or spent an extended amount of time on writ or medical furlough. Table 1 provides a breakdown of inmate subjects by gender, treatment and comparison group assignments, and individual categories within the treatment group.

Table 1

Type of Subject by Gender

Type of Subject	Male		Female	
	Number	Percent	Number	Percent
Treatment	948	51.5	245	51.8
12-month Program Graduate	178	9.7	58	12.3
9-month Program Graduate	585	31.7	113	23.9
Drop-out	36	2.0	22	4.6
Disciplinary discharge	67	3.6	20	4.2
Other reason—incomplete	82	4.5	32	6.8
Comparison	894	48.5	228	48.2
Total	1,842	100.0	473	100.0

Of the 948 male subjects who entered unit-based residential treatment, 80 percent completed the treatment program, 4 percent voluntarily dropped out of the program, 7 percent were removed for disciplinary reasons, and 9 percent did not complete treatment for other reasons (as described above).

Of the 245 women who entered treatment, 70 percent completed the treatment program, 9 percent voluntarily dropped out of the program, 8 percent were removed for disciplinary reasons, and 13 percent did not complete for other reasons. The fact that there is a lower percentage of treatment "completers" among women than men may be related to policy differences between treatment sites and differential enforcement of program rules.

Comparison Subjects

Male and female comparison subjects were drawn from more than 40 institutions, some that offered residential drug abuse treatment programs and some that did not. The comparison subjects consisted of individuals who had histories of moderate or serious drug use and, therefore, would have met the criteria for admission to the residential drug treatment programs. There were 894 male and 228 female comparison subjects.

Outcome Measures

Criminal recidivism and post-release drug use were the primary outcomes of interest in this evaluation. The other outcomes examined were post-release employment and unsuccessful completion of halfway house placement. Because much of the outcome information was obtained from interviews with U.S. probation officers, most of our analyses were conducted with individuals released to supervision. The only analysis which included both supervised and unsupervised subjects was our analysis of one of our indicators of recidivism—arrest for a new offense—because arrest information could be collected on unsupervised subjects from the FBI's National Crime Information Center (NCIC).[10]

Criminal recidivism was defined two ways: 1) an arrest for a new offense or 2) an arrest for a new offense or supervision revocation. Revocation was defined as occurring only when the revocation was solely the result of a technical violation of one or more conditions of supervision (e.g., detected drug use, failure to report to probation officer).[11] Although our primary interest is in arrest for a new offense, revocation for a technical violation is a *competing event*. Unless we include the competing event in our measure of recidivism, our results will be biased. Nonetheless, we also examined results for a new offense both for all subjects as well as for supervised subjects only. Separate analyses of all subjects and supervised subjects was done only with the purpose of determining whether the supervision process itself affects recidivism.

Drug use as a post-release outcome refers to the *first* occurrence of drug or alcohol use. This information consisted of four different categories of a violation of a supervision condition as reported by U.S. probation officers: a positive urinalysis (u/a), refusal to submit to a urinalysis, admission of drug use to the probation officer, or a positive breathalyser test.

Employment information was also obtained through interviews with U.S. probation officers. We used two measures of post-release employment. The first was employment rate, defined as the percent of available time an individual was employed. Each week of post-release supervision was given a value of 40 hours of available work time. The percentage reflects the actual number of hours worked during the supervision period divided by the number of hours available. The second measure was employment level and consisted of the following categories: employed full-time the entire post-release period, employed full-time some portion of the post-release period, employed part-time some or all of the post-release period, and not employed during the post-release period.[12]

The analysis of unsuccessful halfway house completion was limited to those individuals who received halfway house placements. Approximately two-thirds of the subjects received such a placement. Failure to complete a halfway house placement is the result of a disciplinary infraction, either for a violation of halfway house rules or for criminal activity.

Before examining the effects of treatment, it is important to look at the overall rate of failure for each outcome measure for both treatment and comparison inmates. This overall rate of failure is presented by gender in Table 2, and tells us, for example, that the failure rate for arrest on a new offense or revocation for all subjects (both those who received treatment and those who did not receive treatment) is 49 percent for men and 27.8 percent for women. Overall, these results indicate that for each outcome measure, the percentage with a successful outcome is lower for men with the exception of employment.

Table 2

Outcome Measure by Gender: Three-Year Post Release

	Percent	
	Male	Female
Arrest for New Offense: All Offenders	34.7	16.1
Arrest for New Offense: Supervised Subjects Only	33.2	16.7
Arrest for New Offense or Revocation	49.0	27.8
Drug Use	55.0	39.8
Employment Rate (0–100 Percent)	68.0	59.0
Halfway House Placement Failure	23.0	17.0

Analyses

The analyses of the effects of residential drug treatment on the various outcome measures controlled for a wide variety of background factors known to be related to recidivism and treatment outcomes, including a number of factors related to drug-using populations that have seldom been examined in previous evaluation studies. These background measures included type of drug used on a daily basis in the year before arrest, drug treatment history, history of drug problem for spouse, mental health treatment history, psychiatric diagnoses of depression and antisocial personality, criminal history, age, race, ethnic status, educational level, employment history, level of supervision (e.g., halfway house placements before release from custody, release to supervision, frequency of urine testing, frequency of contacts with probation officer, frequency of probation officer collateral contacts), pre-release disciplinary infractions, inprison vocational training, post-release treatment, and post-release living situation.

The most common methodological problem in drug treatment evaluation results from the process of selection into treatment, i.e., selection bias. All inmates with substance abuse problems are strongly encouraged to participate in treatment, but only some agree to do so. Thus, there is an element of self-selecting into the programs. This fact makes it difficult for the researcher to disentangle the effects of treatment from the effects of other differences between the treated and untreated groups (e.g., comparison group) that are reflected in the decision to opt for treatment. Therefore, we used three different methods of analyses to assess treatment effectiveness. One method compares all individuals who were treated to those who were not treated and does not control for selection bias. The second and third methods provide alternative methods of controlling for selection. The results across the three methods were consistent.

All analyses, unlike our preliminary six-month report, were done for males and females separately. With the complete sample and the longer follow-up period, the sample size and failure rate for women was sufficiently large to allow for separate analyses.[13] In addition, our review of the literature suggests that the process of change from a drug using and criminal lifestyle to one without drug use and criminal activity may differ between men and women. Background data on female drug abusers within the Bureau of Prisons corroborated significant gender differences found by other researchers.

Findings—Residential Drug Abuse Treatment

The effects of unit-based residential treatment on post-release outcomes described below are the differences in outcomes between treatment and comparison groups after controlling for various background factors and for self-selection into treatment.

Recidivism

Arrest for new offense—Men who had received unit-based residential treatment had a lower probability of being arrested in the 36-month follow-up period than did comparison subjects. The probability of arrest for all individuals who entered and completed treatment was 30.6 percent as compared to a probability of 37.6 percent for untreated men. However, we found no difference between treated and untreated women: the probability of arrest for both groups was 16 percent. When we analyzed only those offenders released to supervision, we continued to find a difference between treatment and comparison subjects but only for men.

Arrest for new offense or supervision revocation—The primary indicator of recidivism was arrest for new offense or supervision revocation. When outcome was defined as arrest for new offense or supervision revocation, residential drug treatment effects also were found. The probability of arrest for men released to supervision who entered and completed treatment was 44.3 percent as compared to a probability of 52.5 percent for untreated subjects. Men who received and completed residential treatment were 16 percent less likely to recidivate. Although the results for women were not statistically significant, the difference between the treated and comparison group suggests that treatment helped to reduce recidivism among women. Among women who completed residential drug abuse treatment, 24.5 percent were likely to be arrested for a new offense or have supervision revoked within 36 months after release compared to 29.7 percent among untreated inmates; inmates who completed residential drug abuse treatment were 18 percent less likely to recidivate in the first six months following release than those who did not receive treatment.

Drug Use

The results for drug use show that individuals who participated in a residential drug abuse treatment program were less likely to have evidence of post-release drug use than were comparison subjects. Among male inmates who completed residential drug abuse treatment, 49.9 percent were likely to use drugs within 36 months after release compared to 58.5 percent among untreated inmates; that is, those male inmates who completed residential drug abuse treatment were 15 percent less likely to use drugs 36 months following release than those who did not receive treatment. Among female inmates who completed residential drug abuse treatment, 35.0 percent were likely to use drugs within 36 months after release compared to 42.6 percent among untreated inmates; female inmates who completed residential drug abuse treatment were 18 percent less likely to use drugs in the 36 months following release.

Post-Release Employment

We found no significant differences for either measure of post-release employment—employment rate or level of employment—among men when comparing treated to comparison inmates. However, we found significant differences for women for both measures of post-release employment. Women who completed residential treatment were employed 68.6 percent of the post-release period and untreated women were employed 59.1 percent of the time.

CCC Placement Failures

Approximately two-thirds of the individuals received a halfway house placement (CCC) before their release from BOP custody. Results indicate that treatment completion had no effect on whether male or female inmates successfully completed their halfway house stay. However, our ability to assess the effects of residential treatment on halfway house placement completion is hampered because offenders who pose particularly high risks for re-arrest are often not released through a CCC.

Summary

The results of this three-year follow-up of residential drug abuse treatment programs suggest important and exciting possibilities for the treatment of inmates with substance abuse problems. Male inmates who entered, received, and completed residential drug abuse treatment were 16 percent less likely to be re-arrested or have their supervision revoked (and be returned to prison) than inmates who did not receive such treatment; the comparable figure for female inmates is 18 percent. This reduction in recidivism is coupled with the 15 percent reduction in drug use for male treated subjects and the 18 percent reduction in drug use for female treated subjects. We also found improved employment among women after release. Women who completed residential drug abuse treatment were employed 68.6 percent of their post-release period and untreated women were employed 59.1 percent of the time. Although the results for recidivism and drug use are not statistically significant for women, the sample size of women was smaller, their overall failure rate was lower, and there is evidence in the research literature that there are gender differences in treatment needs, treatment processes and relapse. Specifically, it appears that women's drug abuse or dependence is caused by substantially different factors than those for men. Our findings of a lower percentage of women who use drugs and are arrested or revoked after release, despite the greater number of life problems among women, is consistent with results of previous studies.[14] The Bureau of Prisons is now modifying our drug treatment programs for females based upon best practices for treatment of females in public and private sector programs. We will continue to monitor progress around the country in enhancing drug abuse treatment paradigms for female offenders and modify our programs accordingly.

These results strongly suggest that the Bureau of Prisons' residential drug abuse treatment programs make a significant difference in the lives of inmates following their release from custody and return to the community. This evaluation has been methodologically rigorous and has revealed significant positive effects on recidivism, drug use, and employment in post-release outcomes for a three-year follow-up period.

Notes

1. This article forms the Executive Summary of the "Triad Drug Treatment Evaluation Project Final Report of Three-Year Outcomes: Part 1," issued by the Federal Bureau of Prisons, Office of Research and Evaluations, in September 2000. The complete report can be found on the Bureau of Prisons' web site, at www.bop.gov.

2. The Anti-Drug Abuse Act of 1986 laid the groundwork for the drug treatment programs and the Anti-Drug Abuse Act of 1988 contained provisions for the funding of these programs.

3. Among female inmates, while the effect of treatment was not statistically significant, the failure rate for recidivism of treated inmates compared with untreated inmates suggested a positive effect for treatment.

4. The drug failure rates for women suggested a positive effect for treatment but did not reach statistical significance.

5. Community transitional services also are offered to inmates who have not completed any drug abuse treatment in the institution or who have received treatment other than the residential program but still require transitional drug treatment services.

6. The 12-month programs are no longer operational.

7. This early release provision presents issues of disparity for Bureau inmates. The disparity arises when, for example, two inmates convicted of the same offense serve different prison terms because the inmate who has been diagnosed with a substance abuse problem receives a one-year reduction on his/her sentence and the inmate without a substance abuse problem serves the entire sentence. In effect, many perceive this one-year reduction as a reward for drug-abusing behavior.

8. Typically, inmates enter a residential drug abuse treatment program 36 to 24 months before release from BOP custody. This allows inmates to complete treatment and transition into community-based treatment with minimal interruption to their treatment program, and to benefit from the sentence reduction, if eligible.

9. Approximately 12 percent of the subjects were not released to supervision.

10. Thus, in this analysis only our sample size was 2,640 subjects.

11. A violation of a condition of supervision does not always result in a revocation.

12. Individuals not in the work force due to retirement, disability, and homemaking were excluded from this analysis.

13. We were not able to conduct separate analyses for most of the results presented in the 6-month preliminary report.

14. We note that separate analyses of men and women are rare and little is known about the differential impact of treatment on men and women. We refer the reader to the literature review contained in the full report for additional information on gender differences.

Robert Apsler

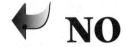

NO

Is Drug Abuse Treatment Effective?

In early February [1994], the Clinton administration spelled out its national antidrug strategy. Much of the debate over the new program will turn on how much federal support should be made available for treating drug addicts. The administration plans to spend $355 million in new grants for the states to use to treat hard-core drug users, while cutting funds for interdiction. Many years of massive federal investment in interdiction—including involvement of the U.S. military—have failed to reduce the availability of low-cost street drugs. And the policy momentum is now toward shifting federal funds from supply reduction to demand reduction, a move that would benefit treatment and prevention programs. Also, news stories about the administration's deliberations often report on drug treatment programs with long waits for new admissions. What is implied if not stated is that the size of the country's drug abusing population, estimated by the Institute of Medicine to be 5.5 million people, would be significantly reduced if more money were spent for drug abuse treatment.

But missing from the news stories and analyses of proposed antidrug strategies is any frank discussion of the underlying assumption that drug abuse treatment is effective. This assumption is based largely on reports from clinicians and recovered drug addicts. It is encouraged by a growing drug treatment industry and accepted by a public that wishes for a solution to the drug problem. The premise may be accurate, but it is not yet supported by hard evidence. We do not know that drug abuse treatment is effective. Clinicians' reports in other areas have not always been reliable. For example, many medical procedures developed through clinical experience alone have been abandoned when researchers showed, through carefully controlled comparisons, that placebos or other alternatives matched their effectiveness.

With a few exceptions, drug abuse treatment has not been subjected to rigorous tests for effectiveness. Good research doesn't exist for a number of reasons. Researchers are hampered by fundamental conceptual issues. Even defining basic ideas is difficult. There are significant practical obstacles that make conducting research difficult as well, and little federal support for drug treatment research has been available for over a decade.

What Is "Drug Abuse Treatment"?

One of the conceptual and practical problems of research is the simple fact that no one process or combination of procedures comprises "drug abuse treatment." Nor do the various types of drug programs have much in common beyond the shared objective of reducing drug abuse.

There are four major types of drug treatment. *Residential therapeutic communities* are highly structured residential settings for drug addicts and typically employ a mixture of psychological and behavioral therapies. Duration of treatment varies widely among these programs. *Inpatient/outpatient chemical dependency treatment* begins with a three- to six-week residential stay in a clinic or hospital that uses the Alcoholics Anonymous philosophy. These clients are then encouraged to attend self-help groups for the rest of their lives. A third type, *outpatient methadone maintenance programs,* involves supervised addiction to methadone hydrochloride as a substitute for addiction to other narcotics, such as heroin. Programs may include counseling and other social services for clients. The fourth category, *outpatient nonmethadone treatment,* joins many different types of programs whose main similarity is that they tend not to treat individuals who are dependent on opiates such as heroin, morphine, and codeine.

This four-group classification is crude because the programs within each category differ markedly from each other. For example, methadone maintenance programs differ in the size of the methadone dose, the number and type of additional services provided, the frequency of urine testing, the strictness of program regulation enforcement, and whether clients are permitted to take their methadone dose home. Some programs focus on illicit drug use and criminal activity, while others target the overall functioning of clients. Some demand abstinence from all illicit drugs; others help clients gain control over their drug use. They differ in whether they concentrate on a particular drug and, if they do, on which drug. Some programs rely heavily on professional practitioners; others employ nonprofessionals, often ex-addicts, as counselors. Programs also differ in the clients they serve: those in the private sector cater mainly to employed drug abusers, whose care is covered by health insurance. The public sector programs serve large numbers of indigent clients.

The differences within each of the four major categories of drug programs are so great that information about the effectiveness of one program in a particular category tells us little about the effectiveness of other programs in the same category. In fact, some differences among programs within a classification group may prove to be more important than the differences among the four groups of programs. For example, new evidence shows that the sheer quantity of treatment provided to clients is crucial to a program's effectiveness. Thus, the amount of counseling and auxiliary services provided by a program may be a more important defining characteristic with respect to efficacy than the types of drug abuse it treats, its treatment philosophy, or whether it operates through a residential or outpatient setting.

What Is "Effective" Treatment?

Just as there is no simple answer to what comprises drug abuse treatment, neither is there an agreed-upon definition of what constitutes *effective* drug abuse treatment. Definitions clash in two important ways. First, strongly held views divide the treatment community on whether abstinence from illicit drug use is necessary. One position holds that successful treatment is synonymous with total abstinence from illicit drugs. The other position holds that treatment is successful if it ends clients' *dependence* on drugs. Continued, moderate drug use is accepted for those clients able to gain control over their drug use and prevent it from interfering with their daily functioning.

Definitions of effectiveness also differ in the number of behaviors they measure. The most common view of effectiveness judges treatment by its ability to reduce the two behaviors most responsible for society's strong reaction against drug abuse: illicit drug use and criminal activity. Others argue that a broader definition of effectiveness is necessary to describe treatment accurately. Advocates of the broader definition believe that treatment should not be considered effective if it can only demonstrate reductions in drug use and illegal activity, since these changes are likely to dissipate rapidly unless clients undergo additional changes. Returning clients who have completed treatment to their previous drug using environment, it is argued, subjects them to the same social and economic forces that contributed to their drug use. According to this view, sustained changes occur only when clients are willing and able to survive and prosper in new environments. To do so, clients must first develop the necessary employment, social, and other skills. Broad definitions of effectiveness usually include: (1) drug abuse, (2) illegal activities, (3) employment, (4) length of stay in treatment, (5) social functioning, (6) intrapersonal functioning, and (7) physical health and longevity.

Motivation and Crisis

Without having resolved even basic definitions about drug abuse treatment, the administration is nevertheless proceeding on the assumption that more money for treatment will mean more help. Doing so ignores the fact that we don't know very much in this area and also ignores the little we do know. We don't know much about client differences, for instance. But we do know that a drug addict's motivation for seeking treatment is crucial. Most clinicians believe that successful treatment is impossible if a client does not want help. Addicts must admit the existence of a serious problem and sincerely want to do something about it. Only then will they accept the assistance of clinicians. However, most experts in the drug abuse field reluctantly acknowledge that almost no drug abusers actually *want* treatment. The news reports implying that thousands of needy addicts would enter treatment and soon be on their way to recovery if the country were willing to spend more money and increase the number of drug programs are inaccurate. While waiting lists exist for some programs, others have trouble attracting addicts.

Furthermore, most drug abusers enter treatment when faced with a crisis, such as threats by a judge, employer, or spouse, or a combination of the three. As a result, the drug abuser's objective may be limited to overcoming the current problem. When the crisis has abated, patients often admit they do not intend all drug use to stop. A national survey of admissions to public drug programs from 1979 to 1981 found that pressure from the criminal justice system was the strongest motivation for seeking treatment. Thus, the existence of long waiting lists may tell us more about judges' efforts to find alternatives to incarceration in overcrowded jails than about the actual intentions of drug abusers or the effectiveness of treatment programs.

The assumption that drug addicts enter treatment at a crisis point has another important ramification for interpreting research on the effectiveness of treatment programs. Studies of treatment effectiveness typically measure clients at least twice: when they enter a program and when they complete treatment. If the first measurement occurs during a time of crisis, it will reflect clients' negative circumstances by showing high levels of drug use, criminal behavior, unemployment, and so on. The second measure of clients, taken at the conclusion of treatment, will likely occur after the precipitating crisis has passed or at least lessened. Consequently, a comparison of the measurements taken at the beginning and end of treatment will show significant improvement for many clients. Is this improvement evidence of effective treatment? Or does it merely reflect the natural cycle of a passing crisis? The main problem is that the research designs used in nearly all drug treatment research cannot separate the effects of treatment from other factors such as these.

Research Problems

Questions about drug treatment effectiveness must be answered the same way as similar questions about treatments for the common cold, AIDS, or other ailments, that is, by obtaining evidence that compares the outcomes of treated and untreated individuals. While this may seem obvious, most drug treatment research has neither compared the necessary groups of drug users nor employed the types of research designs capable of producing strong conclusions. In addition, serious measurement and attrition problems weaken the conclusions of most studies of drug treatment effectiveness.

Research design. Comparisons between drug users who receive treatment and others who do not are almost nonexistent. Researchers study only treated drug users. Yet the observed behavior of drug users who do not enter drug programs reinforces the need for researchers to include untreated addicts in their studies. We have known for years, for instance, that some drug abusers, including heroin addicts, end drug use largely on their own. Researchers have also observed large reductions in drug use among drug abusers waiting for, but not yet receiving, treatment for cocaine abuse.

The phenomenon of people ending their use of highly addictive *legal* substances on their own is well documented. For example, there is mounting evidence that smokers quit on their own at about the same rate as those attending smoking treatment programs. Estimates of remission from alcoholism and alcohol problems without formal treatment range from 45 to 70 percent. No comparable estimate is available for the number of drug users who quit on their own. Until we know the recovery rates for untreated drug abusers, it is impossible to claim that treatment is more effective than the absence of treatment.

Furthermore, the research designs and methods employed in most drug treatment research are so seriously flawed that the results can be considered no more than suggestive. Many investigations study a single group of treated clients and attempt to draw conclusions without a comparison group. Other investigations compare different groups of clients receiving different treatments. In nearly all such cases, the types of clients differ from group to group. Consequently, it is impossible to distinguish between effects caused by treatment differences and effects caused by client differences.

Measuring the outcomes of treatment.   One major need in drug treatment research is for an objective, reliable, and inexpensive method for measuring treatment outcomes. Presently most treatment researchers rely entirely on clients' own reports of past and current behavior. Much of the behavior that clients are asked about is illegal, occurred while they were intoxicated, and may have taken place months, and even years, earlier. As one would expect, clients underreport their drug use and other illegal activities. Yet the drug treatment field continues to rely heavily on these dubious reports because there are no suitable alternatives. Chemical tests, such as urine and hair testing, are important adjuncts for validating clients' reports. But at best these tests confirm use or abstinence; they do not indicate anything about quantity or intervals of use. So they are crude measures that cannot easily track patterns of drug use over long periods after a client leaves a treatment program.

Many treatment studies measure clients at the beginning and end of treatment because it is so difficult and expensive to keep track of them after they have completed a program. Some studies do attempt to assess the impact of treatment six months, a year, or even longer after completion. But investigators can seldom locate more than 70 percent of clients, if that. Clients who cannot be contacted are often deceased, in prison, unemployed, and/or homeless. Leaving them out of the studies may skew the findings, making the conclusions appear more positive than is warranted.

Length of treatment.   The length of drug abuse treatment is a complex and confusing element in the overall picture of treatment effectiveness. To begin with, simply keeping clients in treatment is a major challenge for many drug programs. Most clients are forced into treatment. And many leave shortly thereafter. Therefore, merely remaining in treatment has become a widely accepted measure of treatment effectiveness. While it makes sense that clients can only benefit from treatment if they remain in a program, there is the risk of confusing happenstance for cause and effect.

Addicts who truly want to change their lifestyles are likely to make many changes. Such changes include entering and remaining in a treatment program, reducing drug use, holding a steady job, eschewing illegal activities, and so on. Other individuals not willing to change their lifestyles are more likely to drop out of treatment after being forced into a drug program. They continue using drugs, do not hold steady jobs, engage in illegal activities, and so on. Thus, to prove that drug programs are effective, researchers must show that (1) drug programs help addicts commit to changing their lifestyles, and/or that (2) the resulting improvement among treated clients is greater than the improvement expected anyway from individuals who have already chosen to change their lifestyles.

Another challenge is determining the length of an optimum stay in a drug treatment program. Most private chemical dependency residential programs used to run for 28 days, though cost-reduction pressures have shortened this time. Outpatient nonmethadone treatment averages roughly six months of once-or-twice-a-week counseling sessions. Some therapeutic communities provide treatment for a year or more, while methadone maintenance programs may involve lifetime participation for clients. How much treatment is enough? Some research shows that methadone clients remain in treatment for an unnecessarily long time. This may mean that programs with waiting lists should consider ending treatment for long-term clients to make room for new ones. The impact of treatment may be much greater on someone receiving treatment for the first time than on an individual who has been on methadone for years.

The complex treatment histories of many drug addicts increase the difficulty of judging treatment effectiveness. Over the course of their addiction careers, typical drug addicts enter several different treatment programs. They may enter the same programs on different occasions for different lengths of time. At any point during this involved treatment history, addicts may find themselves participating in a study of treatment effectiveness. However, that study is likely to examine only the most recent treatment episode without taking into account previous treatment stays. Perhaps even small amounts of treatment accumulate over time until they influence an individual. Some drug addicts may try different forms of treatment until they find a type of treatment or a particular counselor that helps them. However, existing treatment research cannot disentangle the effects of multiple treatment episodes in different types of drug programs that last for varying amounts of time.

What We Know About Treatment Programs

Because of research problems, very little is known about the effectiveness of three out of the four categories of drug abuse treatment identified earlier in this article—*residential therapeutic communities, inpatient/outpatient chemical dependency treatment,* and *outpatient nonmethadone maintenance programs.* Surveys of *residential therapeutic communities* have produced promising results, but important questions remain unanswered. Two longitudinal studies of many drug treatment programs reported reductions in drug use and criminal activity among therapeutic community clients who remained in treatment for at least several months. But therapeutic communities are highly selective in at least two ways. First, they appeal only to clients willing to enter a long-term residential setting. Second, most addicts who enter therapeutic communities quickly drop out. Thus, therapeutic communities may influence the drug addiction of only a small and select group of individuals. Furthermore, there is almost no research about the factors that affect success and failure in therapeutic communities.

As for the other two, almost nothing reliable has been produced on *inpatient/outpatient chemical dependency treatment,* though it has become the dominant approach of privately financed inpatient programs. Nor are there reliable findings on *outpatient/nonmethadone treatment.*

The strongest evidence that drug abuse treatment can be effective comes from randomized clinical trials of the remaining category of treatment programs, *methadone maintenance treatment* programs. Randomized clinical trials are powerful studies that randomly assign a pool of subjects to different conditions, such as different types of treatment; researchers are able to conclude that if some groups of subjects improve more than others, the improvement is probably due to the treatment condition, not to preexisting differences among the individuals. The first of three rigorous trials of methadone treatment, a U.S. study conducted in the late 1960s, randomly assigned highly motivated criminal addicts to either a methadone program or a waiting-list group that received no treatment. All 16 addicts on the waiting list quickly became readdicted to heroin, as did 4 addicts in the treatment group who refused treatment. Eighteen of the 20 untreated individuals who became readdicted returned to prison within 1 to 10 months. Only 3 of the 12 addicts who received treatment returned to prison during this period, and their heroin use decreased.

A test in 1984 of a methadone maintenance program in Sweden provides further evidence of treatment effectiveness, though the stringent client selection criteria make it difficult to generalize the findings. Heroin addicts became eligible for this study only after (1) a history of long-term compulsive abuse, and (2) repeated failures to stop, despite documented serious attempts to do so. Thirty-four addicts meeting these eligibility requirements were randomly assigned to either treatment or no-treatment. Two years later, 12 of the 17 drug addicts assigned to treatment had abandoned drug use and started work or studies. The remaining 5 still had drug problems, and 2 had been expelled from the program. Conversely, only 1 of the 17 addicts in the no-treatment group became drug free; 2 were in prison, 2 were dead, and the rest were still abusing heroin.

A very recent randomized clinical trial in the United States compared three levels of methadone treatment: (1) methadone alone without other services, (2) methadone plus counseling, and (3) methadone plus counseling and on-site medical/psychiatric, employment, and family therapy. The results showed that methadone alone was, at most, helpful to only a few clients. The results for clients who received methadone plus counseling were better, and clients who received additional professional services improved most of all. In sum, these three studies demonstrate that methadone treatment has the potential to reduce illicit narcotics use and criminal behavior among narcotics addicts.

To what extent do these findings apply to methadone maintenance programs in general? We do not know, and we must remain skeptical about the level of effectiveness of most methadone programs; their results could be quite different. For example, two of the three studies described above restricted their research to clients who were highly motivated to end their addiction. But methadone programs in this country typically treat individuals who are forced into treatment, many of whom exhibit little desire to change their addict lifestyles. The third study did not restrict the research to highly motivated clients. However, the study took place in a well-funded, stable, hospital-based, university-affiliated setting. Most methadone programs operate on small budgets that severely restrict their ability to provide services and hire qualified staff. Therefore they differ in important ways from the study program.

To learn about the impact of less extraordinary methadone programs, a U.S. General Accounting Office study examined the efficacy of 15 methadone programs in a five-state survey. The survey found that (1) the current use of heroin and other opiates ranged from 2 to 47 percent of clients enrolled in the clinics, (2) many clients had serious alcohol problems, (3) clients received few comprehensive services despite high rates of unemployment, and (4) clinics did not know if clients used the services to which they were referred. Other research has shown that many methadone programs administer doses of methadone smaller than those known to be effective. In sum, typical methadone programs differ significantly from the methadone programs evaluated in the randomized clinical trials discussed above, and they may be less effective.

Conclusions

Drug abuse treatment features prominently in discussions of how the Clinton administration should respond to the country's concern about drug abuse. Yet little hard evidence documents the effectiveness of treatment. Almost nothing is known about (1) the effectiveness of three of the four major treatment modalities, (2) the relative effectiveness of different versions of each major treatment modality, and (3) the prognosis for different types of drug abusers. Instead of answering questions, drug treatment research raises troublesome issues for policymakers. How can treatment work when clinicians claim that success depends on clients wanting help, and we know that most clients are forced into treatment? What happens to drug abusers who never seek treatment?

What can be said with some certainty is that (1) methadone maintenance programs can help clients who are highly motivated to end their drug abuse, and (2) a model program that provides counseling along with methadone has been able to help less well-motivated clients. But there is little good news here since most drug addicts do not want to end their drug use, and typical methadone maintenance programs may not possess the resources to duplicate the impact of the model program.

The absence of convincing evidence about the effectiveness of drug abuse treatment results from the lack of rigorous evaluations. Only a handful of randomized clinical trials have been conducted to date. More need to be done, and valid and comprehensive measures of treatment effectiveness need to be employed in these studies in order to end the reliance of treatment researchers on clients' self-reports of sensitive behaviors. Treatment research also needs more post-treatment follow-ups to show that treatment effects persist once clients leave their programs.

Finally, researchers must learn what happens to untreated drug abusers. Past and current research focuses almost exclusively on drug abusers who enter treatment. This research does not make comparisons between treated and untreated drug abusers and cannot answer the most fundamental question of all: is treatment more cost-effective than no treatment?

POSTSCRIPT

Does Drug Abuse Treatment Work?

Much of the research on the effectiveness of drug treatment is inconclusive. Furthermore, researchers do not agree on how to best measure effectiveness. Determining the effectiveness of drug treatment is extremely important because the federal government and a number of state governments are now contemplating increasing the amount of funding allocated to drug treatment. Many experts in the drug field agree that much of the money that has been used to deal with problems related to drugs has not been spent wisely. To prevent further waste of taxpayer funds, it is essential to find out if drug treatment works before funding for it is increased.

Another concern related to this issue is that addicts who wish to receive treatment often face many barriers. One of the most serious barriers is the lack of available treatment facilities. Compounding the problem is the fact that many communities resist the idea of having a drug treatment center in the neighborhood, even though there is little research on the effects of treatment facilities on property values and neighborhood crime rates. Another barrier to treatment is cost, which, with the exception of self-help groups, is high. Furthermore, some addicts avoid organized treatment altogether for fear that if they go for treatment, they will be identified as drug abusers by law enforcement agencies.

Many addicts in treatment are there because they are given a choice of entering either prison or treatment. Are people who are required to enter treatment likely to succeed more or less than people who enter treatment voluntarily? Early studies showed that treatment was more effective for voluntary clients. However, a study conducted by the U.S. federal government of 12,000 clients enrolled in 41 publicly funded treatment centers found that clients referred by the criminal justice system fared as well as if not better than voluntary clients in terms of reduced criminal activity and drug use.

Donna Lyons examines whether drug addicts should be sent to prison or to treatment in "Conviction for Addiction," *State Legislatures* (June 2002). In "Report Sheds Light on Drug Abuse," *Counseling Today* (January 2001), Jennifer Simmons discusses recommendations by the federal government to improve success rates for drug treatment. Two articles that look at the effectiveness of methadone maintenance programs are "Methadone Maintenance and HIV Prevention: A Cost-Effectiveness Analysis," by Gregory Zaric, Margaret Brandeau, and Paul Barnett, *Management Science* (August 2000) and "Revisiting the Effectiveness of Methadone Treatment on Crime Reduction in the 1990s," by Aileen Rothbard et al., *Journal of Substance Abuse Treatment* (June 1999). A national poll by Peter Hart Research Associates found that more people support drug treatment over drug interdiction. See "Survey Finds Public Support for Treatment Over Interdiction," *Alcoholism and Drug Abuse Weekly* (July 24, 2000).

ISSUE 19

Do Alcohol Advertisements Influence Young People to Drink More?

YES: Sandi W. Smith, Charles K. Atkin, and Thomas Fediuk, from "Youth Reactions to Televised Liquor Commercials," Letter to the Editor, *Journal of Alcohol and Drug Education* (Winter 2000)

NO: Secretary of Health and Human Services, from *Tenth Special Report to the U.S. Congress on Alcohol and Health* (June 2000)

ISSUE SUMMARY

YES: Professors of communication Sandi W. Smith and Charles K. Atkin and Ph.D. candidate Thomas Fediuk assert that advertisements for alcoholic beverages are perceived as appealing and influential by young people. The ads consistently portray alcohol use as humorous and fun, and actors in the advertisements are perceived as masculine, sociable, romantic, elegant, adventurous, and relaxed.

NO: The secretary of health and human services contends that the research demonstrating a link between alcohol advertisements and actual drinking behavior among young people is inconsistent. Young people whose alcohol use is affected by alcohol advertisements may be predisposed to alcohol use in the first place, says the secretary, concluding that alcohol advertisements essentially reinforce behavior.

Over 90 percent of students will have consumed alcohol by the time they graduate from high school. Alcohol use by young people, especially binge drinking, has increased steadily over the past decade. Ironically, as the number of young people who binge drink goes up, the number of young people who totally abstain from alcohol also goes up. A conclusion could be drawn that young people either drink to excess or do not drink at all. Drinking in moderation does not appear to be the norm.

Some critics maintain that the preponderance of alcohol advertisements has contributed to an increase in alcohol consumption. Yet how much do these advertisements actually affect a young person's decision to drink? If young people are easily swayed to drink by advertisements, then that implies that young people lack reasoning skills.

Alcohol advertisements are apparently designed to appeal to young people. For example, almost all people in television and print advertisements are young and active. It is not only in advertisements that alcohol is portrayed in a fun way. Alcohol consumption is commonly portrayed in music videos. There are plenty of television programs that show college students on spring break, and these shows are replete with scenes of students imbibing alcohol. Very few older people are depicted in these programs or advertisements. In addition, seldom does one see any of the problems that occur due to drinking.

According to the alcohol industry, the point of advertisements is to promote brand loyalty, not to promote drinking. Many companies state that they make a concerted effort to promote responsible alcohol use. One trend that has developed in recent years is the advertising of distilled spirits. In the past, alcohol companies did not advertise distilled spirits. Congress is now debating whether or not advertisements for distilled spirits should be allowed.

Besides alcohol advertisements, there are other factors that contribute to alcohol use and abuse by young people. It has been argued that teenagers drink because they are bored and need more alternative activities, especially on weekends. Some young people drink because their friends drink. Others drink because they lack social skills and because alcohol gives them a false sense of confidence. If these are reasons young people drink, then how much blame should be directed toward companies that advertise alcohol?

In the following selections, Sandi W. Smith, Charles K. Atkin, and Thomas Fediuk argue that alcohol advertisements send the wrong message to young people—that alcohol use is humorous, adventurous, and romantic. The secretary of health and human services indicates that alcohol advertisements have not been shown unequivocally to cause young people to drink more alcohol. The secretary concludes that although some young people with a propensity to drink may be influenced by these advertisements, this does not apply to most youths.

Sandi W. Smith, Charles K. Atkin, and Thomas Fediuk

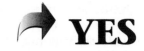 **YES**

Youth Reactions to Televised Liquor Commercials

Dear Editor:

Liquor ads have been appearing in magazines and on billboards for most of the past century, and beer companies have been advertising on TV since the earliest days of this medium. However, liquor commercials were traditionally considered to be too sensitive for television. After a decade of declining sales, the liquor companies began to actively consider the advantages of television in the mid-1990s. The self-imposed distilled spirits industry restriction on televised commercials was formally broken in 1996 when liquor commercials began airing on certain cable channels and local stations. By 1998, liquor advertisers were spending $15 million to place ads in the broadcast media. These ads represent another media channel through which youth may be influenced to engage in alcohol consumption.

This change in policy suggests some important questions that are the focus of this research. How will youths respond to these televised liquor commercials, in terms of their affective reactions, opinions about appeal of the ads, perceived targeting of ads, the effectiveness of the ads, and the number of drinks they believed the characters had consumed? The questions will be answered by use of the focus group method with underage youth. Both the methodology and the results of the study have important implications for media literacy training and alcohol education. In addition, the answers to these questions are critical as the Distilled Spirits Council of the United States (DISCUS) claims in their Code of Good Practice for Distilled Spirits Advertising and Marketing that they will continue to avoid targeting individuals below the legal purchase age in their advertisements (DISCUS, 2000).

Alcohol advertisers have consistently asserted that the main purpose of advertisements is either to retain product loyalty or to induce customers of the competition to switch brands, not to lure new customers. DISCUS argues that advertising does not cause an individual to consume alcohol and claims that parents and peers are the most influential factors in determining adolescent alcohol consumption. Research evidence on advertising impact is mixed; some experts conclude that alcohol advertisements do not increase consumption (Saffer, 1996; Smart, 1988), while other researchers find that adolescent drinking intentions and consumption patterns are influenced by alcohol ads and that the ads serve as an important source of information about drinking (Atkin, Hocking & Block, 1984; Kelly & Edwards, 1998; Wyllie, Zhang, & Casswell, 1998).

Liquor industry codes assert that advertising should not appeal to underage audiences. DISCUS, in its Code of Good Practice, states that: "Distilled spirits should not be advertised or marketed in any manner directed or primarily intended to appeal to persons below the legal purchase age." They also claim that "The content of distilled spirits advertising and marketing material should not be intended to appeal to individuals below the legal purchase age," and state "DISCUS has always encouraged those adults who choose to drink to do so responsibly. For individuals under the legal purchase age, the only responsible use is zero use" (DISCUS, 2000).

While the effects of alcohol advertising on consumption of alcohol are in dispute, there is ample evidence that alcohol ads produce cognitive effects among youth. Grube (1993) concludes that as children age, they become more aware of and more engaged in alcohol advertisements, particularly ads that portray fun lifestyles, celebrity endorsements, humor, animation and rock music (Grube, 1993). The most susceptible adolescents are those who are favorably disposed to alcohol, but have not yet begun to drink, and it is at this point that adolescents may develop brand preferences (Kelly & Edwards, 1998).

With the introduction of televised liquor commercials in the late 1990's, there are widespread concerns that these ads may influence adolescent audiences. A national poll shows that 48% of adults agree that "liquor companies are trying to influence teenagers to drink liquor" (Atkin & Smith, 1998). Fully 74% of adults said that it is likely that "teenagers who see a lot of TV liquor commercials . . . will be encouraged to start drinking liquor," and 63% said that teenagers "will drink a greater amount of liquor" after being exposed to liquor commercials. These beliefs among the general public are clearly at odds with the assertions of the liquor industry, but research is needed with samples of youth to shed more light on their own reactions to these ads. This research effort attempts to begin to address this issue.

The current study included results from 16 focus groups with young people at the middle school and high school age levels. The questions examined their reactions to the ads, opinions about appeal of the ads, perceived targeting of ads, the effectiveness of the ads, and perceived alcohol consumption by characters in the ads. This method could be used by educators to increase the media literacy of youth because knowing how to read messages conveyed through visual images, music, and advertising translates into power by giving control over personal beliefs and behaviors (Potter, 1998).

Image advertising focuses on the lifestyle of the user of the product rather than on the values of the product. Content analyses of alcohol ads link drinking to highly valued attributes, such as sociability, elegance, physical attractiveness, success, relaxation, romance and adventure (Grube, 1993). Zinser, Freeman, & Ginnings (1999) found that ads are seen as adventurous, appealing, eye-catching, informative, believable, portray good times, athletic, romantic, and recreational.

Image advertisements tend to be more influential with adolescents than with adults; those who do not drink, but think they may in the future, like the image ads (Kelly & Edwards, 1998). Content analyses reveal that ads portray drinkers in a favorable and desirable manner. Actors in the ads tend to be young adults who are perceived as: masculine, sociable, romantic, elegant, adventurous and relaxed. Such portrayals may be desirable to adolescents as well.

Focus group interviews were used to provide answers to the research questions posed in this study. Participants in each group were relatively homogeneous with respect to age, sex, and ethnicity. Six of the groups were composed of pre-teens and younger teenagers between the 5th and the 8th grades, and ten groups of high school students were assembled. There were a total of 140 participants in these groups, primarily in Michigan, Missouri, Connecticut, and California. The assembled participants were shown videotaped commercials to stimulate reactions. Three specimen TV ads were selected from among the initial array of 10 liquor commercials aired during the first year that television stations permitted such advertising: Crown Royal whiskey *Graduation Dogs* spot (featuring two attractive dogs and graduation music; one dog has a diploma while the "valedictorian" dog holds the whiskey bottle in a velvet sack); Kahlua *Mudslide Village* (showing the brown liqueur flowing like lava through a foreign village, with young adults partying and playing pool in the local bar); Cuervo Gold *Paradise Island* (rapid-fire scenes of extreme sports and beach fun by youthful characters).

A supplemental technique used in these sessions was the use of self-administered questionnaire sheets: following exposure to each of the three commercials, every participant marked a one-page survey instrument with close-ended items asking for their individual reactions to the commercial.

The affective reaction to the specimen ads was measured with both survey and open-end items measuring liking of each message, enjoyment of the music, and the experience of having fun while watching the ads. Questions included: "Do you like or dislike watching these ads? Why?" "Do you like or dislike this commercial? . . . Why?" (*Graduation Dogs*) "Do you think the dogs in this commercial are cute? Do you like the graduation music in the commercial?" (*Mudslide Village*) "Do you like the song in the commercial?" (*Mudslide Village* & *Paradise Island*) "Do you think this ad is fun to watch?"

Middle school viewers in all five groups expressed positive comments about the "cute" and "likeable" dogs after seeing the *Graduation Dogs* commercial. The *Mudslide Village* spot generated divergent responses. Half liked it and half did not like the commercial. One student commented that the liquor "looked like a nice glass of gold milk" while another said that the liquor "looked nasty." The characters were seen as youthful and attractive, with comments such as "beautiful women," "strong men," "good-looking people," and "people looked younger than 21." Several noted that people were enjoying the activities such as playing pool: "everyone was having fun" and "socializing with alcohol." Stylistically, several regarded the ad as "boring," "stupid," and "unrealistic," but one pointed out that the ad "looked like a Starburst commercial" and several stated that they like the Rolling Stones music. In the survey, three-fifths reported liking for the song in the ad. Three-fifths thought the ad was fun to watch.

Half liked the *Paradise Island* TV spot, and three-fifths thought it was fun to watch. The positive reactions to the commercial focused on the attractive setting: "guys on the beach," "looks like spring break," "paradise island is fun." In regard to the behavior portrayed, one student [said] that "boys and girls are together sexually," and several commented that the alcohol consumption involved "binge drinking" and "glorified getting drunk."

In the high school groups, two-fifths of the students expressed liking for the *Graduation Dogs* spot. The main reasons for enjoying the messages were the "cute dogs" (which were appreciated by most participants), the humor, and the graduation music. Nevertheless, a solid majority disliked the commercial, criticizing it as "boring" and "stupid"; in several cases, they felt the theme disrespected academic excellence.

A slight majority liked the *Village Mudslide* commercial; it was particularly well received by the black focus groups. The positives were the "catchy music," the "fun party" portrayal, the interesting actions, and the "pretty women." The results from the survey questions showed that three-fifths liked the song played throughout the commercial, and three-fifths replied that it was fun to watch.

There were mixed reactions to the *Paradise Island* ad, but positive comments clearly outnumbered the negative comments. Most participants appreciated the high-energy extreme sports clips, and many liked the tropical beach and "spring break feel." The attractive women and party scene also received favorable responses from several participants. Based on survey answers, three-fifths like the ad, and the same proportion said it was fun to watch.

Participants were asked about their perceptions of the amount of liquor being consumed by the characters in the two specimen ads depicting characters in drinking contexts (in accordance with conventional practice, none were actually portrayed in the act of drinking). The viewers could make inferences based on the presence of bottles and glasses, the behavior of the characters, and the expected consumption norms associated with beach or bar settings. This analysis focused on the proportion who perceived that "binge drinking" quantity (five or more drinks) was being consumed. The survey questionnaire asked viewers to "Think about the people on the beach/playing pool in the bar. About how many drinks do you think each character in this commercial will drink altogether?"

In judging the number of drinks consumed by characters in the *Village Mudslide* bar scene, half of the middle school participants estimated five or more drinks. For the *Paradise Island* spot, three-fifths believe at least five drinks were being consumed by characters on the beach. One-third of the high school students estimated that the bar patrons were consuming at least five drinks, and two-thirds thought that the beach drinkers were consuming that much alcohol.

The next issue examined in the study is the perceived teen targeting by liquor advertisers. Questions included "Who do you think this liquor commercial is supposed to influence?," "Does Seagram/Kahlua/Cuervo want teenagers to watch this ad?," "What part of the ad makes you think it's aimed at teenagers?,", "Are there certain things in the commercial that might appeal to teenagers?," and "How old do you think the Seagram/Kahlua/Cuervo Company wants people to be before they start drinking liquor?"

All five middle school groups felt that the *Graduation Dog* commercial was aimed at high school students; the main reasons offered were the cute dogs and the use of the graduation music. When asked to estimate the age when the Seagram company wants people to start drinking liquor, four-fifths of the middle school students picked an age under 21 years old (two-thirds of them said age 18 or under).

After seeing the Kahlua *Village Mudslide* commercial, about half of the students said the ad was aimed at middle and late teenagers. Key cues suggesting that the ad was aimed at teenagers were the sexy characters, the party scene, the rock music, and the people "having a fun and wild time." When asked to estimate the initial drinking age sought by the Kahlua company, half of the middle school students indicated an age under 21 years old (including one-third who said age 18 or under).

The Cuervo Gold *Paradise Island* spot was almost universally regarded as targeted to teenagers, based on the youthful characters, the extreme sports activities, and the spring break beach party atmosphere. Almost all of these younger students felt that the Cuervo company wants liquor consumption to occur before 21 years old. . . .

In the high school groups, most participants mentioned teenagers as a secondary target audience for the *Graduation Dogs* spot, but the initial responses emphasized older people, those with higher income, and sophisticated drinkers. For the *Village Mudslide* spot, a majority said that the message was aimed at teenagers. About two-thirds thought Kahlua wants teenagers to watch the ad, because of the "music and partying and hanging out" that was considered to be popular with their age group. Half of the high school students said that the Kahlua Company wants those under age 21 to drink liquor.

Almost all of the teenagers believe that the Cuervo *Paradise Island* ad was targeted to their age group because of the beach scenes and the rebellious attitude expressed in the message. Almost all of the high school students felt that the Cuervo Company wants liquor consumption to occur before 21 years old (two-thirds said age 18 or under).

Another set of questions sought to discover the message features that young people perceived as cues that a commercial was aimed at teenage audiences. The moderator began with general questions "How can you tell whether a TV commercial is aimed at teenagers?" "What are the features that help you decide if ads might appeal to teenagers instead of older adults?," and then specified examples (music, pacing, humor, animals, youthful characters) to prompt further assessment by the participants.

For the middle school participants, one key cue was the portrayal of "cool" people, because it was recognized that high school students want to be seen as "cool." Another factor was the depiction of people doing "extreme things," which was appealing to younger aged groups where "everyone tries everything." More generally, alcohol advertising portrayals of young-looking performers, animals, "good-looking babes," "people having fun," "exciting action" and "cool sports" were seen as teen-oriented. Teenage audiences were thought to be attracted by the use of upbeat "hip" music, bright colors, and fast pacing of camera shots.

For the high school groups, the two leading features suggesting that ads were aimed at teens were type of music (such as rap, ska, rock) and the youthfulness of the performers. Another key factor was humor, followed by portrayals of people having fun or playing games. Depiction of animals, and "cool sports," use of vivid color, and fast paced action were also mentioned by some participants.

The survey questions also sought to measure subjective and hypothetical impact of specimen ads: After all three specimen commercials, participants answered a yes-no question about favorability toward the advertised brand of liquor; after the two spots that depicted party action with attractive characters, the question asked if the ad gave the impression that drinking was "cool." A closing pair of yes-no items asked participants if a heavier schedule of commercials such as these would increase their likelihood [of] trying new brands . . . and drinking a greater quantity of liquor: "Suppose liquor advertisers start showing lots more ads on TV next year . . . if you often saw liquor commercials like these, do you think you would be more likely to try different brands of liquor that you don't usually drink?," and ". . . would you be more likely to drink a greater amount of liquor than you usually drink?"

Across the three spots, about one-fourth of the middle school participants replied that the first ad made them feel more favorable toward the liquor product, and about the same proportion said the two lifestyle ads made them think drinking was cool. Two-fifths said they would more often try new brands and one-quarter said they would consume more liquor if an increased number of ads were to be presented on TV in the next year.

Almost one-third of the high school students reported that they became more favorable toward each of the three liquor brands. Half felt that the *Mudslide Village* ad conveyed a "cool" image, and one-third felt that this was the case for the *Paradise Island* portrayal of drinking. Three-fifths expect an increased likelihood of trying new brands and one-third expect they would drink more liquor if more ads were on TV.

After seeing the full set of the specimen commercials, participants responded to three questions dealing with the appropriateness of allowing liquor ads on TV, and the acceptability of teenagers and children seeing these ads. Each student marked yes-no items on the survey, and was asked to elaborate their opinions on each question in the focus group discussion. "Think about [the] three commercials that you just saw. Do you think that these ads should be allowed on TV?" "Should ads be shown on programs that lots of teenagers watch?" "Is it OK for teenagers to see these ads?" "Is it OK for children under age 12 to see these ads?"

Two-thirds of the students said that the liquor commercials should be allowed on television, but more negative opinions were expressed when the questions focused on underage audiences. Regarding teenage audiences, two-thirds thought that it is acceptable for underage viewers to see these ads. Three-fourths did not feel it's appropriate for children to see the ads, but some thought that children would not understand the subject of drinking, so it would [be] acceptable for them to see the ads.

Three-quarters of high school students believe that liquor ads should be allowed on TV, because "it's a free country," "the ads are shown late at night," "people [are] free to make their own choice," and "young people do what they want anyway." Those who opposed allowing ads said that the messages have a "bad influence on young people." Three-fourths felt that it was OK for teenagers to see the ads in their programs. A large majority was opposed to children seeing the ads, primarily due to the "bad influence" on young viewers who are impressionable or unable to understand the concept of drinking. Comments included "these ads give young people the wrong idea of what is a good time" and "the younger you are the more curious and easily influenced."

In conclusion, the focus group discussions show that most youth perceive that liquor commercials are aimed at underage audiences, and many regard the ads as personally appealing and influential. Moreover, the youthful viewers perceive that the characters are drinking heavily in the two spots depicting party scenes. These findings indicate that television liquor ads pose potential problems among adolescents unless the advertisers act more responsibly in targeting the messages and portraying the drinking experience, and that media literacy and alcohol education programs should teach youth how to critically evaluate liquor advertising.

References

Atkin, C.A., Hocking, J., & Block, M. (1984). Teenage drinking: Does advertising make a difference? *Journal of communication, 34,* 157–167.

Atkin, C.K., & Smith, S.W. *Studying audience responses to televised liquor advertising.* Paper presented to the Health Communication Division of the Western State Communication Association, Denver, February, 1998.

DISCUS (2000). *Code of Good Practice for Distilled Spirits Advertising and Marketing, and Distilled Spirits Council of the United States (DISCUS).* Available: http://discus.health.org.

Grube, J.W. (1993). Alcohol portrayals and alcohol advertising on television. *Alcohol Health and Research World, 17,* 61–66.

Kelly, K.J., & Edwards, R.W. (1998). Image advertisements for alcohol products: Is their appeal associated with adolescents' intention to consume alcohol? *Adolescence, 33,* 47–59.

Potter, J.W. (1998). *Media Literacy.* Thousand Oaks, CA: Sage.

Saffer, H. (1996). Studying the effect of alcohol advertising on consumption. *Alcohol Health and Research World, 20,* 266–272.

Smart, R.G. (1998). Does alcohol advertising affect overall consumption? A review of empirical studies. *Journal of Studies on Alcohol, 49,* 314–23.

Wyllie, A., Zhang, J.F., & Casswell, S. (1998). Responses to televised alcohol advertisements associated with drinking behaviors of 10–17-year-olds. *Addiction, 93,* 361–371.

Zinser, O., Freeman, J.E., & Ginnings, D.K. (1999). A comparison of memory for and attitudes about alcohol, cigarette, and other product advertisements in college students. *Journal of Drug Education, 29,* 175–185.

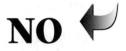
Alcohol Advertising: What Are the Effects?

Does alcohol advertising increase the overall level of alcohol consumption? Does it predispose children and adolescents to drinking? Although these and other related questions have been raised by public health advocates and echoed in public opinion surveys, the evidence from research to date is mixed and far from conclusive. In general, studies based on economic analyses suggest that advertising does not increase overall consumption, but instead may encourage people to switch beverage brands or types. At the same time, research based on survey data indicates that children who like alcohol advertisements intend to drink more frequently as adults. While these findings might offer some grounds for both reassurance and concern, the limitations of the research methods that have been used hinder the ability to draw firm conclusions about cause and effect in either case.

In recent years, public health advocates have called for strict regulation or elimination of alcohol advertising (Mosher 1994), and community-level action has focused on reducing local alcohol advertising (Woodruff 1996). Particular attention has been devoted to how alcohol advertising might affect young people (Atkin 1993) and to the targeting of minority communities (Abramson 1992; Alaniz and Wilkes 1995; Scott et al. 1992). A poll of public attitudes found that 57 percent of the public support prohibiting alcoholic beverage advertisements on television, 64 percent support advertising to counteract alcohol advertisements, and 41 percent support prohibiting sports sponsorship by the alcohol industry (Kaskutas 1993).

As described in this section, researchers have examined the effects of alcohol advertising through four main types of studies: experimental research in controlled settings; econometric analyses, which apply economic research techniques; surveys; and intervention studies of "media literacy" programs that encourage skepticism about advertisements. In general, experimental studies based in laboratory settings provide little consistent evidence that alcohol advertising influences people's drinking behaviors or beliefs about alcohol and its effects (Kohn and Smart 1984; Kohn et al. 1984; Lipsitz 1993; Slater et al. 1997; Sobell et al. 1986). In addition, econometric studies of market data have produced mixed results, with most showing no significant relationship between

From Secretary of Health and Human Services, *Tenth Special Report to the U.S. Congress on Alcohol and Health* (June 2000). Washington, DC: U.S. Government Printing Office, 2000.

advertising and overall consumption levels (Fisher and Cook 1995; Gius 1996; Goel and Morey 1995; Nelson and Moran 1995).

Survey research of children and adolescents, however, provides some evidence of links between alcohol advertising and greater intentions to drink, favorable beliefs about alcohol, and a greater likelihood of drinking (Austin and Meili 1994; Austin and Nach-Ferguson 1995; Grube 1995; Grube and Wallack 1994; Wyllie et al. 1998a,b). Still, the survey study designs employed thus far have not been able to establish whether, for example, the advertisements caused the beliefs and behaviors, or whether preexisting beliefs and behaviors led to an increased awareness of the advertisements. Media literacy training may increase the ability of children and adolescents to offer counterarguments to messages in alcohol advertisements (Austin and Johnson 1997a,b; Slater et al. 1996a), but studies have not yet measured whether these effects persist beyond a short term.

The following is a review of the evidence, from each of these research areas, about the effects of alcohol advertising on alcohol consumption, alcohol-related problems, and drinking-related beliefs and attitudes. Studies have been drawn from such diverse fields as drug and alcohol studies, communications, psychology, sociology marketing and advertising, and economics.

Background: The Frequency and Content of Advertising Messages

Concerns about alcohol advertising stem at least in part from its pervasiveness. The alcohol industry spent $1.03 billion on alcohol advertising in 1996, with the expenditures concentrated on television commercials and beer advertising (Besen 1997). Thus alcohol advertising, especially for beer, appears relatively frequently on television. Moreover, this advertising tends to appear most often during sports programming. While about one alcohol commercial appears in every 4 hours of prime-time fictional programming, one appears for every 25 minutes of programming for major professional sports (football, baseball, and basketball) and one for every 50 minutes of college sports programming (Grube 1993, 1995; Madden and Grube 1994). Overall, alcohol commercials make up 1.5 percent of all advertisements on prime-time television and 7.0 percent of all advertisements in sports programming.

Standard commercials, however, are not the only way in which alcohol is marketed on television. Alcohol advertisers use other types of promotions embedded in sports programming to place their product names, slogans, and symbols before the television viewing audience. Stadium signs, brief sponsorships (such as "This half-time report is brought to you by . . . "), and on-site promotions (such as product symbols and names on race cars) are broadcast to the television viewing audience at a rate of 3.3 per hour in major professional sports programming, 3.0 per hour in other professional sports programming, and 0.3 per hour in college sports programming (Grube 1993, 1995; Madden and Grube 1994).

The engaging images and messages in alcohol commercials may add to the perception, among critics, that advertisements contribute to increased drinking and drinking problems. What is engaging about the advertisements? Although no recent research has investigated this question, older content analysis studies of alcohol advertisements show that alcohol ads link drinking with highly valued personal attributes, such as sociability, elegance, and physical attractiveness, as well as with desirable outcomes, such as success, relaxation, romance, and adventure (see, for example, Atkin and Block 1980; Strickland et al. 1982).

Researchers have been particularly interested in the degree to which children and adolescents pay attention to these commercials. In one survey of fifth- and sixth-grade children, 59 percent of the children could correctly identify the brand of beer being promoted from an edited, still photograph taken from a television commercial featuring Spuds McKenzie (Grube 1995). A vast majority of the children (82 percent) in the same survey correctly matched the advertising slogan, "Spuds McKenzie, the original party animal" with Budweiser.

Alcohol advertising with celebrity endorsers, humor, animation and rock music has been shown to be especially appealing to adolescents (Atkin and Block 1983; Grube 1995). In addition, a study of adolescent boys confirmed that they were particularly attracted to alcohol advertisements depicting sports (Slater et al. 1996c, 1997). In one recent study, adolescents perceived that a significant number of alcohol advertisements portray people under 21 years of age (Slater et al. 1996b). Other research has indicated, however, that adolescents' identification with the actors in the ads, or their desire to be like the actors, is relatively low (Austin and Meili 1994). Lifestyle- or image-oriented alcohol advertising has been shown to be more appealing to both adults and adolescents than is alcohol advertising that promotes only product quality (Covell et al. 1994).

Besides the frequency of advertisements and their appeal to minors, concerns have also stemmed from advertising content that raises safety questions. One study found that 33 percent of television beer advertisements (16 of 49) contained scenes of people drinking and either driving or engaging in water activities such as swimming or boating (Grube 1995). Moreover, messages to drink safely and moderately (such as "Know when to say when") appear in less than 1 percent of alcohol advertisements and have been criticized for not clearly defining responsible drinking (DeJong et al. 1992).

Does Alcohol Advertising Affect Drinking or Drinking Problems?

Earlier reviews have concluded that the effects of alcohol advertising on people's drinking beliefs and behaviors are limited, at best (Atkin 1995: Calfee and Scheraga 1994; Fisher 1993; Smart 1988). More recent research has not markedly changed this conclusion.

The two key questions that frame most of the current studies are whether alcohol advertising (1) increases overall drinking and drinking problems in the population or (2) increases drinking among children and adolescents or favorably predisposes them toward alcohol. A third important question about the possible effects of alcohol advertising on minority populations, who have been targets of advertising for particular alcohol products, has received little or no quantitative research to date and therefore is not covered in this review.

In the descriptions below, alcohol advertising research is grouped into four types of studies: experimental studies, econometric studies, survey research, and media literacy interventions.

Experimental Studies

Experimental studies have investigated how short-term exposure to alcohol advertising affects people's drinking beliefs and behaviors under controlled conditions. Typically, a group of participants is exposed to one or more alcohol advertisements embedded in a television program, among a series of neutral advertisements, or, in the case of print advertising, in a booklet or magazine. The investigators then compare the experimental group's beliefs or behaviors related to drinking with those of a control group that views the same items without the embedded alcohol advertisements. The results of earlier experimental studies have been mixed, with some studies finding no effects (Kohn et al. 1984; Sobell et al. 1986) and others finding small or short-term effects for some study participants (Kohn and Smart 1984).

A later study applied this approach to examine the effects of television beer advertising on the drinking beliefs of young people who were not regular drinkers (Lipsitz et al. 1993). The researcher showed three groups of fifth- and eighth-grade students videotapes containing 40 television commercials. One group saw videotapes containing 5 beer commercials scattered among 35 other commercials. Another group saw videotapes with the same five beer commercials plus two antidrinking public service announcements (PSA's). The control group saw videotapes with five soft-drink commercials in place of the beer commercials. The remaining 35 commercials were the same for all groups and advertised a variety of products, such as foods and automobiles.

After viewing the videotapes, the children completed a memory task that showed they attended to the advertisements and remembered seeing the beer and soft-drink commercials. Then they completed an "alcohol expectancy" questionnaire that measured the extent to which they believed drinking would lead to a number of desirable outcomes, such as enhancing social behavior or promoting relaxation. Neither exposure to the beer advertisements nor to the antidrinking PSA's affected the children's expectancies about the outcomes of drinking.

More recently, an experimental study examined young people's responses to variations in the placement of alcohol advertisements. The researchers exposed a sample of 244 high school students to videotaped television beer advertisements embedded in either a sports program or an entertainment program (Slater et al. 1997). The researchers asked the students to complete a questionnaire that measured their reactions after viewing each advertisement. The research team also asked the students about their present alcohol use and their future drinking intentions.

The responses were split along gender lines. The female students responded more negatively to the beer advertisements and offered more counterarguments than did the male students, particularly when the programs they watched had sports content.

In addition, adolescents of Anglo-American descent who responded favorably toward the beer advertisements were more likely to report current drinking and future intentions to drink. This finding might be interpreted as suggesting that alcohol advertising increases drinking predisposition. The effects were relatively small, however, and the finding did not hold for Latino students. Moreover, the design of this study did not allow the researchers to determine whether a favorable orientation toward alcohol advertisements predisposed the young people to drinking, or whether being predisposed to drinking made the young people more favorable toward alcohol advertisements. Nevertheless, the Latino-Anglo difference is an interesting finding. Although the Latino students liked the advertisements, they may have seen them as less personally relevant. Factors such as identification or perceived similarity with actors in television advertisements may influence the relationship between a person's attitude toward alcohol advertisements and his or her beliefs and behaviors related to drinking.

Experimental studies: Methodological considerations   Overall, the results of these experimental studies offer only limited support, at best, for effects of alcohol advertising on drinking beliefs and intentions (Atkin 1995; Grube and Wallack 1994; Lastovicka 1995; Thorson 1995). Although laboratory experimental studies can control for extraneous factors and can allow for strong causal inferences, they often lack realism. In a typical study, respondents are exposed to alcohol advertising in an artificial setting such as a schoolroom. The stimulus advertisements are often embedded among a very large number of "neutral" advertisements shown one after another. This style of presentation does not reflect the natural situation in which viewers are usually exposed to advertising. As a result, it is difficult to draw conclusions about the "real world" effects of alcohol advertising on beliefs and behaviors on the basis of these laboratory studies.

Furthermore, advertisers target specific audiences with particular advertisements (Thorson 1995). If the stimulus advertisements do not contain images, themes, or music that appeal to the participants in a specific study, it is less likely that any effects will be observed. In most cases, including the study described previously involving third and fifth graders (Lipsitz et al. 1993), the stimulus advertisements are not described in enough detail to ascertain if they were appropriate for the experimental participants. Additionally, these laboratory experiments can only address the effects of short-term exposure to a limited number of alcohol advertisements. The relevance of such studies for understanding the cumulative effects of exposure to hundreds or thousands of alcohol advertisements over many years is questionable. This research paradigm may be most relevant to understanding which ads appeal to viewers and whether or nor exposure to alcohol advertising elicits immediate and short-term increases in consumption among those already favorably predisposed to drinking (Kohn and Smart 1984).

Econometric Studies

A number of studies have applied the theoretical and statistical techniques of economic research to analyze issues relating to alcoholic beverage advertising.

Generally these econometric studies have focused on the relationship between the advertising expenditures of the alcohol industry and the average amount of alcohol consumed per person (per capita consumption) or the amount of alcohol sales, with price and other factors taken into account. A few studies have investigated whether alcohol advertising affects rates of traffic fatalities and other alcohol-related problems such as liver cirrhosis.

Overall, the econometric studies conducted to date provide little consistent support for a relationship between alcohol advertising and alcohol consumption and related problems. They do provide indirect support, however, for the hypothesis that alcohol advertising leads to changes in brand or beverage preferences without increasing total consumption. To follow is a summary of recent studies as well as criticisms related to methodological issues.

The question of consumption The overall conclusion from econometric studies conducted prior to 1990 is that alcohol advertising exerts a negligible effect on overall alcohol consumption (for reviews, see Calfee and Scheraga 1994; Fisher 1993; Saffer 1995a,b, 1996). These early studies suggest that a 1-percent decrease in alcohol advertising would be associated, at most, with a 0.1-percent decrease in consumption (Godfrey 1994).

Since then, two econometric studies have departed from the previous findings in that they reported substantive and statistically significant effects of alcohol advertising on alcohol-related problems (Saffer 1991, 1997). The first of these studies reported that countries with restrictions on broadcast alcohol advertisements had lower rates of both alcohol consumption and traffic fatalities (Saffer 1991, 1993b). Using data from 17 European and North American countries for the years 1970 through 1983, the researcher determined that countries with partial restrictions on television alcohol advertising, such as prohibitions on commercials for liquor, had 16-percent lower alcohol consumption rates and 10-percent lower motor vehicle fatality rates than did countries with no restrictions. In turn, countries with complete bans on television alcohol advertisements had 11-percent lower consumption rates and 23-percent lower motor vehicle fatalities rates than did countries with partial restrictions.

Controversy about these findings arose with the publication of a reanalysis (Young 1993) that criticized the original study (Saffer 1991) on a number of grounds. The reanalysis indicated that countries with low rates of alcohol problems were more likely to adopt bans on alcohol advertising because of preexisting, conservative drinking styles and attitudes. The reanalysis also suggested that partial alcohol advertising bans might actually *increase* alcohol consumption, a counterintuitive outcome. Questions about these findings, in turn, were raised by the author of the original study, who reported that the reanalysis suffered from methodological flaws that rendered the results inconsistent (Saffer 1993b).

More recently, another study reported significant advertising effects on drinking problems (Saffer 1997). The study has a number of methodological strengths and, although it cannot establish causation, it offers the strongest econometric evidence to date that alcohol advertising might influence drinking problems. The researcher looked at the relationship between motor vehicle fatalities and variations in local alcohol advertising in the top 75 media markets in the United States from 1986 through 1989. Alcohol advertising was represented as the sum of industry expenditures for producing and broadcasting television, radio, and outdoor advertisements, weighted for their relative impact based on the estimated number of people exposed to each.

After accounting for regional price differences and population variables such as income and religion, the researcher found that increases in alcohol advertising were significantly related to increases in total and nighttime vehicle fatalities. The effects appeared to be greater for older drivers than younger drivers (18 through 20 years old). On the basis of these analyses, the researcher estimated that a total ban on alcohol advertising might reduce motor vehicle fatalities by as much as 5,000 to 10,000 lives per year.

A separate analysis examined how variations in prices paid by the alcohol industry for advertising might influence rates of motor vehicle fatalities. The researcher found that higher advertising prices were associated with lower fatality rates, apparently because higher prices reduced the amount of advertising and consequently the rate of alcohol consumption. These results indicated that eliminating the advertising tax credit for the alcohol industry would reduce motor vehicle fatalities by as many as 1,300 lives per year (Saffer 1997).

The divergence of the findings of this study from some earlier econometric studies may, in part, be a result of improvements in methodology. Investigating local variations in advertising and adjusting for the relative impact of different media types are two important innovations that have not been duplicated in other econometric studies. Nonetheless, establishing a cause-and-effect relationship based on this study is problematic. Even though important background and demographic variables were controlled, the possibility that the observed relationship between alcohol advertising and motor vehicle fatalities resulted from some third variable, such as social norms, cannot at this point be discounted.

Reallocating market shares   All of the remaining recent econometric studies produced primarily negative findings, and they support earlier conclusions that alcohol advertising has little or no effect on overall consumption levels.

In the most thorough econometric investigation of alcohol advertising to date, researchers used U.S. data from 1970 through 1990 to analyze changes in per capita consumption as a function of changes in advertising. In addition, they looked for "cross-sectional associations," or links between consumption and advertising at specific, narrow time frames over the two decades (Fisher and Cook 1995).

Considering the cross-sectional links first, the researchers found that increased alcohol industry expenditures for magazine advertisements were associated with increased liquor consumption. This finding is consistent with the fact that liquor advertising in the United States occurs primarily in magazines. Although alcohol consumption dropped overall during the two decades, the researchers found that the years with higher total wine and liquor advertising (across all media) also had higher relative consumption levels not only for wine and liquor, but also for beer, and thus, total alcohol. Interestingly, increases in total beer advertising were associated with decreased liquor consumption, as would be expected if market shares were being shifted. These cross-sectional findings provided some support for the effects of advertising on alcohol consumption.

When the researchers analyzed the data using method that accounted for changes over time rather than a static, cross-sectional model, however, there was no evidence that changes in advertising were related to changes in consumption. The reanalysis did indicate that increased advertising of spirits was linked to a drop in the market share for wine. Overall, the findings of this study provide little or no evidence that alcohol advertising increases overall alcohol consumption, although they suggest that such advertising may realign market share.

Other studies have taken different paths to arrive at similar conclusions. One team used four different estimation procedures on annual U.S. data from 1964 through 1990 to investigate the effects of "real" (that is, inflation-adjusted) advertising expenditures for beer, wine, and spirits on the consumption of these beverages (Nelson and Moran 1995). The researchers examined "same-beverage effects," such as the effects of beer advertising expenditures on beer consumption, as well as "cross-beverage effects," such as the effects of beer advertising expenditures on wine consumption. They found that alcohol advertising expenditures were unrelated to total alcohol consumption once the researchers accounted for differences in price, population, income, and age and for advertising for all other goods. Their results also supported the claim that advertising reallocates market shares among brands and, to a lesser degree, beverage types.

Another study examined the effects of brand-level advertising on spirits consumed in the United States from 1976 through 1989 (Gius 1996). Advertising for a given brand of spirits was positively related to consumption of that "own brand" of spirits, whereas rival-brand advertising was not significantly related to own-brand consumption. This pattern was interpreted as indicating that alcohol advertising does not change overall consumption of spirits but rather leads simply to a reallocation of market shares.

It is not clear, however, that this conclusion necessarily follows from the pattern of findings. If own-brand advertising *increases* own-brand consumption but does not significantly *reduce* rival-brand consumption, then it might be having an overall market effect of increasing total consumption of spirits. This is a concern especially because successful advertising campaigns may elicit extensive counteradvertising by rival brands. Additional research would be needed to bear this theory out, as well as to investigate whether such campaigns build brand loyalty among underage drinkers that is then associated with underage consumption.

An additional study investigated the effects of advertising on alcohol and tobacco consumption in selected States for the years 1959 through 1982 (Goel and Morey 1995). The researchers found mixed results for the effects of advertising on consumption. Some of their findings showed that either the current or the previous year's advertisements for alcohol appeared to *decrease* consumption. As a possible explanation for this counterintuitive finding, the authors suggested that advertising might induce brand switching without increasing overall demand, which may force firms to advertise more to maintain their market shares. Other studies support the proposition that advertising may be a function of sales, as well as sales a function of advertising (Saffer 1995*b*, 1996). The models used in this study (Goel and Morey 1995), and in most econometric studies of alcohol advertising conducted to date, do not capture these potential reciprocal effects.

Econometric studies: Methodological considerations Econometric studies on alcohol advertising have been criticized on a number of grounds (Calfee and Scheraga 1994; Fisher 1993; Saffer 1995*a,b*). One recurring limitation is that the studies tend to combine, or aggregate, the advertising data across the different media types, which prevents researchers from detecting the effects of individual media types. In a related issue, the use of data that are aggregated at the yearly level may hide the short-term effects of "pulsed" advertising campaigns that have peaks and valleys in the concentration of advertisements over the year (Saffer 1995*a*). It has also been argued that econometric studies have not taken into consideration the possible cumulative effects of advertising over many years; as a result, they could underestimate advertising effects (Saffer 1995*a*).

Another important caution in interpreting these studies concerns conclusions about cause and effect. Some of the studies have relied on cross-sectional analyses, which take a "snapshot" of the status of many variables at specific, narrow points in time. With this method, even if significant links were to be found between advertising and other variables, it is not possible to draw strong conclusions about cause-and-effect relationships. Although researchers strive to adjust the data for the key factors that might cloud the findings, an apparent relationship between two variables may actually be due to a third, omitted variable in the model. Moreover, the causal direction may be the opposite of that assumed.

Finally, another limitation of the existing econometric studies is that they have focused on per capita consumption, problems, or sales rather than on individuals. As a result, interpretations of results from these studies are susceptible to the "ecological fallacy," that is, erroneously drawing conclusions about individuals on the basis of aggregated data. Thus, the finding that alcohol advertising has no *aggregate* effect on consumption does not mean that there is no effect for any *individual*. Not enough is known about how alcohol advertising might affect specific populations that may be more susceptible or more exposed to the advertising. In particular, it has been argued that young people may be especially influenced by alcohol advertisements (Atkin 1993) and that minority populations have been specially targeted by alcohol advertising (Abramson 1992; Scott et al. 1992). In addition, studies have yet to explore whether advertising has a greater impact on individuals during the initiation or early stages of drinking behavior than after drinking patterns have been established.

Survey Studies

For the most part, survey studies of alcohol advertising have focused on children and adolescents. Many of the early survey studies found significant, positive relationships between exposure to or awareness of alcohol advertising and drinking beliefs and behaviors among young people (Aitken et al. 1988; Atkin and Block 1980; Atkin et al. 1983, 1984). These effects were small, however, and a few studies found no significant relationships (Adlaf and Kohn 1989; Strickland 1982, 1983).

More recent studies using survey or questionnaire methods, . . . have continued to find significant, though still small, associations between alcohol advertisements and drinking beliefs and behaviors. Almost all of the studies are cross-sectional snapshots of the study groups, however, so they can show associations between variables but cannot confirm cause-and-effect relationships.

References

Abramson, H. *Booze Makers Buy Into Racial/Ethnic Communities*. San Rafael, CA: Marin Institute for the Prevention of Alcohol and Other Drug Problems, 1992.

Adlaf, E.M. and Kohn, P.M. Alcohol advertising, consumption and abuse: A covariance-structural modeling look at Strickland's data. *Br J Addict* 84(7):749–757, 1989.

Aitken, P.P.; Eadie, D.R.; Leathar, D.S.; McNeill, R.E.; and Scott, A.C. Television advertisements for alcoholic drinks do reinforce under-age drinking. *Br J Addict* 83(12):1399–1419, 1988.

Alaniz, M.L., and Wilkes, C. Reinterpreting Latino culture in the commodity form: The case of alcohol advertising in the Mexican-American community. *Hispanic J Behav Sci* 17(4):430–451, 1995.

Atkin, C.K. Effects of media alcohol messages on adolescent audiences. *Adolesc Med* 4(3):527–542, 1993.

Atkin, C.K. Survey and experimental research on effects of alcohol advertising. In: Martin, S.E., and Mail, P., eds. *Effects of the Mass Media on the Use and Abuse of Alcohol*. NIAAA Research Monograph No. 28, NIH Pub. No. 95-3743. Bethesda, MD: National Institute on Alcohol Abuse and Alcoholism, 1995. pp. 39–68.

Atkin, C.K., and Block, M. *Content and Effects of Alcohol Advertising*. Washington, DC: Bureau of Tobacco, Alcohol, and Firearms, 1980.

Atkin, C.K.; Hocking, J.; and Block, M. Teenage drinking: Does advertising make a difference? *J Commun* 34(2):157–167, 1984.

Atkin, C.K.; Neuendorf, K.; and McDermott S. The role of alcohol advertising in excessive and hazardous drinking. *J Drug Educ* 13(4):313–324, 1983.

Austin, E.W., and Johnson, K.K. Effects of general and alcohol-specific media literacy training on children's decision making about alcohol. *J Health Commun* 2(1):17–42, 1997a.

Austin, E.W., and Johnson, K.K. Immediate and delayed effects of media literacy training on third grader's decision making for alcohol. *J Health Commun* 9(4):323–349, 1997b.

Austin, E.W., and Meili, H.K. Effects of interpretations of televised alcohol portrayals on children's alcohol beliefs. *J Broadcasting Electronic Media* 38(4):417–435, 1994.

Austin, E.W., and Nach-Ferguson. B. Sources and influences of young school-age children's general and brand-specific knowledge about alcohol. *J Health Commun* 7(1):1–20, 1995.

Besen, D. US alcohol beverage advertisers sharpen their focus on core brands. *Impact* 27:1–5, 1997.

Calfee, J.E., and Scheraga, C. The influence of alcohol advertising on alcohol consumption: A literature review and an econometric analysis of four European nations. *Int J Advertising* 13:287–310, 1994.

Covell, K.; Dion, K.L.; and Dion, K.K. Gender differences in evaluations of tobacco and alcohol advertisements. *Can J Behav Sci* 26(3):404–420, 1994.

DeJong, W.; Atkin, C.K.; and Wallack, L. A critical analysis of "moderation" advertising sponsored by the beer industry: Are "responsible drinking" commercials done responsibly? *Milbank Q* 70(4):661–678, 1992.

Fisher, J.C. *Advertising, Alcohol Consumption, and Abuse: A Worldwide Survey.* Contributions to the Study of Mass Media and Communications No. 41. Westport, CT: Greenwood Press, 1993.

Fisher, J.C., and Cook, P.A. *Advertising, Alcohol Consumption, and Mortality: An Empirical Investigation.* Westport, CT: Greenwood Press, 1995.

Gius, M.P. Using panel data to determine the effect of advertising on brand-level distilled spirits sales. *J Stud Alcohol* 57(1):73–76, 1996.

Godfrey, C. Economic influence on change in population and personal substance behavior. In: Edwards, G., and Lader M., eds. *Addiction: Process of Change.* Society for the Study of Addiction Monograph No. 3. New York, NY: Oxford University Press, 1994. pp. 163–187.

Goel, R.K., and Morey, M.J. The interdependence of cigarette and liquor demand. *South Econ J* 62(2):451–459, 1995.

Grube, J.W. Alcohol portrayals and alcohol advertising on television: Contents and effects on children and adolescents. *Alcohol Health Res World* 17(1):54–60, 1993.

Grube, J.W. Television alcohol portrayals, alcohol advertising, and alcohol expectancies among children and adolescents. In: Martin, S.E., and Mail, P., eds. *Effects of the Mass Media on the Use and Abuse of Alcohol.* NIAAA Research Monograph No. 28. NIH Pub. No. 95-3743. Bethesda, MD: National Institute on Alcohol Abuse and Alcoholism, 1995. pp. 105–121.

Grube, J.W., and Wallack, L. Television beer advertising and drinking knowledge, beliefs, and intentions among schoolchildren. *Am J Public Health* 84(2):254–259, 1994.

Kaskutas, L.A. Changes in public attitudes toward alcohol control policies since the warning label mandate of 1988. *J Public Policy Marketing* 12(1):30–37, 1993.

Kohn, P.M., and Smart, R.G. The impact of television advertising on alcohol consumption: An experiment. *J Stud Alcohol* 5(4):295–301, 1984.

Kohn, P.M.; Smart, R.G.; and Ogborne, A.C. Effects of two kinds of alcohol advertising on subsequent consumption. *J Advertising* 13(1):34–40, 48, 1984.

Lastovicka, J.L. Methodological interpretation of the experimental and survey research evidence concerning alcohol advertising effects. In: Martin, S.E., and Mail, P., eds. *Effects of the Mass Media on the Use and Abuse of Alcohol.* NIAAA Research Monograph No. 28. NIH Pub. No. 95-3743. Bethesda, MD: National Institute on Alcohol Abuse and Alcoholism, 1995. pp. 69–81.

Lipsitz, A.; Brake, G.; Vincent, E.J.; and Winters, M. Another round for the brewers: Television ads and children's alcohol expectancies. *J Appl Soc Psychol* 23(6):439–450, 1993.

Madden, P.A., and Grube, J.W. The frequency and nature of alcohol and tobacco advertising in televised sports, 1990 through 1992. *Am J Public Health* 84(2):297–299, 1994.

Mosher, J.F. Alcohol advertising and public health: An urgent call for action. *Am J Public Health* 84(2):180–181, 1994.

Nelson, J.P., and Moran, J.R. Advertising and US alcoholic beverage demand: System-wide estimates. *Appl Econ* 27(12):1225–1236, 1995.

Saffer, H. Alcohol advertising bans and alcohol abuse: An international perspective. *J Health Econ* 10(1):65–79, 1991.

Saffer, H. Advertising under the influence. In: Hilton, M.E., and Bloss, G., eds. *Economics and the Prevention of Alcohol-Related Problems: Proceedings of a Workshop on Economic and Socioeconomic Issues in the Prevention of Alcohol-Related Problems, October 10–11, 1991, Bethesda, MD.* NIAAA Research Monograph No. 25. Rockville, MD: National Institute on Alcohol Abuse and Alcoholism, 1995*a*. pp. 125–140.

Saffer, H. Alcohol advertising bans and alcohol abuse: Reply. *J Health Econ* 12(2):229–234, 1993*b*.

Saffer, H. Alcohol advertising and alcohol consumption: Econometric studies. In: Martin, S.E., and Mail, P., eds. *Effects of the Mass Media on the Use and Abuse of Alcohol.* NIAAA Research Monograph No. 28. NIH Pub. No. 95-3743. Bethesda, MD: National Institute on Abuse and Alcoholism. 1995*b*. pp. 83–99.

Saffer, H. Studying the effects of alcohol advertising on consumption. *Alcohol Health Res World* 20(4):266–272, 1996.

Saffer, H. Alcohol advertising and motor vehicle fatalities. *Rev Econ Stat* 79(3): 431–442, 1997.

Scott, B.M.; Denniston, R.W.; and Magruder, K.M. Alcohol advertising in the African-American community. *J Drug Issues* 22(2):455–469, 1992.

Slater, M.D.; Rouner, D.; Murphy, K.; Beauvais, F.; Van Leuven, J.; and Domenech-Rodriguez, M.M. Adolescent counter-arguing of TV beer advertisements: Evidence for effectiveness of alcohol education and critical viewing discussions. *J Drug Educ* 26(2):143–158 1996*a*.

Slater, M.D.; Rouner, D.; Beauvais, F.; Murphy, K.; Domenech-Rodriquez, M.; and Van Leuven, J.K. Adolescent perceptions of underage drinkers in TV beer ads. *J Alcohol Drug Educ* 42(1):43–56, 1996*b*.

Slater, M.D.; Rouner, D.; Domenech-Rodriquez, M.; Beauvais, F.; Murphy, K.; and Van Leuven, J.K. Adolescent responses to TV beer ads and sports content/context: Gender and ethnic differences. *J Mass Commun Q* 74(1):108–122, 1997.

Slater, M.D.; Rouner, D.; Murphy, K.; Beauvais, F.; Van Leuven, J.K.; and Domenech-Rodriguez, M. Male adolescent reactions to TV beer advertisements: The effects of sports content and programming context. *J Stud Alcohol* 57(4):425–433, 1996*c*.

Smart, R.G. Does alcohol advertising affect overall consumption? A review of empirical studies. *J Stud Alcohol* 49(4):314–323, 1988.

Sobell, L.C.; Sobell, M.B.; Riley, D.M.; Klajner, F.; Leo, G.I.; Pavan, D.; and Cancilla, A. Effect of television programming and advertising on alcohol consumption in normal drinkers. *J Stud Alcohol* 47(4):333–340, 1986.

Strickland, D.E. Alcohol advertising: Orientations and influence. *J Advertising* 1:307–319, 1982.

Strickland, D.E. Advertising exposure, alcohol consumption and misuse of alcohol. In: Grant, M.; Plant, M.; and Williams, A., eds. *Economics and Alcohol: Consumption and Control.* New York, NY: Gardner Press, 1983. pp. 201–222.

Thorson, E. Studies of the effects of alcohol advertising: Two underexplored aspects. In: Martin, S.E., and Mail, P., eds. *Effects of the Mass Media on the Use and Abuse of Alcohol.* NIAAA Research Monograph No. 28. NIH Pub. No. 95-3743. Bethesda, MD: National Institute on Alcohol Abuse and Alcoholism, 1995. pp. 159–195.

Woodruff, K. Alcohol advertising and violence against women: A media advocacy case study. *Health Educ Q* 23(3):330–345, 1996.

Wyllie, A.; Zhang, J.F; and Casswell, S. Responses to televised alcohol advertisements associated with drinking behavior of 10–17-year-olds. *Addiction* 93(3):361–371, 1998*a*.

Wyllie, A.; Zhang, J.F.; and Casswell, S. Positive responses to televised beer advertisements associated with drinking and problems reported by 18- to 29-year-olds. *Addiction* 93(5):749–760, 1998*b*.

Young, D.J. Alcohol advertising bans and alcohol abuse [Comment]. *J Health Econ* 12(2):213–228, 1993.

POSTSCRIPT

Do Alcohol Advertisements Influence Young People to Drink More?

In the United States, companies spend billions of dollars advertising on television and in the print media to promote use of their products. One would assume, therefore, that advertisements are an effective way to encourage the use of products. If advertisements did not work, then companies would be wasting their money. Yet can one be sure that advertising—in this case, of alcohol—actually increases the use of a product?

One could argue that even if alcohol advertisements do increase alcohol consumption by young people, companies still have the right to promote their products as they wish. Freedom of speech is protected by the Constitution. Advertising could be viewed as a form of free speech. If one believes that alcohol advertisements influence behavior, does that mean that these advertisements should be banned, or should they simply be more closely regulated?

One dilemma in determining whether or not alcohol advertisements influence drinking behavior is that many young people who drink might be inclined to consume alcohol in the first place. In other words, alcohol advertising may reinforce existing beliefs and behaviors rather than alter those beliefs and behaviors. Attitudes and behaviors in the home might also have a powerful effect. It is likely that children who see their parents abstain from alcohol, drink moderately, or drink to excess will be affected by what they see. The drinking behavior of older siblings affects behavior as well.

One organization that is devoted to antidrug advertisements is the Partnership for a Drug-Free America (PDFA). Although the federal government provides funding to the PDFA, it is a private organization that receives money from charitable organizations as well as from pharmaceutical companies, beer manufacturers, and tobacco companies. One criticism of PDFA advertisements is that they do not address cigarette and alcohol use by young people because the organization is afraid of losing income from the beer and tobacco companies. Thus, rather than ban alcohol advertisements, one could argue that more effective media campaigns regarding the hazards of alcohol use by young people should be implemented.

Two organizations that provide research on the topic of alcohol and young people are the Center on Alcohol Marketing and Youth at Georgetown University and the Center for Science in the Public Interest. Their Web sites are http://camy.org and http://www.cspinet.org, respectively. Two articles that look at this issue are "Alcohol Advertising and Youth," by Henry Saffer, *Journal of Studies on Alcohol* (March 2002) and "Alcohol Counter-Advertising and the Media: A Review of Recent Research," by Gina Agostinelli and Joel W. Grube, *Alcohol Research and Health* (vol. 26, no. 1, 2002).

Contributors to This Volume

EDITOR

RAYMOND GOLDBERG is a professor of health education at the State University of New York College at Cortland. Since 1977 he has served as coordinator for graduate programs in the School of Professional Studies. He received a B.S. in health and physical education from the University of North Carolina at Pembroke in 1969, an M.Ed. in health education from the University of South Carolina in 1971, and a Ph.D. in health education from the University of Toledo in 1981. He is the author of *Drugs Across the Spectrum,* 3rd ed. (Morton, 2000) and the author or coauthor of many articles on health-related issues, and he has made many presentations on the topic of drug education. He has received over $750,000 in grants for his research in health and drug education.

STAFF

Jeffrey L. Hahn   Vice President/Publisher
Theodore Knight   Managing Editor
David Brackley   Senior Developmental Editor
Juliana Gribbins   Developmental Editor
Rose Gleich   Permissions Assistant
Brenda S. Filley   Director of Production/Manufacturing
Julie Marsh   Project Editor
Juliana Arbo   Typesetting Supervisor
Richard Tietjen   Publishing Systems Manager
Charles Vitelli   Designer

AUTHORS

ROBERT APSLER is an assistant professor of psychology in the Department of Psychiatry at Harvard Medical School in Boston, Massachusetts, and president of Social Science Research and Evaluation, Inc.

CHARLES K. ATKIN is the University Distinguished Professor of Communication at Michigan State University and a member of the university's Alcohol and Other Drug Network. He holds a Ph.D. from the University of Wisconsin, and he is coeditor, with Ronald E. Rice, of *Public Communication Campaigns* (Sage, 2001).

MICHAEL S. BAHRKE is an acquisitions editor in the Scientific, Technical, and Medical Division of Human Kinetics in Champaign, Illinois. He has also been an assistant professor at the University of Kansas, director of research for the U.S. Army Physical Fitness School, and fitness area coordinator at the University of Wisconsin. A fellow of the American College of Sports Medicine, he is coauthor, with Charles E. Yesalis, of *Performance-Enhancing Substances in Sport and Exercise* (Human Kinetics, 2002). He holds a master's degree in exercise physiology and a doctorate in sport psychology from the University of Wisconsin–Madison.

DENNIS BERNSTEIN is an investigative reporter, a radio host, a human rights advocate, and a poet. He is a regular contributor to Pacifica's *Democracy Now* and an associate editor for Pacific News Service. Also, he is currently cohost and associate producer of KPFA's *Flashpoints News Magazine,* and he is a frequent commentator on WBAI airwaves. His articles have appeared in numerous publications, including *The Nation, Mother Jones,* and *The Progressive,* and he is coauthor, with Leslie Kean, of *Henry Hyde's Moral Universe: Where More Than Space and Time Are Warped* (Common Courage Press, 1999).

ANN BOUCHOUX is director of communications for the International Food Information Council.

NELL BOYCE, formerly a Washington correspondent for the London-based weekly *New Scientist,* is now an associate editor for *U.S. News & World Report,* where she covers biomedicine, genetics, and other scientific topics. She was awarded the Evert Clark/Seth Payne Award in 1998.

ANNE B. BROWN, a writer, has reported on such subjects as posttraumatic stress disorder, bipolar disorder, and adolescent depressive disorders.

THOMAS BYRD, now retired, was an instructor in the Division of Biological and Health Sciences at De Anza College in Cupertino, California.

TED GALEN CARPENTER is vice president for defense and foreign policy studies at the Cato Institute. He is at the forefront of efforts to develop a new U.S. security strategy that minimizes costs and risks to the American people. His writing has appeared in such publications as the *New York Times,* the *Wall Street Journal,* and the *Boston Globe,* and he is a frequent guest on radio and television programs around the world. He has written over 200 articles and 13 books, including *Bad Neighbor Policy: Washington's Futile War on*

Drugs in Latin America (Palgrave Macmillan, 2003). He holds a doctorate in U.S. diplomatic history from the University of Texas.

BRUCE M. COHEN is a clinical instructor of psychiatry and behavioral sciences at the University of Arkansas for Medical Sciences. He is director of the Child Study Center Clinic and Community Outreach Program in the Division of Pediatric Psychiatry as well as clinical director of Arkansas CARES. His clinical work has focused on children and adolescents with ADHD, learning problems, and depression, and he has extensive experience in school consultation. He earned his B.S. in psychology and his M.S. in clinical psychology (child clinical specialty) from Memphis State University.

J. B. COPAS is a professor in the Department of Statistics at the University of Warwick in Coventry, United Kingdom. His research interests include enhancements in regression modeling and risk scoring, and he is currently researching methods of performing statistical sensitivity analysis.

THOMAS S. DEE is an assistant professor in the Department of Economics at Swarthmore College and a faculty research fellow of the National Bureau of Economic Research in Cambridge, Massachusetts. A member of the American Economic Association and the American Educational Research Association, he has also taught in the School of Economics at the Georgia Institute of Technology. His research interests include public finance, health, education, and applied econometrics. He earned his M.A. in economics and his Ph.D. in economics from the University of Maryland in 1994 and 1997, respectively.

RONALD W. DWORKIN is a physician in the Department of Anesthesiology at the Greater Baltimore Medical Center and a senior fellow of the Hudson Institute in Washington, D.C. He is also cofounder of the Calvert Institute for Policy Research, a public policy center directed at looking at the entire range of state and local public policy issues. He is a regular contributor to the op-ed page of the *Baltimore Sun,* and his writings have also appeared in *The Public Interest.* He is the author of *The Rise of the Imperial Self: America's Culture Wars in Augustinian Perspective* (Rowman & Littlefield, 1996).

THOMAS FEDIUK is a doctoral candidate in the Department of Communication at Michigan State University. He earned his master's degree in communication from Illinois State University in 1999. His doctoral research interests include strategic communication and organizational communication, especially in public relations; crisis communication; and information campaigns.

MICHAEL FUMENTO is an author, journalist, and attorney specializing in science and health issues. He is a science columnist for Scripps-Howard and a senior fellow of the Hudson Institute in Washington, D.C. He has also been a legal writer for the *Washington Times* and an editorial writer for the *Rocky Mountain News* in Denver, and he was the first "National Issues" reporter for *Investor's Business Daily.* Fumento has lectured on science and health issues throughout the world, including Great Britain, France, the Czech Republic, Greece, Austria, China, and South America. His publications include

BioEvolution: How Biotechnology Is Changing Our World (Encounter Books, 2003).

GENERAL ACCOUNTING OFFICE (GAO) is the investigative arm of the U.S. Congress. The GAO examines the use of public funds, evaluates federal programs and activities, and provides analyses, options, recommendations, and other assistance to help Congress make effective oversight, policy, and funding decisions.

LESTER GRINSPOON is chair of the board of directors for the National Organization for the Reform of Marijuana Laws. He is also executive director of the Massachusetts Mental Health Research Corporation and an associate professor of psychiatry at Harvard Medical School in Boston, Massachusetts. He has been involved in marijuana research for over 20 years, and he received the Norman E. Zinberg Award for marijuana research in 1990.

EDITH HOWARD HOGAN is the owner of Nutrition Consulting Services on Capitol Hill in Washington, D.C., where she provides private and corporate clients with nutrition counseling and nutritional expertise. She has been actively involved in nutrition and food issues, including caffeine and food safety. In addition to her longstanding involvement with the American Dietetic Association (ADA) and her local district, she currently serves as an ADA national media spokesperson and makes frequent radio and television appearances.

BETSY A. HORNICK is a nutrition writer and consultant based in Poplar Grove, Illinois. She is also a state media representative for the Illinois Dietetic Association.

DREW HUMPHRIES is a professor of sociology in the Department of Sociology, Anthropology, and Criminal Justice at Rutgers University, where she is director of the Criminal Justice Program. She teaches a variety of criminal justice courses, including police, deviance, gender and crime, domestic violence, and drugs and society. She is also coeditor of *Women, Violence, and the Media,* a special issue of *Violence Against Women.*

BENJAMIN JUNGE is senior research coordinator with the Department of Epidemiology at the Johns Hopkins School of Hygiene and Public Health. He is also evaluation director for the Baltimore Needle Exchange Program.

LESLIE KEAN, formally the full-time director of the Burma Project USA, a human rights and media advocacy group, is now an investigative journalist and associate producer of KPFA's *Flashpoints News Magazine.* Her articles have appeared in numerous publications, including the *Boston Globe, The Kyoto Journal,* and *The Progressive,* and she is coauthor, with Dennis Bernstein, of *Henry Hyde's Moral Universe: Where More Than Space and Time Are Warped* (Common Courage Press, 1999).

JONATHAN LEO is an associate professor of anatomy in the College of Osteopathic Medicine of the Pacific at the Western University of Health Sciences, where he teaches courses in gross anatomy, neuroscience, and histology. He has also served as editor-in-chief of the journal *Ethical Human Sciences* *and Services.* He earned his Ph.D. in anatomy from the University of Iowa in 1995.

ALAN I. LESHNER, former director of the National Institute on Drug Abuse at the National Institutes of Health, now serves as chief executive officer for the American Association for the Advancement of Science, where he is also executive publisher of the association's journal *Science.* His areas of expertise include science for society, cloning, international research, and health care reform. Leshner holds a Ph.D. in psychology and neuroscience, and he began his career as a professor of psychology at Bucknell University. He has held leadership positions at the National Science Foundation and the National Institute of Mental Health, and he is credited with helping to clarify to the public the health aspects of addiction and its biological bases.

ROBERT A. LEVY is a senior fellow in constitutional studies at the Cato Institute. He is also an adjunct professor at the Georgetown University Law Center, director of the Institute for Justice, a member of the Board of Visitors of the Federalist Society, and a trustee of the Objectivist Center. He has discussed public policy on many national radio and TV programs, including CNN's *Crossfire* and ABC's *Nightline,* and his writings have appeared in such publications as the *New York Times* and the *Wall Street Journal.* He earned his Ph.D. in business from the American University in 1966 and his J.D. from George Mason University in 1994.

PAUL A. LOGLI is state's attorney for Winnebago County, Illinois, and a lecturer at the National College of District Attorneys. A member of the Illinois State Bar since 1974, he is a nationally recognized advocate for prosecutorial involvement in the issue of substance-abused infants. He earned his J.D. from the University of Illinois.

ALICIA M. LUKACHKO is assistant director of public health at the American Council on Science and Health.

ROSALIND B. MARIMONT is a retired mathematician and scientist, having done research and development for the National Institute of Standards and Technology (formerly the Bureau of Standards) for 18 years and for the National Institute of Health (NIH) for another 19. She started in electronics defense work during World War II, then went into the logical design of the early digital computers during the 1950s. At the NIH she studied and published papers on human vision, speech, and other biomathematical subjects. Since her retirement she has been active in health policy issues, particularly the war on smoking.

MERRILL MATTHEWS, JR., is a public policy analyst specializing in health care, Social Security, welfare, and Internet issues, and the author of numerous studies in health policy, as well as other public policy issues. Currently a visiting scholar with the Institute for Policy Innovation, he is former president of the Health Economics Roundtable for the National Association for Business Economics and former health policy adviser for the American Legislative Exchange Council. Matthews also serves as the medical ethicist for the University of Texas Southwestern Medical Center's Institutional Review

Board for Human Experimentation. He earned his Ph.D. in philosophy and humanities from the University of Texas at Dallas.

BARRY R. McCAFFREY is former director of the Office of National Drug Control Policy at the White House, where he served as the senior drug policy official in the executive branch and as the president's chief drug policy spokesman. He is also a member of the National Security Council. Upon his retirement from the U.S. Army, he was the most highly decorated officer and the youngest four-star general.

JAMES R. McDONOUGH is director of the Florida Office of Drug Control. From 1996 to 1999, he was director of strategy for the Office of National Drug Control Policy, and he was also an officer in the U.S. Army. In addition, he has served as an associate professor of political science and international affairs at the U.S. Military Academy, as an analyst with the Defense Nuclear Agency, and as a detailee to the U.S. State Department. His publications include *Platoon Leader* (Presidio Press, 1996).

ETHAN A. NADELMANN is director of the Lindesmith Center, a New York–based drug-policy research institute, and an assistant professor of politics and public affairs in the Woodrow Wilson School of Public and International Affairs at Princeton University in Princeton, New Jersey. He was the founding coordinator of the Harvard Study Group on Organized Crime, and he has been a consultant to the Department of State's Bureau of International Narcotics Matters. He is also an assistant editor of the *Journal of Drug Issues* and a contributing editor of the *International Journal on Drug Policy.*

TODD NIGHSWONGER reports on safety issues for the journal *Occupational Hazards.*

OFFICE OF NATIONAL DRUG CONTROL POLICY (ONDCP) was created by the Anti-Drug Abuse Act of 1988 to advise the president on a national drug control strategy, a consolidated drug control budget, and other management and organizational issues. The principal purpose of the ONDCP is to establish policies, priorities, and objectives for the nation's drug control program, with the overall goal of significantly reducing the production, availability, and use of illegal drugs both in the United States and abroad.

HEATHER OGILVIE, a writer and journalist, has edited several health-related books. She is also coauthor, with A. Thomas Horvath and Frederick Rotgers, of *Alternatives to Abstinence: A New Look at Alcoholism and the Choices in Treatment* (Hatherleigh Press, 2001).

BERNADETTE PELISSIER is chief of research at the Federal Correctional Institution in Butner, North Carolina, where she directs the evaluation of the Federal Bureau of Prisons' drug treatment program. She also chairs the board of directors of the Orange Water and Sewer Authority in Carrboro, North Carolina, and serves on the Budget and Financial Planning Committee. She earned her master's degree in sociology from Virginia Commonwealth University and her doctorate in sociology from the University of North Carolina at Chapel Hill.

JEFFREY A. SCHALER has been a psychologist and therapist in private practice since 1973. He is also an adjunct professor of justice, law, and society at American University's School of Public Affairs, where he has taught courses on drugs, psychiatry, liberty, justice, law, and public policy since 1990. He writes a regular column for *The Interpsych Newsletter,* and he is the author of *Smoking: Who Has the Right?* (Prometheus Books, 1998).

J. Q. SHI is a research associate for the Mining and Environmental Research Group in the T. H. Huxley School of Environment, Earth Sciences and Engineering at the Imperial College of Science, Technology and Medicine in London, United Kingdom. In addition to publishing a number of research papers, he is coauthor, with B. C. Wei and G. P. Lu, of *Introduction of Statistical Diagnostics* (Southeast University Press, 1991). He earned his Ph.D. from the University of Southampton.

ERIC SIGEL, a pediatrician and adolescent medicine specialist, is an assistant professor of pediatrics at the University of Colorado School of Medicine in Denver, Colorado, and medical director of the Eating Disorders Clinic at the Children's Hospital of Denver. He also serves as chair of the Eating Disorders Committee of the Society of Adolescent Medicine.

SANDI W. SMITH is a professor of communication at Michigan State University, where she teaches courses in interpersonal communication, relational communication, communication theory, and persuasion. She has also been a faculty member at Purdue University, and she has received several awards for outstanding scholarship and teaching, including the Outstanding Young Teacher Award from the Central States Communication Association. Her research has appeared in such journals as *The American Behavioral Scientist, Human Communication Research, Communication Studies,* and *Journal of Applied Communication Research.* She holds a Ph.D. in communication from the University of Southern California.

JACOB SULLUM is a senior editor at *Reason* magazine. In addition to drug policy, he has written about gun control, censorship, and religious freedom, and his articles have been published in *National Review,* the *Wall Street Journal,* and the *New York Times.* A fellow of the Knight Center for Specialized Journalism, he has been a featured speaker at the International Conference on Drug Policy Reform. He is the author of *Saying Yes: In Defense of Drug Use* (J. P. Tarcher/Putnam, 2003).

WILLIAM N. TAYLOR is a doctor who has been studying the anabolic steroid issue for over 20 years. He is the author of a number of books, including *Anabolic Therapy in Modern Medicine* (McFarland, 2002) and *Osteoporosis: Medical Blunders and Treatment Strategies* (McFarland, 1996)

U.S. DEPARTMENT OF HEALTH AND HUMAN SERVICES (HHS) is the principal agency for protecting health and providing essential human services to Americans. Administering some 250 separate programs, the HHS provides services that protect and advance the quality of life for all Americans.

DAVID VLAHOV is a professor of epidemiology and medicine at the Johns Hopkins School of Hygiene and Public Health. He is also principal investigator of the evaluation of the Baltimore Needle Exchange Program.

ERIC A. VOTH is chairman of the International Drug Strategy Institute and a clinical assistant professor in the Department of Medicine at the University of Kansas School of Medicine. He is also medical director of Chemical Dependency Services at St. Francis Hospital in Topeka, Kansas. He has testified for the Drug Enforcement Administration in opposition to legalizing marijuana, and he is recognized as an international authority on drug abuse.

ELIZABETH M. WHELAN is president and cofounder of the American Council on Science and Health. She holds master's and doctoral degrees in public health from the Yale School of Medicine and the Harvard School of Public Health. She has published a number of books, including *Fad-Free Nutrition*, coauthored by Fredrick J. Stare (Hunter House, 1998).

JAMES E. WRIGHT, a military officer and research scientist, is the senior science editor for *Flex* and the editor of *Muscle & Fitness*. An authority on exercise program design, specific exercise techniques, and diets and nutrition for optimal physical and mental performance, he has spent most of his professional life studying ways to improve body composition, physical capacities, and performance. He has written hundreds of articles for popular health and fitness magazines, and he is coauthor, with Virginia S. Cowart, of *Altered States: The Use and Abuse of Anabolic Steroids* (Masters Press, 1994).

CHARLES E. YESALIS is a professor of health policy and administration and of exercise and sport science at Pennsylvania State University. His research focuses on the nonmedical use of anabolic-androgenic steroids and other performance-enhancing drugs. His other research interests include chemical dependency, drug use, and hormones. He holds a master's of public health from the University of Michigan and a doctoral degree from the Johns Hopkins University School of Hygiene and Public Health. He is coauthor, with Virginia S. Cowart, of *The Steroids Game* (Human Kinetics, 1998) and coeditor, with Michael S. Bahrke, of *Performance-Enhancing Substances in Sport and Exercise* (Human Kinetics, 2002).

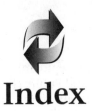

Index